Immuno-globulins

Conference on

Biologic Aspects and Clinical Uses

Ohio State University College of Medicine
and
Division of Medical Sciences
National Research Council

Edited by EZIO MERLER

NATIONAL ACADEMY OF SCIENCES Washington, D.C.   1970

ISBN 0-309-01850-1

Available from

Printing and Publishing Office
National Academy of Sciences
2101 Constitution Avenue
Washington, D.C. 20418

Library of Congress Catalog Card Number 74-607554

Printed in the United States of America

Preface

The National Research Council, organized in 1916 by the National Academy of Sciences at the request of President Woodrow Wilson, has as one of its principal functions the promotion of the effective application of science and engineering for the benefit of society. Within the Council, the Division of Medical Sciences has responsibility for promoting the application of medical science for this purpose. In this respect, the Division has a longstanding interest in basic and developmental research on human blood and blood products and has maintained a series of scientific advisory committees to assist with its undertakings in the field. This function is currently vested in the Committee on Plasma and Plasma Substitutes.

In the early 1960's, this Committee was called upon to evaluate the current and proposed uses of what was then referred to as "gamma globulin," for which therapeutic efficacy was supported by valid data. Many of the originally proposed uses of gamma globulin in the prevention and treatment of infectious diseases had been obviated by vaccines, the sulfonamides, and the antibiotics. The Committee found that gamma globulin was used principally in the prevention and amelioration of measles and viral hepatitis and in the management of hypogammaglobu-

iii

linemia, but that its use in measles might decline if a vaccine then under study became available.

It was evident that both basic and applied research on gamma globulin had lagged in the 1950's. However, enthusiasm was developing in the study of the physicochemical nature of immunoglobulins as an area of basic research, and, although it was premature to consider the possible application of the data from these early research efforts, the Committee felt that there was an inherent promise of useful application. It therefore determined to review the field later. In 1967, the Committee, noting the rapid progress that was being made, particularly in the field of immunoglobulin physicochemistry, proposed that a meeting be held before the close of the decade to review the status of this research. In so proposing, the Committee pointed out that the work was being done principally by persons in basic research fields having specialized interests and viewpoints. In the normal course of events, the emerging data would be published in a variety of scientific journals, and its application in medical practice would be delayed and piecemeal. The Committee was of the opinion that a meeting and a publication for the purpose of acquainting clinicians with the research and the researchers with the potential clinical application of their work would expedite the flow of scientific and technical information from the laboratory to the bedside.

Dr. Charles L. Dunham, Chairman, Division of Medical Sciences, invited the Ohio State University College of Medicine to conduct such a meeting, and Dr. Richard L. Meiling, Dean of the College, accepted the invitation with enthusiasm. As mutually agreed, the Division established a National Research Council committee to plan the scientific program, and the College assumed responsibility for all other tasks related to the planning and conduct of the meeting. The meeting, attended by over 150 scientists and medical practitioners from the United States and abroad, was held March 31 through April 2, 1969, in Columbus, Ohio.

The emphasis of this conference on the biology of immunoglobulins, rather than their immunochemistry (as in the previous conference, held in October 1962), reflected the growth of immunology in the intervening eight years. Once it had been learned what, in a broad sense, immunoglobulins were, it was reasonable to ask how they behave, what they do, and how they could be used in solving medical problems. This conference tried to summarize some relevant facts along these lines. The cellular aspects of immunology, only briefly alluded to here, may well form the basis of another conference eight years hence.

These proceedings contain the reports of all but one of the authors who contributed to the conference. The contributions have been arranged, not necessarily in the order of their presentation or overall importance, but rather to cover areas of common interest, beginning with scientific essays on the classes of immunoglobulins and closing with more general discussions of the standardization and surveillance of immunoglobulins and their uses.

Each author has emphasized his own interests to create a variegated, slightly opinionated, but readable account of his particular field. The presentations are not overburdened with the experimental details that often tend to narrow scientific reporting, but instead are brief overviews of a broad, complex, and at times frightfully confused field of endeavors. Although details often change, broad lines of thought appear immutable, by virtue of the scientific approach that we follow.

The conference appears to have served its purpose well, and the information it produced should be helpful in defining steps that should be taken to increase the value of immunoglobulins in preventing and alleviating human disease.

ROBERT L. WALL, M.D., *Chairman*
Conference on Biologic Aspects
and Clinical Uses of Immunoglobulins

A NOTE ON THE NOMENCLATURE OF
HUMAN IMMUNOGLOBULINS

Because the study and application of the human immunoglobulins are expanding rapidly, their nomenclature is often inconsistent. Most of this volume reflects an attempt to impose a degree of needed consistency. The main points of the nomenclature used here are:

1. The symbol Ig (usually) or γ followed immediately by a capital letter (A, D, E, G, M) is reserved for chemically pure proteins.

2. The word "immunoglobulin" is used chiefly to indicate the normal distribution of the proteins IgG, IgA, IgM, and so on, as they occur in serum.

3. Cohn's fraction II+III (which is 95% IgG, but also contains notable amounts of IgA, IgM, and albumin), the material used clinically for prophylaxis and therapy, is called "gamma globulin."

4. A gamma globulin preparation with known antibody activity is referred to as an "immune globulin."

5. Immune globulins are sometimes called "antibodies"; the serum from which an antibody (or an immune globulin) is derived can be called either an "immune serum" or an "antiserum."

6. Immunoglobulin chains are designated by the symbols κ and λ for L chains and γ, a, μ, etc., for H chains.

Acknowledgments

When an invitation was received by the Ohio State University from Dr. Charles L. Dunham, Chairman, Division of Medical Sciences of the National Research Council, to host this conference, a "seed fund" contribution from the College of Medicine was made available to further the planning of the meeting. This in turn made it possible to receive a generous grant from the Office of Naval Research, Department of the Navy, necessary for the actual conduct of the conference, for which we are deeply grateful. Additional financial support for the conduct of the meeting, including its social aspects and accommodations for the European participants, was made available by generous contributions from Ortho Pharmaceutical Corporation, Pitman-Moore Biological Laboratories, Behringwerke A.G., Armour Pharmaceutical Co., Osterreiches Institut für Haemoderivate, American Association of Blood Banks, Lederle Laboratories, Hyland Division of Travenol Laboratories, Abbott Laboratories, Parke, Davis and Co., Merck Institute for Therapeutic Research, and Hoffman-LaRoche Inc. We express our appreciation for their understanding and generosity.

This volume itself could not have been made available except for a most generous grant (DADA17-69-G-9287) from the U.S. Army Medical Research and Development Command; that grant, entirely and exclusively for support of the preparation and publication of this book, is gratefully acknowledged.

The content of the conference was established by a planning committee, which included Drs. Harlan D. Anderson, Marcel E. Conrad, John L. Fahey, Henry T. Gannon, Elvin A. Kabat, Robert B. Pennell, Fred S. Rosen, and Robert L. Wall.

Local planning for the conference was facilitated by the Center for Continuing Medical Education of the Ohio State University College of Medicine and the local planning committee, consisting of Drs. Samuel G. Murphy, Albert S. Klainer, and Robert L. Wall.

For valuable help and assistance during the conference, we are indebted to Dr. Robert B. Schweikart of the Center for Continuing Medical Education and his staff.

We are especially grateful to Dr. Ezio Merler, of the Laboratory of Immunology of Harvard Medical School, and Mr. Norman Grossblatt, editor for the Division of Medical Sciences of the National Research Council, for their anxious attention to the details of the scientific and literary content of this book.

RICHARD L. MEILING, M.D., *Dean*
Ohio State University College of Medicine

Contents

I
INTRODUCTION

CHARLES A. JANEWAY

The Development of Clinical Uses of Immunoglobulins: A Review

The history of the immunoglobulins is one of the mainstreams of the science of immunology over the last 30 years. Immunology had its first golden age in the late nineteenth and early twentieth centuries, when antibodies were discovered and first used in the treatment and prevention of disease, when complement was recognized by Ehrlich, and when the concept of allergy, which had been foreshadowed by the work of Koch, was elaborated by von Pirquet. For the first 25 years of this century, a great deal of quiet work went on, which led up to the biochemical era of immunology. Credit must be given to a biologist, my old teacher, Hans Zinsser, who, with Julia Parker, first described the specific soluble substance of the pneumococcus in the early 1920's. This set off the great studies at the Rockefeller Institute and at Columbia University by Avery, Heidelberger, and Goebbel, which led to the chemical characterization of the pneumococcal polysaccharides and the quantitation of their reactions with specific antisera—logical extensions of the pioneering studies of Landsteiner on the chemical nature of the specificity of antigens.

At about the same time, Felton introduced purification of antibody from type-specific antipneumococcal serum for therapeutic use by salt fractionation; this was the conceptual forerunner of the purification of human gamma globulin. It was no accident that Dubos called immunology the science of pneumococcal polysaccharide in the late 1930's; the definition lost its meaning almost immediately with the introduction of sulfapyridine and penicillin. Felton's technique for preparing partially purified antipneumococcal antibody by salt fractionation had two major drawbacks: a long period was required for removal of the ammonium sulfate by dialysis, frequently permitting contamination and consequent pyrogenic reactions in clinical use; and the starting material was horse serum, much of whose antibody had a high molecular weight. With the introduction of antibody purified from rabbit antiserum, a preparation much more like human antibody in its physicochemical characteristics became available. But this preparation sometimes produced severe reactions when administered intravenously. One of Albert Sabin's first major contributions to medicine was to show that, if rabbit antibody were absorbed with Fuller's earth, the incidence of such reactions, presumably due to high-molecular-weight complexes, was diminished. Thus, the tremendous amount of work on the treatment of pneumococcal pneumonia with purified heterologous antibody during the 1930's by the Rockefeller Institute group and by White, Robinson, and Finland in Massachusetts provided an important background of knowledge for the development of human gamma globulin.

The first application of these techniques to human source material came in the 1930's, when Charles F. McKhann, a pediatrician, and Arda Green, a physical chemist, developed a globulin extract of ground human placentas as a source of human antibody for the prevention and modification of measles in susceptible children. Although the theory—that the placental tissue was probably the source of antibodies, was contaminated with tissue proteins and tissue breakdown products, and gave rise to occasional immediate reactions—was wrong, placental extract was an extremely useful therapeutic agent for several years.

In the late 1930's, Tiselius developed the technique of electrophoresis and was able to demonstrate, with Elvin Kabat, that the antibodies were associated with the gamma globulin fraction. At the same time, Edwin J. Cohn was developing a new system of plasma fractionation to meet his exacting standards for separation of proteins from mixtures in high purity and without denaturation so that their chemical and biologic properties could be studied accurately. This work came to fruition just as the National Research Council was looking for ways to obtain a stable blood substitute that would be an improvement over the gum acacia solutions used in the First World War. Cohn rapidly organized a team and started to develop his method for industrial use, with beef plasma as the starting material. Owen Wangensteen had already shown that beef plasma was effective in alleviating hypovolemic shock but was prone to produce immediate reactions, as well as serum sickness. In addition, Cohn began a parallel study of the fractionation of human plasma; this ultimately became the sole starting material, when it was found that highly purified bovine albumin, although almost never causing immediate reactions after intravenous injection, still could give rise to severe serum sickness in some recipients. The great advantages of the method developed by Cohn and his group were: (1) The use of a cheap, volatile compound (ethyl alcohol) as precipitant permitted the work to be done below the freezing point of water, thus minimizing the risk of microbial multiplication or denaturation. (2) The alcohol could be removed rapidly from the relatively small volume of precipitated protein by using the newly developed lyophile process, which had already been applied to the preservation of plasma by Strumia. (3) It was possible to manipulate five different variables, thus allowing maximal opportunities for separating one protein from another on the basis of solubility differences.

Blood plasma was supplied to Cohn's group by the American National Red Cross; research funds were provided by the Office of Scientific Research and Development, acting on behalf of the Navy, which wanted a stable, compact blood substitute, which it soon obtained in human serum albumin. But Cohn could see beyond albumin. His system of fractionation must be inclusive; no one of the precious human proteins present in plasma was to be wasted. However, the government was interested only in albumin, so, using an unrestricted grant to his laboratory from the Rockefeller Foundation, Cohn set teams to work on the various other proteins. Joseph Stokes and his co-workers in Philadelphia quickly proved that fraction II+III, which contained most of the gamma globulins and in which Enders had demonstrated antibodies to various common infections, would protect susceptible persons against measles. Oncley then began work on the subfractionation of fraction II+III, and, with the aid of Enders's laboratory assays and clinical studies by Stokes's group and ours, each of us assisted by a large group of collaborating pediatric practitioners, he quickly developed the process that is still used for the production of human gamma globulin.

Later, as the demand for gamma globulin grew larger, additional source materials besides surplus Red Cross plasma and plasma from out-dated blood were needed, and placentas began to be collected on an increasing scale under carefully controlled conditions. Gamma globulin derived from the blood included in the placenta has proved safe and efficacious for intramuscular use, although immunologic studies by Maurer first showed that it contains small amounts of antigenic components that are not present when gamma globulin is prepared from venous blood; the presentation in this volume by Dauber *et al.* indicates the problem of contamination with blood-group substances.

The development of human gamma globulin has had important consequences for public health, for medicine, and for research. It is primarily responsible for a tightening of standards for biologic products in our country, and for the application of chemical, as well as biologic, criteria to their standardization. The availability of large amounts of pooled human antibody in a safe form has provided material for many types of clinical and biologic investigation, and it has served medicine well as a means of preventing or modifying measles and infectious hepatitis in large numbers of susceptible persons. By providing a way to protect patients with the antibody deficiency syndrome against infection, it has minimized morbidity and prolonged life in what previously had been a fatal condition; at the same time, we have learned much about resistance to infectious disease.

All studies of the gamma globulins from human plasma have indicated their heterogeneity, but only in the last few years has the full extent of this heterogeneity become apparent. This has been due to the introduction of new tools—principally the gel-diffusion methods, developed by Oudin, Ouchterlony, and Grabar and Williams. It was Gitlin and Hitzig's application of Grabar and Williams's technique of immunoelectrophoresis to the sera of patients with agammaglobulinemia that first established clearly that three globulin components, rather than just one, were missing from these sera. From this recognition of three immunologically distinct antibody globulins in human plasma came the concept of the immunoglobulins, which has been so closely associated with the name of Joseph F. Heremans (a participant in this conference) and which has

stimulated many further advances. Much of the present knowledge of
gamma globulin structure, of functional and metabolic differences between the various immunoglobulins, and of their behavior in disease has
arisen from application of immunochemical techniques whereby these
classes of proteins in sera and in cells have been distinguished. I am
happy that Dr. Ishizaka is participating in this conference to discuss in
detail the newest addition to the family of immunoglobulins—IgE, for
whose recognition he is responsible—and that Drs. Kunkel and Fahey,
who have made major contributions to our knowledge of the genetic,
chemical, and biologic complexity of the immunoglobulin system, are
also participating.

A technical advance that has had an important impact both on our
understanding of the immunoglobulins and on their clinical use occupies
another important segment of this conference: fragmentation by proteolytic enzymes. This goes back at least 30 years, to the development
of improved preparations of antitoxic sera from antidiphtheritic and
antitetanic horse gamma globulins by a combination of digestion with
pepsin and differential denaturation and precipitation of the remaining
proteins with heat. When the plasma fractionation program began during the Second World War and Stokes and Enders had proved that fraction II + III contained protective antibodies in a concentration approximately 10 times that in whole plasma and Oncley had gone to work on
purifying the antibodies in this fraction further, Cohn called on his col-
league, John Williams, from the University of Wisconsin, to collaborate
in the study of this problem. Williams and Harold Deutsch (also participating in this conference) studied the effect of various proteolytic enzymes on the gamma globulins of fraction III-1, the portion of fraction
II + III that remained after the prothrombin in fraction III-2 and the
major portion of the antibodies in fraction II had been removed by
Oncley's method of subfractionation. Williams and Deutsch characterized the products obtained after digestion of gamma globulin with pepsin, papain, and bromelin, and we used an excellent preparation of
pepsin-digested fraction III-1 antibodies clinically after its antibody
activity had been confirmed in Enders's laboratory. It is of interest that,
by immunizing guinea pigs with pepsin and then giving them an intravenous challenge with this preparation, we were able to produce anaphylaxis in these animals, indicating the difficulty of removing all traces of
pepsin.

Since that time, Porter in England, Cebra in this country, and others have used enzymatic digestion to analyze the molecular structure of the gamma globulins, and enzymatic digestion has made it possible to overcome the problem of reactions to intravenously injected gamma globulin.

Early in the clinical use of gamma globulin, it became apparent that intravenous injection into acutely ill children was fraught with danger, leading to very acute vasomotor reactions followed within 15–20 min by chills and fever. Similar reactions have been observed when larger doses have been injected into persons who were not acutely ill. Finally, the Swiss have reported that there is a greater frequency of reactions in subjects with hypogammaglobulinemia. The reason for these reactions is not clear, although they appear to be associated with the formation of complexes in the gamma globulin solution; this is reminiscent of Sabin's work on antipneumococcal rabbit sera.

A personal digression may be of historical interest. Cohn, advised by Elliot F. Robinson, Director of the Massachusetts State Laboratories, insisted on clinical tests of all preparations of plasma fractions that were intended for use in patients, before their distribution for investigation elsewhere. Because gamma globulin was an excellent and highly purified preparation of human protein, we felt that it would be perfectly safe. As the first preparations from commercial sources began to come through, each of us in the laboratory took his turn as recipient of an intravenous injection of 2 cc. Things went well until the first preparation from a new producer arrived. It was my turn. The injection went uneventfully, as had all the others; but within about 30 min, acute gastrointestinal symptoms, chills, fever, and mild shock developed, which put me in the hospital for 2 days and gave my associates and my wife an anxious 12 hours. This episode clearly illustrates Cohn's wisdom, as well as my own naïveté at the time. The lot was withdrawn, and investigation revealed that it had been produced before the coldrooms for processing were completed. Although the preparation was sterile and passed the usual pyrogen tests in rabbits, it contained a considerable amount of staphylococcal enterotoxin that could be demonstrated only in kittens and man. Intravenous testing of our laboratory personnel ceased, and a test of each subsequent preparation was made in kittens before clinical trials, until a year had elapsed without further trouble.

Other serious reactions to human gamma globulin were not seen until it began to be used intravenously for the treatment of sick children. Both

Stokes's group and ours were interested to learn whether gamma globulin could be given in large doses to abort the symptoms of severe measles. For this purpose, intravenous administration seemed desirable. At about the same time, Stokes gave a large dose to a child with measles encephalitis, and we treated an adolescent with a very early but severe case of measles. Marked hyperpyrexia and convulsions in the child with encephalitis and vasomotor collapse, restlessness, chills, and hyperpyrexia in our patient made us put *Not for Intravenous Use* on every vial, to prevent further intravenous injections of gamma globulin except under strict experimentally controlled conditions. A long series of studies with Oncley, Otto Krayer at the Harvard Medical School, and my associate, Dr. William Berenberg, failed to solve this problem. Efforts to eliminate the reactive material by further purification of the gamma globulin and attempts to develop an adequate screening test in animals for detection of reactive preparations all ended in failure. In fact, the severity of the reactions to doses as low as 3 cc when gamma globulin was given to children with scarlet fever or early severe measles, in whom we felt its trial was indicated, was so great that our group did not feel justified in carrying out any further clinical investigation of this problem.

There the problem lay until, with the recognition of agammaglobulinemia in 1953 and of the need of its victims for regular prophylactic injections of large doses, Swiss workers found that these patients, like children with acute infections, seemed to be peculiarly susceptible to these reactions. As a result of the work of Isliker, Barandun, and others, the association of these reactions with complexes was recognized, and methods were found for their elimination. H. G. Schwick will discuss a pepsin-digested preparation for intravenous use, and James T. Sgouris and Crain *et al.* will discuss preparations digested with human plasmin, whose effect in the usual gamma globulin preparation was first pointed out by Dr. Škvařil in Czechoslovakia and Dr. Painter from Toronto (both of whom are contributors to this conference). The development of safe preparations for intravenous use constitutes important progress for the clinician.

The biologic advances made possible by the development of human gamma globulin preparations are numerous. Our understanding of the metabolism of the gamma globulins in health and in a variety of diseases, of the behavior of their various fragments, of the rate of transfer of IgG across the placenta, and of the urinary and secretory immunoglobulins has been derived from the use of purified immunoglobulins labeled either with radioisotopes or by their specific antibody activity. The availability of purified immunoglobulins and of myeloma proteins for the production and absorption of specific antisera has meant that very sensitive, specific immunochemical reagents could be prepared for quantitative analysis of biologic fluids and for localization of various immunoglobulins in the cells in which they are produced or stored by using the technique of immunofluorescence developed by Coons and first applied so effectively in clinical studies by Gitlin.

Another aspect of the practical use of the immunoglobulins concerns the problem of homologous serum hepatitis. The risk of transmission of this disease by plasma fractions prepared from plasma pooled from hundreds or even thousands of donors was recognized from the start. Follow-up studies of large numbers of children who had received gamma globulin for measles prevention or modification seemed to show that, for some as yet unknown reason, this infection was not transmitted, although it occurred after local application of thrombin (also a derivative of fraction II + III) and later was shown to be transmitted by fraction IV-1, as well as by fraction I. That experience suggested to Stokes that gamma globulin might contain antibodies to the virus of epidemic (infectious) hepatitis and led him and his associates to test its value in an unusually severe outbreak of this disease in its waterborne form at a summer camp. The results were unequivocally positive and have been confirmed in a series of later studies in both civilian and military life; their application to the protection of our Peace Corps volunteers has been generally successful.

During the Second World War, work with human volunteers and a limited number of virus strains by Stokes, Neefe, Havens, and others seemed to indicate that hepatitis could be produced by two types of virus—one with a short (average, 30 days) incubation period, transmissible by the fecal–oral route and by injection of blood taken during a brief period of prodromal viremia (epidemic or type A hepatitis), and the other with a long (60–180 days) incubation period, transmissible only by injection of blood, in which virus obviously circulated over a long period, often when the carrier was totally asymptomatic (serum or type B hepatitis). Inasmuch as the diseases produced by these two agents (and several others, which have since been incriminated in rare cases in infancy) were clinically indistinguishable, the situation was complicated, but not nearly as complicated as it has become as a result of various epi-

demiologic observations and the work of Krugman and his group with
the Willowbrook strain of virus.

Unfortunately, progress with this major public-health problem has
been severely hampered by a decision that research supported with
federal funds could not use human volunteers. I feel that that decision
was understandable but unfortunate. Not only has it deprived prisoners
of one of the few ways in which they could serve the interests of human-
ity, but it has also blocked the development of blood derivatives and
greatly slowed advances in our comprehension of the complex problem
of hepatitis. Moreover, it has confused the use of human volunteers
under legitimate and ethical circumstances in this country with the
flagrant abuse of helpless prisoners by Nazi doctors, and it has allowed
the toll of death and disability from serum hepatitis to continue for
many years. As examples of the results of the decision, we do not now
know how many strains of hepatitis virus there are, or what the serologic differences between them are. We do not yet know whether two
promising possibilities—the substitution of well-washed erythrocytes in
serum albumin solution for whole blood and the administration of
gamma globulin with each transfusion—will diminish the incidence of
homologous serum hepatitis. Nor has it been possible to test the applicability (to the treatment of plasma destined for fractionation) of
LoGrippo's work on the sterilization of plasma with ultraviolet light
in combination with betapropiolactone.

The therapeutic and prophylactic applications of gamma globulin
have continued to develop. One of Cohn's major contributions, in addition to the development of a safe, relatively stable preparation of human
antibody for clinical use, was his insistence on chemical thinking in a
field that had been dominated by those with primarily biologic training.
This resulted in a degree of quantitative chemical standardization, a
delicacy and elegance in methods used for the separation and preservation of biologically active proteins, and an insistence on sterility and
care throughout—a far cry from the practices of the old-timers, who
knew their business well but covered their potential slips with a good
dose of phenol in the final product.

Cohn was more than a preparative protein chemist. He had a remarkably broad view of the potential significance of his discoveries. Early
in the game he saw that, although his chemical controls could guarantee
a 25-fold concentration of the gamma globulins, they could not guar-

antee uniformity of the levels of various antibodies in the starting plasma. Thus, he insisted on careful records of the source of starting plasma for each lot and careful examination of the antibody content of gamma globulin prepared from plasma collected in various parts of the country. He suggested the use of convalescent plasma as source material for specific antibodies. The first two practical attempts were made during the Second World War. Convalescent scarlatinal plasma was collected by William Thalhimer in New York, and the gamma globulin from it was tested by Dr. John Landon in a clinical experiment that died a-borning because of the introduction of penicillin. Convalescent mumps plasma collected by Stokes's group was tested by McGuiness and Peters in an epidemic of mumps among soldiers in Wisconsin; it was shown not only to have a much higher antibody content than normal plasma, but to be fairly effective in the prevention of testicular involvement, compared with standard gamma globulin. Another concept that Cohn promoted vigorously was the banking of gamma globulin preparations at various times and from various sources to permit surveys of immunity in population groups as new infectious agents were discovered. This concept was never put into practice as he envisioned it, but was later made a reality by the serum bank established at Yale by John Paul. This foresight has recently been vindicated by Evans, the bank's present curator, who has been able to prove that students who contracted infectious mononucleosis at Yale uniformly changed from seronegative to seropositive with the EB virus present in tissue cultures of Burkitt lymphoma cells.

In the second major phase of his practical work, stimulated by the Korean War, Cohn saw, as one of the principal uses of his automated mechanical system of blood collection and separation, the possibility of repeated plasmapheresis of specially selected donors. The practicability of this was demonstrated by Stokes and Smolens, using donors hyperimmunized with mumps and pertussis vaccine. Plasmapheresis by various techniques has since been widely used for the commercial preparation of human hyperimmune and convalescent gamma globulin preparations. The latest and perhaps most significant of these developments is the production of anti-Rh gamma globulin to block the antigenic stimulation of parturient Rh-negative women by cells from their Rh-positive infants.

This calls to mind Stokes's division of gamma globulin usage into passive–active and active–passive immunization. By this he meant that a patient exposed to an infectious disease and then given gamma globulin to modify it undergoes active–passive immunization, because he becomes actively immunized by the infection, which one hopes to keep subclinical by the subsequent administration of antibody. The patient to whom antibody is given first and who then develops active immunity as a result of infection, which may occur as the concentration of antibody falls to low levels, undergoes passive–active immunization. This principle applies to infants in the early months of life and is used in the administration of gamma globulin to Peace Corps volunteers as they depart for service in tropical areas. It is hoped that they will acquire inapparent hepatitis as they catabolize the passively administered antibodies. The use of anti-Rh gamma globulin is a special case of active–passive immunization, in which immunization is actually prevented, probably because one is dealing with a nonmultiplying antigen that can all be removed after combination with antibody. The same effect can be obtained with a multiplying antigen, such as measles virus, if an adequately large dose of antibody is administered before the fifth or sixth day of incubation.

A final point, of great importance for those using gamma globulin, is that our experience with its prophylactic administration to patients with agammaglobulinemia has proved beyond question that antibody to a number of infections, which is present before exposure, can be protective, even when its administration in active–passive immunization may be totally ineffective. We have never seen rubella, varicella, mumps, polio, or any of a considerable number of other viral infections develop while children are receiving regular and adequate injections at a dose that is known not to be protective against mumps, varicella, and possibly rubella if given after exposure.

If I seem to have overstressed Cohn's contributions, it is only because I do not believe that we would be having this conference (which follows the format of a collaborative enterprise such as those he liked to organize) if it had not been for his pioneering work and for the broad vision he had of its implications. One reason he was able to see so far ahead was that he insisted on discussing his work and enlisting the help of the very best person he could find anywhere in whatever field he was working in. He would settle for nothing but the best, so that he was the beneficiary of the collective wisdom of some of this country's top scientists. And we should not forget the backing given to him by A. N. Richards, A. Baird Hastings, and A. R. Dochez of the Office of Scientific Research and Development; by the National Research Council's Subcommittee on Blood Substitutes, headed by Dr. Robert Loeb as Chairman; by those in the National Research Council's Division of Medical Sciences, such as Lewis Weed and R. Keith Cannan; and by many in the National Institutes of Health, such as Kenneth Endicott, who later were enormously helpful.*

This conference is to review many of the practical implications for medicine and health of the theoretical and clinical studies that have been carried on in laboratories and clinics here and abroad since the last conference held in Washington, several years ago. We are deeply grateful to Dr. Robert L. Wall and his staff in Columbus, to the Organizing Committee, to Ohio State University, to Dr. Robert B. Pennell's Committee of the National Research Council, and to the staff of its Division of Medical Sciences, represented by Dr. Henry T. Gannon, for the splendid meeting that lies ahead of us.

In closing, I would like to do a little looking ahead myself. While work has been going ahead on the immunoglobulins, the immunologists and clinicians in this country and abroad—notably in England and in Dr. Good's and a few other laboratories in America—have been concentrating increasingly on the cellular aspects of immunity. Although recent work indicates that there is indeed a two-component immunologic system in man—the system of the thymus and its dependent lymphocytes, which mediates delayed hypersensitivity and allograft rejection, and the system consisting of germinal centers, lymphoid follicles, and plasma cells, which mediates humoral immunity by synthesizing immunoglobulins—present work, nevertheless, is tending to bring these two systems together through the multiple potentialities of the lymphocytes arising in hematopoietic tissues and through the importance of lymphocytes that bear immunologic memory, not only for delayed hypersensitivity but also for the anamnestic synthesis of antibodies specific for plasma IgG. I hope that by the time our next conference is held, the mysteries of the cellular responses to antigenic stimulation will have been solved in clear biochemical terms, as have so many aspects of the immunoglobulins during the last decade. This is a real challenge for future work.

*Several other persons played an important role in making the plasma fractionation program an administrative reality: Admiral Ross J. McIntyre, Surgeon General, and Capt. Lloyd R. Newhouser, of the U.S. Navy, and Basil O'Connor and later General George C. Marshall, as presidents, and G. Foard McGinnes, as medical director, of the American National Red Cross.

JOHN L. FAHEY

Developments in Fundamental Research Related to Clinical Uses of Immunoglobulins

INTRODUCTION

Immunoglobulin Classes

The human immunoglobulin system is characterized by its diversity. Yet this diversity has considerable order. The human immunoglobulin system is composed of major classes (IgG, IgA, IgM, IgD, and IgE) and subclasses within them. Parallel to the major structural categories are functional categories; these are summarized in Table 1. In brief, IgM represents antibody that is promptly formed, remains largely intravascular, is catabolized relatively rapidly, and has high agglutinating efficiency and complement-fixation capacity. IgG seems to accumulate with repeated exposure to antigen and is slowly catabolized; it is largely extravascular and is transported across the placenta. IgA is secretory antibody, being transported into saliva, tears, the gastrointestinal tract, the urinary tract, and colostrum. IgE is a reaginic antibody.

The various classes of antibody molecules represent different functional groups that are required to meet different types of antigen challenges. The concept that diversity permits optimal response to a

15

TABLE 1 Functional Features of Human Immunoglobulin Classes[a]

Feature	Immunoglobulin Class			
	IgG	IgM	IgA	IgE
Prompt appearance after first antigen exposure	−	+	−	−
Largely intravascular	−	+	−	−
High agglutination efficiency	−	+	−	−
High complement-fixation (cytotoxicity) efficiency	−	+	−	−
Bulk of antibody after repeated antigen exposures	+	−	−	−
Largely extravascular	+	−	−	−
Placental transport	+	−	−	−
Slow catabolism	+	−	−	−
Secretory antibody	−	−	+	−
Reaginic antibody	−	−	−	+

[a]At this writing, immunoglobulin D (IgD) has no apparent biologic activity.

variety of challenges is supported by the existence of the major immunoglobulin classes in many different species. Because multiple distinct immunoglobulin classes probably developed relatively early in evolution and have been retained in most species, the various classes must be assumed to serve important and, probably, functional needs. If that is so, it hardly seems likely that all the possible therapeutic uses of immunoglobulins have been exhausted by parenteral administration of preparations that largely represent one immunoglobulin class. Certainly, therapeutic investigations with immunoglobulin classes other than IgG are warranted.

Most therapeutic efforts have used the (relatively) long-lived IgG antibodies, which form the bulk of the plasma immunoglobulins. It is not known what special value serum IgM (or IgA or IgE) antibodies might have if they could be separated from IgG antibodies. Because blocking antibodies are characteristically IgG molecules, the effect of administering purified preparations of antibody in other molecular forms, such as IgM, cannot be predicted from experience with immune serum or fractions that contain large quantities of IgG. Means are now available for purification or partial purification of the various immunoglobulin classes. Perhaps these could be improved both qualitatively and quantitatively. Then antibody preparations representing the various immunoglobulin classes could be used and assessed separately.

Immunoglobulin Catabolism

Two metabolic characteristics of immunoglobulins are especially relevant to their clinical use: (1) the classes of immunoglobulins are catabolized at different rates, and (2) immunoglobulins can change during
fractionation and storage so that they are rapidly catabolized when
they are reinjected into a host. The first of these is reviewed by Waldmann *et al.* elsewhere in these proceedings. The second warrants discussion here.

Prophylactic use of gamma globulin requires that the administered
antibody activity be present during exposure to the infectious agent.
Thus, the catabolic behavior (i.e., survival) of antibody in the circulation is critical to the usefulness of gamma globulin preparations that
contain antibodies (immune globulins). Some degraded gamma globulin
preparations have been reported to have half-lives of hours, in contrast
with the 21-day half-life of carefully prepared human IgG. Clearly, the
antibody content and stability, as well as sterility, of the gamma
globulin preparation are important. Metabolic properties, however,
are probably equally important if gamma globulins are to be used in
patients with congenital hypogammaglobulinemia or those exposed to
endemic infectious hepatitis.

It should be feasible to find out which steps in the purification and
storage processes are deleterious to immunoglobulin survival after injection. Screening tests for catabolic properties could probably be done
satisfactorily in mice or other small animals after intravenous injection
of radioiodine-labeled protein. Whole-body counting is relatively easy,
and the essential data can be obtained in the 5–7 days (or more) that
elapse before the immune response of the animal would accelerate the
catabolic rate of the labeled human gamma globulin.

Immune Amplification

The immune system depends on amplification of the antibody action
for some of the major effects of immune reactions. For instance, activation of the complement system causes cytolysis, and complement par-
ticipates in some agglutination and adherence phenomena. The phago-
cytic system removes bacteria and damaged cells after reaction with
antibody within the body. It is not clear, however, what, if any,

amplification systems are present in the mouth, in the gastrointestinal and urinary tracts, or on body surfaces. Perhaps maximal effectiveness of immunotherapy of diseases in those areas will require addition of an amplification system, as well as a supply of antibody molecules.

Areas of Uncertain Clinical Significance

Several findings on the structure of human immunoglobulins have not yet been shown to have clinical relevance. One of these is the discovery of IgD, an immunoglobulin component in the serum of most persons. The immune function of IgD is not known. This lack of information about physiologic significance makes IgD stand in marked contrast with other immunoglobulin classes, such as IgG, IgA, and IgE.

κ and λ L chains are present in all classes of immunoglobulins, but the contribution of this dual system is not clear. Specific antibody activity apparently can be found in molecules with either κ or λ chains. Molecules with κ or λ chains are metabolized at the same rate. No comprehensive scheme, however, has been evolved to indicate the value of having two major types of L chains, although it seems reasonable to suppose that having two types of L chains is important. Everyone has them; we have tested over 1,000 sera without finding an example of severe selective κ or λ deficiency. Indeed, many animal species have κ and λ chains. Evidently, development of the two L-chain groups has survival value in the environment that animals and man face on earth.

It is conceivable that immunoglobulin molecules have exploitable effects that are unrelated to their immune function. In Waldenström's macroglobulinemia, for example, the disease manifestations attributable to the hyperviscosity syndrome are not due to any immune feature of the molecules, but rather to size, shape, and concentration. In another situation, Herberman has found that human IgM (from normal or Waldenström macroglobulinemic serum) can facilitate the growth of human lymphoid tissue-culture cells implanted in rabbits. The mechanism is uncertain, but antibody activity of the IgM molecules is probably not responsible for the effect. A mind open to the unexpected and nonantibody effects of immunoglobulins may lead to new clinical uses of these proteins.

THERAPEUTIC USE OF SPECIFIC CLASSES
OF IMMUNOGLOBULIN

Secretory Immunoglobulin A (IgA)

The finding that IgA is secreted in saliva, tears, milk, and gastrointestinal and urinary tracts has emphasized an important new focus on the functions of the immunoglobulin system. Immunoglobulins had been viewed largely in terms of protection against invasive infection. The finding of a major secretory immunoglobulin system raises questions about the means by which this system can be augmented if deficient, or supplemented if there will be delay in the normal response.

The good correlation between secretory antibody levels and protection against respiratory infection indicates that these immunoglobulins are significant. Attempts to demonstrate that administration of antibody to the respiratory tract surfaces will reduce infections are logical next investigations. Also, it will be of interest to know whether antibodies of other immunoglobulin classes are as effective as secretory antibody in this situation.

There may be some merit in considering the various secretory organ systems separately—respiratory, gastrointestinal, and so on—especially because administration of antibody in the different areas may require different techniques.

The possibility of benefit from treatment or prevention of respiratory infections can be translated into a series of questions: Would local antibody reduce the hazard of respiratory infection in persons with chronic pulmonary or cardiac disease? Would patients with agammaglobulinemia benefit by addition of local antibody to the upper (or lower) respiratory tract? Will persons with selective deficiency of IgA benefit from local respiratory antibody administrations? Would such persons as astronauts and submarine crewmen, who are in a restricted environment for long periods, benefit (and would costly delays be avoided) by preventive antibody treatment before departure? And, of course, what toxicity or undesirable side effects might develop from repeated administration of antibody to the respiratory tract?

Cholera has received some thought as a gastrointestinal disease that might benefit from immune therapy. Here a devastating gastrointestinal infection causes marked change because of the exotoxin liberated from the vibrio organism. As long as a vaccine is lacking, it would be advantageous to have an antibody that could be effectively administered orally. Secretory IgA might be especially useful because of the protection that secretory piece apparently provides against enzymatic degradation. I believe efforts are being made to obtain secretory antibody of high potency and that therapeutic trials in cholera are planned. Such investigations are needed, and this new focus on antibody in the gastrointestinal and respiratory tracts and on other body surfaces indicates new dimensions for immunoglobulin therapy.

Immunoglobulin G (IgG)

Normal human IgG contains four subclasses: IgG1, IgG2, IgG3, and IgG4. Should gamma globulin preparations contain all four subclasses for maximal therapeutic value? Do currently available immune globulin preparations contain the four subclasses? These are relevant questions, especially in view of the differences in functional features already known to exist in the IgG subclasses (see the review by Kunkel and Yount).

Many patients with normal IgG levels suffer from recurrent infections. One possible cause is deficiency of an IgG subclass. Deficiency of a subclass, however, has not yet been related to disease. Quantitative techniques for measuring serum IgG subclass levels are required in conjunction with suitable clinical observation. If a clinical syndrome associated with IgG subclass deficiency is found, this would be helpful in developing a better understanding of the functional roles of these subclasses.

An alternative to subclass deficiency (in patients with repeated infections or other immune-related disorders) is specific antibody deficiency. Current evidence is compatible with a germ-line theory indicating that antibody specificity may be encoded in the genetic material of germinal cells. There is no reason to believe that everyone will be equally endowed with genetic information for production of all antibodies. If individuals vary in their capacity to respond to antigenic challenge, then those with restricted antibody deficiencies may provide more important

leads for obtaining new information than those with gross immunoglobulin deficiency. Immunologic fingerprinting in any detail is not yet
possible. But such fingerprinting (or phenotyping) of antibody capacity
should become possible and would eventually allow genotyping of
immune competence. Identification of deficiency would allow compen-
sation by avoidance of the harmful agents or by prophylaxis.

MORE AGGRESSIVE CLINICAL USE OF ANTIBODIES

The usual view of clinical gamma globulin use involves prophylaxis and
therapy of infection or replacement of antibody deficiency, generally
because normal antibody synthetic function is impaired, as in patients
with agammaglobulinemia. These are important uses. A more aggressive
intervention in clinical disease, however, may also be appropriate. Antibodies can be used to attack physiologic or pathologic processes within
the patient. This concept goes beyond treating or preventing infection.
It calls for immune manipulation of the body's own cells.

An example of interference with normal body processes for a desirable effect is the use of antibodies against the Rh antigens of fetal
erythrocytes to prevent erythroblastosis fetalis (see the review by
Diamond). In the absence of antibody therapy, erythrocytes carrying
Rh antigens leak from the fetus into the maternal circulation and excite
an antibody response. Administration of Rh antibodies to the mother
at the time of delivery, however, can neutralize the Rh antigens on the
(foreign) erythrocytes of the fetus when they enter the mother's circulation. The immune system of the mother is thus prevented from reacting strongly against the erythrocytes of the fetus, and a destructive
hemolytic process that would seriously affect the fetus in a future pregnancy is averted. Antibody is given in the potential Rh-sensitization
situation to interfere with the normal immune mechanism. Presumably,
the administered antibody combines with antigen before the antigen can
activate the immune system of the mother. This is an example of direct
interference with an entirely normal process. An undesirable result is
avoided. Furthermore, the interference is restricted to the response
against a single antigen; the remainder of the immune system continues
to function normally.

Transplantation Antibodies

A similar approach might very well be useful in transplantation research. The major problem in tissue transplantation is the homograft-rejection process. The rejection process is initiated by histocompatibility antigens on the transplanted tissue.

In man, both the ABH(O) and HL-A systems are strong histocompatibility-antigen systems represented on most tissues. The ABH antigens are easily identified on erythrocytes but are also present on other tissues. The HL-A antigens are not present on erythrocytes but are found on the nucleated cells of most tissues. Other histocompatibility systems probably exist in man, but those are the two that are identifiable now. The ABH genetic locus has three major alleles that are readily identified as A, B, and H. The HL-A gene locus has many more alleles, and HL-A matching of random donors is extremely difficult. Matching in families is feasible in some instances, but most organ transplantation will have to be done without complete HL-A matching. Thus, control of the immune response to HL-A (and possibly other) histocompatibility antigens is, and will continue to be, a major requirement for successful tissue transplantation in man.

Essentially, there is a need to avert the normal immune response against a group of histocompatibility antigens. At present, this is done by the very nonselective and broadly immunosuppressive action of cytotoxic drugs, such as Imuran, and such other agents as corticosteroids. As a consequence, infection and possibly tumor development complicate chronic nonspecific immunosuppression.

A more specific form of immunosuppression might be developed if antibodies for specific HL-A antigens could be administered in such a way as to reduce the immune response—preferably with a result similar to that seen when Rh antibodies are administered to avert maternal Rh sensitization. HL-A and Rh immunity are not entirely equivalent. The Rh immunity is a humoral immunity involving circulating antibody. HL-A immunity, at least for the homograft rejection, is primarily a manifestation of cellular immunity. This difference may influence the effectiveness and manner of antibody use in transplantation immunology. Administration of HL-A antibodies alone may not be sufficient to block a homograft response. Antiserum, however, administered in

conjunction with immunosuppressive therapy of other types, might
very well be useful in reducing or even helping to suppress completely
the homograft reaction. The results of animal studies support this
approach.

What is delaying the clinical trial of HL-A antibodies in tissue transplantation? One problem is the need to be able to identify the HL-A
antibodies and to obtain large quantities of alloantisera—i.e., human sera
that have plentiful amounts of antibody against the HL-A antigens.
Today, the serum is obtained from women who have had multiple pregnancies and from men who have been intentionally immunized. For obvious reasons, potential donors who have had hepatitis or who have
unsuitable blood-group antibodies have to be excluded. Furthermore,
sera have been collected in relatively small quantities for reagent purposes, rather than in the large amounts needed for therapeutic trials.
Another problem is the large number of HL-A antigens, and the need to
administer a variety of HL-A antibodies. Donor and recipient usually
differ in several HL-A antigens. A single antiserum may not contain antibodies against all the antigens. Batteries of antisera may be required,
from which sera could be selected so as to provide each patient with the
antibodies needed to affect the antigens from his particular tissue donor.
A further problem is the toxicity that can occur with these potent antisera. Some antisera cause severe thrombocytopenia. Pulmonary complications were observed in the course of other HL-A antiserum
administrations.

In summary, clinical use of HL-A antibodies in transplantation immunology is an important area for research with beneficial, as well as
hazardous, potential.

Antitumor Antibodies

The possible benefit from the use of blocking or enhancing antibodies
has been emphasized up to this point. It is worth considering, however,
that cytotoxic serum antibodies may be exploitable, particularly in
relation to tumors. The premise in cancer chemotherapy is that the neoplastic cell is more susceptible to chemical damage than is the normal
cell. It is also possible that neoplastic cells are more susceptible to antibody damage than normal cells. Two general categories of antibodies

can be considered: antibodies against normal-cell determinants, and antibodies against tumor-specific antigens.

Lymphoid cells seem to be particularly susceptible to cytotoxic antisera against histocompatibility antigens. Antisera directed against HL-A histocompatibility antigens have been administered to patients with lymphoid malignancies, especially in chronic lymphocytic leukemia. Increased peripheral lymphocytic counts and enlarged lymph nodes can be reduced temporarily by administration of HL-A antiserum alone. Administration of such antiserum in connection with other modes of therapy might enhance the benefits of multiphasic attacks on the neoplastic cells.

Even more hopeful from the standpoint of tumor immunotherapy is the evidence that many tumors in animals have tumor-specific antigens on their surfaces. By extrapolation, at least some human tumors would be expected to be similarly distinctive. The use of tumor-specific antiserum to damage tumor cells selectively seems logical.

There are some difficulties in immediate application of these ideas. One is methodologic: the difficulty of identifying tumor-specific antigens (and antibodies) in man. Lacking a reliable means of identifying human tumor-specific antibodies, it is hard to be sure that one has the right antisera for appropriate investigation. And how is antiserum with plentiful antibodies against tumor-specific antigens to be obtained? Until tumor-specific antigens and antibodies are identified with certainty, studies in this area will be empiric indeed.

Cytotoxic versus Blocking Antibodies

The immunologic complexity of antisera presents another problem. Antisera commonly contain both cytotoxic and blocking antibodies. Their coexistence can be demonstrated by testing at various dilutions and with and without complement. There is still no physical means of separating these two categories of antibody. Perhaps such laboratory procedures will be developed, or biologic means can be found so that immunization will selectively yield either enhancing or cytotoxic antibodies and avoid the simultaneous production of the two forms. Both approaches are worthy of investigation. In cancer immunotherapy, we would like to avoid enhancing antibody and concentrate on cytotoxic antibody.

Heterologous Antibodies

The foregoing discussion of both transplantation and tumor immunology was conceived in a context of using homologous (human) antibodies against body cells. More radical would be the use of heterologous antibodies. Recently, heterologous antiserum against human lymphocytes (ALS) was introduced into clinical transplantation immunology. These antisera, prepared largely in horses, and the derived fractions, such as antilymphocyte globulin (ALG), represent, in part, a return to older concepts of serum (antiserum) therapy and, in part, the new view of interfering with normal body processes.

The use of a heterologous animal source instead of allogeneic (i.e., human) antisera offers several advantages: greater potency and quantity, availability of tissue-specific antibodies, and freedom from hepatitis virus. There are hazards, too, with heterologous antisera, such as anaphylactic reactions, foreign-protein nephritis, and other forms of immune pathology. In the case of ALS, furthermore, there appears to be a high incidence of neoplasms in those subjected to this form of immunosuppression. In spite of the hazards, the experience with heterologous ALS (ALG) and the potential for other useful applications make it appropriate to consider heterologous antibody in some detail.

1. Heterologous ALS works. The immune system can be suppressed, at least temporarily. Immune response to newly administered antigens can be reduced, and induction of immune tolerance can be facilitated.

2. High titers of antibody can be prepared in animals by intentional repeated immunization. Potent adjuvants that might not be appropriate in man can be used to boost antibody response. Side effects of repeated immunization, such as amyloidosis, which would be unacceptable in man, can be disregarded in immunized animals.

3. Large quantities of potent antisera can be obtained by repeated bleeding of the immunized animals. These can be pooled and calibrated so that clinical effects can be reliably predicted.

4. Fractionation techniques permit the purification of undegraded IgG. Such a fraction should contain most of the antibody that is in IgG. This reduces the chances of developing foreign-protein allergic reactions by freeing active IgG from unnecessary, nonimmunoglobulin contaminant proteins.

5. Specific immunologic tolerance to heterologous gamma globulin has been induced in adult animals. Presumably, it could be induced in man. Attempts would be facilitated by the use of purified, undegraded IgG preparations, as noted above. If tolerance were induced, it would be specific for the administered protein and would not apply to other foreign agents; resistance to bacterial infection would remain intact (assuming that the administered IgG did not contain an immunosuppressive agent, such as antilymphocyte antibodies).

6. Tissue-specific antisera can be prepared in heterologous species. An extensive absorption process is usually required to remove antibodies against species-specific (in contrast with tissue-specific) antibodies. By taking advantage of specific tolerance, however, it might be possible to obtain tissue-specific antisera without using absorption procedures.

The introduction of heterologous antibodies into clinical research to achieve a kind of immune surgery puts another question squarely to the immunologist. Can the heterologous molecules be made nontoxic while retaining full activity?

MORE AGGRESSIVE CHEMICAL MODIFICATION OF ANTIBODIES

Gamma globulin fractions for clinical use have been evaluated largely in terms of antibody activity. Certainly, antibody content, as well as sterility, stability, and lack of toxicity, is a major concern in preparing plasma globulin for therapeutic use. But antibody activity is only part of the activity of the molecule. From a molecular standpoint, furthermore, the antibody-active part represents only the portion of the immunoglobulin molecule that contains the L chains and about half the H chains (left half of Figure 1). The functional significance of the other portion (right half of Figure 1), composed of approximately the Fc parts of two H chains, however, has been receiving increasing attention. This part of the molecule is responsible for such characteristics as complement fixation, placental transfer, determination of polymer formation, and rate of catabolism.

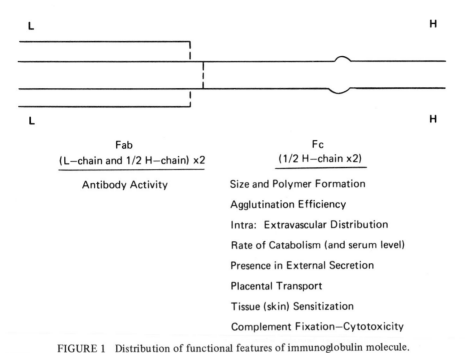

FIGURE 1   Distribution of functional features of immunoglobulin molecule.

Modification of Immunoglobulin Molecules

Manipulation of the immunoglobulin molecule need not wait—indeed, has not waited—for further separation of the immunoglobulin classes. More direct attack on the antibody molecule can be undertaken to modify its functional characteristics. Enzymatic treatment of gamma globulins represents such an attempt to modify the protein to avoid undesirable effects.

The functions to be modified should be separated in the molecule from the site of antibody activity. This appears to be the case for many functional features represented in the Fc part of the molecule (see Figure 1). With progressive work toward solving the primary structure of the H chains, specific chemical components with individual biologic functions will be identified. With this knowledge, it certainly should be possible to modify selected parts of the molecule chemically. For example, this modification might prevent complement fixation so as to reduce undesired side effects and, perhaps, increase the effectiveness of a blocking (enhancing) antibody preparation.

Alternatively, where cytotoxicity is desired, the complement-fixation capacity of antibody preparations could be increased. Reaction of such modified antibodies with antigen could take full advantage of this immune amplification system to achieve important cytotoxic effects. In another example, the transport part of the IgG molecule could be masked. Antibodies modified in this way could be administered to pregnant women, without fear of harmful effect on the fetus.

Modification of immunoglobulins to prolong their survival might be a fruitful area for clinical investigation; it would have clinical relevance in allowing the long survival of passively transferred antibody. This would reduce the need for frequent administration and would increase the value of these important protective materials.

The chemical manipulation of the immunoglobulin molecules has hardly begun. Modification to obtain specific desired effects should be pursued.

Large-Scale Industrial Production of Human Antibody

All preparation of human antibody has depended on the collection of serum from persons who have been exposed to the appropriate antigen and have developed an antibody response. In all such sera, the desired antibody constitutes a very small fraction of the total immunoglobulin population. The other proteins are administered, as well as the desired antibody, because separation of specific antibody is not satisfactorily accomplished. Preparation of large quantities of the required antigens would constitute a major problem. Furthermore, purified antibodies solubilized by current techniques probably would have a low affinity for antigen, because high-affinity antibodies are very hard to isolate in a pure form. It does not now seem feasible or necessary to obtain pure antibody separated from other immunoglobulins. Nevertheless, it seems certain that antibody levels will not be very great in pools from convalescent or random blood donors.

Recent advances in tissue culture of human cells indicate that antibody synthesis in large quantities in the laboratory will become possible. Three steps are necessary to achieve *in vitro* production of human antibody: establishment of human lymphoid or plasma cells in continuous culture, maintenance of immunoglobulin production capacity in these cells, and retention or introduction of capacity to make specific antibody.

The first two of these three steps have been achieved. In studies for an entirely different purpose (to isolate virus from human tumors), lymphoid cells were established in cultures from patients with a variety of neoplasms. At first it was thought that these cells in culture represented the Burkitt tumor or leukemia of the patient, and these were termed "Burkitt cultures" or "leukemic cultures." Similar lymphoid-cell cultures were later started from normal persons, and many observations indicated that most of the cultures might indeed represent cells from the normal lymphoid-cell population.

Further studies revealed that many of these cell lines produce immunoglobulins. IgG, IgA, and IgM have been identified. Some cell lines produce immunoglobulin in appreciable quantity. Immunoglobulin production generally remains stable for several years, as do other characteristics of the cell lines.

The major problem now remaining is to find means of obtaining antibody-producing clones in culture. This might be done by improved culture techniques, which would permit selecting desired antibody-producing clones of cells and establishing them in continuous culture. Alternative approaches are also being explored, with efforts to modify existing clones so that they will produce antibody against desired antigen. These are important areas of investigation, for both fundamental and applied immunology.

There are other problems to be overcome. Optimal growth of human lymphoid-cell lines requires that some protein be present in the medium, but this might have to be separated from the newly synthesized immunoglobulin. Human serum can be substituted for the presently used 10% fetal calf serum. Ideally, of course, growth of cell lines that produce antibody in a protein-free medium, or at least in a medium that differs from the immunoglobulin in protein size, would permit isolation of large quantities of specific antibody—and antibody free of hepatitis virus. Human lymphoid cells are already being grown in large amounts. When antibody-producing cells are grown in such quantities, specific antibody will be available as milligrams or grams per day.

The availability of large quantities of antibody will introduce a new era of immune therapy. It is not possible to anticipate all that might be accomplished by having specific antibody in amounts undreamed of today. By analogy, antibody use today can be viewed as being in the horse-and-buggy era; the jet age lies ahead.

CONCLUSION

As Dr. Janeway has indicated, the clinical uses of gamma globulins in the last 15 years have largely been refinements and extensions of materials and concepts introduced about 20 years ago. Meanwhile, progress in immunochemistry and other relevant sciences has continued at a fundamental level. New opportunities for clinical uses of antibody are now apparent.

More attention to applied research with antibodies is certainly appropriate. But this "applied" research is going to continue to depend on advances in "basic" sciences. Both need continued support. Both are part of the effort to reach common goals—understanding the immune system and preventing disorder or correcting or abolishing human disease.

A third area, lying between fundamental research and clinical trials, deserves special note: the technology needed to provide adequate materials for clinical trials. Clinical studies with gamma globulins require plasma fractionation—and on a large scale. The use of specific immunoglobulin components (IgA and IgM, for instance) requires more sophisticated separation techniques. The use of specific kinds of antibody (cytotoxic, blocking or enhancing, and so on) will require further innovation. Large-scale trials and therapy will be expensive. This is part of the high cost of applied research, and high cost is one of the reasons why close communication between scientists concerned with fundamental, technologic, and clinical aspects of antibodies and immunoglobulins is important. The present conference represents such an effort to achieve close communication and collaboration.

II
IMMUNOGLOBULIN
CLASSES

THOMAS A. WALDMANN, WARREN STROBER,
and R. MICHAEL BLAESE

Variations in the Metabolism of Immunoglobulins Measured by Turnover Rates

The serum concentration of immunoglobulins reflects a balance among the rates of synthesis and catabolism and the patterns of distribution of these molecules. Immunoglobulin-turnover studies allow the measurement of these metabolic characteristics and thus provide information necessary for the rational use of gamma globulin or its subunits as therapeutic tools. Such turnover studies have also been valuable in elucidating the physiologic and pathophysiologic factors controlling the rates of immunoglobulin synthesis, catabolism, and transport. Finally, turnover studies have led to the delineation of new classes of immunologic deficiency diseases. In the present study, radioiodinated purified immunoglobulins of each of the major classes were used to determine values for the various metabolic factors of the immunoglobulins in normal man, to determine physiologic factors controlling immunoglobulin metabolism, and to study the pathogenesis of the reduced immunoglobulin concentrations seen in various human diseases.

METHODS

The IgG, IgA, IgM, IgD, and IgE immunoglobulins and their fragments used in the turnover studies were prepared from freshly obtained serum

33

or, in the case of the fragments, from urine, using fractionation procedures described previously.[3,27,29,34] The purified proteins were labeled with ^{131}I or ^{125}I by the iodine monochloride method of McFarlane.[23] The radiolabeled proteins were administered intravenously in tracer amounts measured to contain 20–50 microcuries (μc) of iodine to patients who were receiving saturated solution of potassium iodide to prevent thyroidal uptake of the radioiodine. The radioiodine released after protein catabolism was rapidly excreted in the urine. The time course of decline of radioactivity in the serum and the whole body was used to determine the protein-pool sizes, fractional catabolic rates, and, in the steady state, rates of synthesis of the various proteins, according to the methods of Matthews[22] and others.

METABOLISM OF IMMUNOGLOBULINS IN CONTROL SUBJECTS

Each of the major classes of immunoglobulins has a unique pathway and rate of catabolism. The data obtained from the studies of the metabolism of immunoglobulins in 10–20 control subjects are recorded in Table 1. The total body pool size ranged from 0.037 mg/kg of body weight for IgE to 1,100 mg/kg of body weight for IgG. The fraction of the intravascular pool catabolized per day ranged from 6.7% for IgG to almost 90% for IgE. The rate of synthesis of IgG is 33 mg/kg of body

TABLE 1   Metabolic Characteristics of the Immunoglobulins

Characteristic	IgG	IgA	IgM	IgD	IgE
Serum level, mg/ml	12.1	2.5	0.93	0.023	0.0005
Distribution, % total body pool intravascular	45.0	42.0	76.0	75.0	51.0
Total circulating pool, mg/kg of body weight	494.0	95.0	37.0	1.1	0.019
Fractional catabolic rate, % of intravascular pool/day	6.7	25.0	18.0	37.0	89.0
Half-life, days	23.0	5.8	5.1	2.8	2.5
Rate of synthesis, mg/kg of body weight per day	33.0	24.0	6.7	0.4	0.016

TABLE 2 Metabolic Characteristics of Intact IgG and IgG Subunits

Characteristic	Intact IgG	Fc	Fab	L Chain
Half-life, days	23	10–20	0.18	0.14
Maternofetal transport	+	+	−	−
Survival affected by concentration	+	+	−	−

weight per day, similar to that of IgA but about 5 times that of IgM, about 80 times that of IgD, and over 2,000 times that of IgE. In addition to the differences in catabolic rates between the classes of immunoglobulins, there are differences between the subclasses of IgG[24, 31]: IgG1, IgG2, and IgG4 have catabolic rates similar to that of IgG isolated from normal serum by O-[diethylaminoethyl] cellulose (DEAE) chromatography, whereas IgG3 has a shorter survival, with a half-life of 7.5–9 days in control subjects, compared with 23 days for all other subclasses.

By studying the metabolism of naturally occurring subunits, or those experimentally produced by treating IgG with papain or pepsin, it has been shown that the differences in metabolic behavior between different immunoglobulin classes are determined by the Fc fragment.[13, 32, 49] As seen in Table 2, the metabolism of the Fc fragment is similar to that of the intact immunoglobulin. The half-life of the Fc fragment obtained either by digestion with papain or from the urine of patients with heavy-chain disease is over 50 times longer than that of L chains or Fab fragment and is nearly half that of intact IgG of the same subclass. In mice, intravenous infusion of Fc fragment, but not L chains or Fab fragment, shortens the survival of intact IgG, and infusion of IgG shortens the survival of Fc fragment. Both IgG molecules and Fc fragment are preferentially transferred across the gut wall of newborn rodents. The Fc fragment will competitively inhibit the transport of intact IgG molecules in this system. Thus, the Fc fragment determines the catabolic rate and the transport of the entire molecule. It is clear that immunoglobulin fragments that will be useful for prophylaxis in man will have to retain the part of the Fc fragment that controls the survival of the protein, inasmuch as modes of treatment of proteins that result in the production of such antibody fragments as the Fab and the $F(ab')_2$ lead to too short a biologic survival for proteins so treated to be of use.

VARIATIONS IN THE METABOLISM OF IMMUNOGLOBULINS

A number of physiologic factors can be shown to influence immunoglobulin synthesis and catabolism. Central lymphoid organs, such as the bursa of Fabricius of birds, have been shown to be of major importance in the development of immunologic capabilities. If its bursa of Fabricius is removed surgically *in ovo* or after hatching with subsequent wholebody irradiation, a bird will produce no plasma cells, germinal centers, antibodies (to antigenic challenge), or immunoglobulin molecules.[10] In immunologically competent animals, the primary factor that controls immunoglobulin synthesis is antigenic stimulation. The rates of synthesis of the different classes of immunoglobulin molecules in mice raised in a germ-free environment vary from less than 1/300 to 1/50 of normal.[15,28] In contrast, mice hyperimmunized with hemocyanin or raised in an environment with high bacterial count have rates of synthesis of immunoglobulins 5–10 times those seen in normal animals. There is at least a 500-fold range in the rate of synthesis of immunoglobulin molecules between germfree and infected mice. There is no truly normal serum immunoglobulin level; the rates of synthesis of the immunoglobulins are not controlled by their serum concentration or pool size but are determined by the bacterial environment and the magnitude of antigenic exposure. Other factors influencing immunoglobulin synthesis are the age of the animal[12]; the level of antibody, which acts as a specific self-regulator of antibody synthesis[37]; the genetic background of the animal; and various hormonal factors.

The catabolism of intact immunoglobulin molecules is determined in part by factors that affect all serum proteins, such as the metabolic rate,[16] and in part by factors that are specific for one or more of the immunoglobulin classes. An example of a factor that specifically affects one immunoglobulin class is the relationship between serum immunoglobulin concentration and immunoglobulin catabolism. The different classes of immunoglobulins differ significantly in relationship between fractional catabolic rate and concentration in the plasma. In one pattern,

exemplified by IgM and IgA, the catabolic rate is independent of the
serum concentration. The catabolic rate of IgM, for example, is the same
in normal control subjects as in patients with agammaglobulinemia and
markedly reduced IgM concentrations or in patients with Waldenström's
macroglobulinemia and markedly increased concentrations.[3] Another
pattern of concentration–catabolism relationship is observed with IgG,
whose fractional rate of catabolism varies in direct proportion to its
concentration in plasma. The survival of IgG is generally prolonged (fractional catabolic rate reduced) in patients with reduced IgG concentration
secondary to decreased synthesis. In these cases, the half-life may be as
long as 70 days.[29,43] Conversely, the half-life of IgG shortens progressively until a limit of approximately 11 days is reached at a serum IgG
concentration of approximately 30 mg/ml.[17,21,29,43,46] Further increases
in the serum IgG concentration do not result in further shortening of
the IgG half-life (Figure 1). It has been elegantly shown by Fahey and
co-workers[14,15] that the effect of IgG catabolism is specifically related
to the serum IgG concentration or the concentration of the Fc fragment.
The survival of IgG is not affected by the concentration of the other
classes of immunoglobulins in the serum. We have developed a mathe-
matical model that can be used to predict the IgG survival if the serum
IgG concentration is known.[46]

Mechanisms have been proposed to explain the concentration–
catabolism relationship observed with IgG. These postulate a mechanism similar to that proposed to explain the selective transport of IgG
across the placenta, yolk-sac, or intestinal epithelium: a saturable
protection system specific for IgG.[8]

DISORDERS OF IMMUNOGLOBULIN METABOLISM IN PATHOLOGIC STATES

Abnormalities of the serum immunoglobulin concentration are secondary
to a variety of pathophysiologic conditions. Hypogammaglobulinemia
may result from defective synthesis of any or all of the five immunoglobulins. It may be secondary to an abnormality in the endogenous protein degradative mechanisms, which would lead to an increase in the rate
of immunoglobulin catabolism. The concentration of immunoglobulins
may also be decreased because of excessive loss of immunoglobulins into

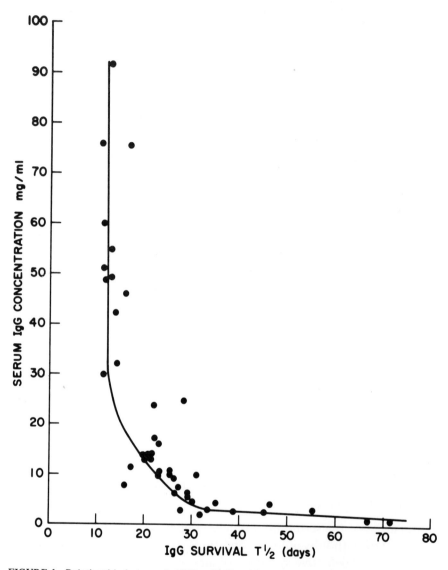

FIGURE 1   Relationship between half-life of IgG and its serum concentration, obtained from turnover studies performed in patients with a wide range of IgG concentrations.

the urinary or gastrointestinal tract. Some major examples of these
causes of reduced serum immunoglobulin concentration are discussed
in the following pages.

Hypogammaglobulinemia Secondary to Decreased Immunoglobulin Synthesis

A major mechanism of hypogammaglobulinemia is decreased synthesis
of one or more classes of immunoglobulins. We have studied the metabolism of immunoglobulins in 15 patients who had sex-linked agammaglobulinemia, idiopathic acquired hypogammaglobulinemia, or hypogammaglobulinemia associated with thymic tumors, and in whom all
immunoglobulins were reduced.[43,47] In each case, the rate of synthesis
of IgG, IgA, and IgM was reduced to 2–20% of normal. In patients without associated gastrointestinal protein loss, the survival of IgA and IgM
was normal, but the survival of IgG was prolonged, with a mean half-
life of 38 days (compared with 23 days in controls) and a fractional
catabolic rate of 3.9% of the intravascular pool per day (compared with
6.7% per day in controls). This prolonged IgG survival appears to be an
example of a concentration–catabolism relationship.

Of adults with hypogammaglobulinemia due to decreased immunoglobulin synthesis, 20–40% also have gastrointestinal disorders. About
half the patients with hypogammaglobulinemia and gastrointestinal disorders have excessive loss of serum proteins into the gastrointestinal
tract.[2,40,43] In these patients, decreased synthesis was the primary defect,
and excessive loss of immunoglobulins into the gastrointestinal lumen
was secondary. When the gastrointestinal disorder was successfully
treated, the survival of serum proteins returned to normal, but hypogammaglobulinemia and the decreased rate of IgG synthesis persisted.

A defect of immunoglobulin synthesis may be restricted to one or
two classes of immunoglobulins, as in patients with dysgammaglobulinemia or ataxia-telangiectasia. The latter syndrome is an autosomal
recessive disease characterized by cerebellar ataxia and oculocutaneous
telangiectasia. It has been associated in some patients with recurrent
sinopulmonary infections, reticuloendothelial neoplasms, and a variety
of immunologic defects.[25,36,50] The immunologic defects have included
delayed skin-homograft rejection, decreased circulating-antibody response to antigenic stimulation, lymphocytopenia, thymic abnormali-

ties, and a somewhat heterogeneous dysgammaglobulinemia. About 70% of patients with ataxia-telangiectasia have a marked reduction in or absence of serum IgA.

We have studied the metabolism of IgA in 12 patients with ataxia-telangiectasia.[34] No IgA was detectable in the serum of eight of them. There was a defect in IgA synthesis in each of the eight patients; calculated maximal IgA synthetic rates were all less than 2.5% of normal. In addition to this primary defect in IgA synthesis, the survival of IgA was short in two patients, with fractional catabolic rates up to 20 times those seen in control subjects. The short IgA survivals were shown to be due to antibodies to IgA in the patients' serum. These antibodies were demonstrated by radioimmunoelectrophoresis and by the C1A fixation and transfer test of Borsos and Rapp.[7] In addition, labeled IgA that was incubated *in vitro* in the serum of one of these patients and then injected into control patients was very rapidly catabolized.

Although the syndrome of ataxia-telangiectasia is rare, absence of IgA from the serum is relatively common, reportedly occurring in one in 700 persons.[1] We and others have demonstrated antibodies to IgA and very short IgA half-lives in some patients who lack serum IgA. Some of these patients have experienced severe reactions to infusions of small quantities of blood products from donors if the donors were not IgA-deficient.

These findings, as well as the demonstration that intravenously administered IgA does not readily enter the external secretions, suggest that parenteral therapy with materials that contain IgA may not be of value in patients with isolated IgA deficiency and may, in fact, be very dangerous in such patients, who have the capacity to produce antibodies to IgA.

Hypogammaglobulinemia Secondary to Disorders of Immunoglobulin Catabolism

A second major pathophysiologic mechanism of hypogammaglobulinemia is hypercatabolism of one or more classes of immunoglobulins. Such hypercatabolism may affect many different protein classes, as in patients with familial idiopathic hypercatabolic hypoproteinemia or the Wiskott-Aldrich syndrome. Or it may be specific for one class of immunoglobulins, as IgG in patients with myotonic dystrophy or abnormal immunoglobulin interactions, as occur in patients with complex cryogels.

Familial Idiopathic Hypercatabolic Hypoproteinemia We have recently
noted a disorder involving hypercatabolism of different classes of serum
proteins, including IgG and albumin.[41] The 34-year-old daughter and
17-year-old son of married first cousins were shown to have marked reductions in serum IgG (1.3 and 4.4 mg/ml, respectively) and serum albumin (19 and 21 mg/ml, respectively). The concentrations of IgM and
IgA were essentially normal or slightly higher. The total body pools of
IgG and albumin were markedly reduced. The rate of synthesis of these
proteins was normal. The fractional catabolic rate was, however, markedly increased. The catabolic rate for IgG was increased fivefold to 34%
and 35% of the intravascular pool per day for these two patients. Both
had normal clearance of ^{51}Cr-labeled albumin, excluding excessive gastrointestinal protein loss as the cause of their protein abnormality. There
was no proteinuria or abnormality of thyroid, renal, or liver function.
These patients were felt to have a new syndrome involving a defect in
the endogenous catabolism of serum proteins as a familial disorder.

Wiskott-Aldrich Syndrome We have also recently noted hypercatabolism of several serum proteins in patients with the Wiskott-Aldrich syndrome.[4] The Wiskott-Aldrich syndrome is a sex-linked recessive disease,
in which patients exhibit thrombocytopenia, eczema, and an increased
number of infections. Patients have a marked inability to manifest delayed hypersensitivity and homograft rejection, although they have
nearly normal levels of lymphocytes that transform normally to phytohemagglutinin *in vitro*.[4,9] Similarly, they have markedly lowered antibody responses to antigenic challenge and low levels of many natural
antibodies, in spite of the presence of normal amounts of serum immunoglobulins.[4,9] The basic defect in this disease has been considered to
be in antigen recognition and processing—an abnormality of the afferent
loop of immunity.[4,9]

The metabolism of IgG, IgA, IgM, and albumin was studied in five
patients, using purified radioiodinated proteins.[5] The serum level of IgM
in the patients was moderately but significantly decreased, owing to de-
pressed synthesis. The patients' serum concentrations of IgG, IgA, and
albumin were the same as or higher than those of age-matched controls.
The survival of each of these proteins, however, was significantly shortened, with half-lives of 7.5 days for IgG (normal, 23 days), 2.9 days for
IgA (normal, 5.8 days), and 9.3 days for albumin (normal, 17 days).
These results indicate that increased rates of synthesis are masking sig-

nificant hypercatabolism. In the case of IgA, the synthetic rate averaged almost five times normal. Gastrointestinal albumin-clearance studies using ^{51}Cr-labeled albumin showed slight gastrointestinal protein loss, but that could account for only a small fraction of the observed hypercatabolism. There was no proteinuria or abnormality of thyroid, adrenal, renal, or liver function. Therefore, these patients also appear to have abnormally high endogenous protein catabolism involving most of the classes of immunoglobulins and albumin.

Myotonic Dystrophy   Myotonic dystrophy is a hereditary progressive muscular abnormality with dominant transmittance. Patients have muscle weakness, wasting, and myotonia. Other associated abnormalities include frontal alopecia, cataracts, gonadal atrophy, low basal metabolic rate, and ECG abnormalities. The albumin, IgM, IgA, and IgD concentrations and metabolism in 19 patients with myotonic dystrophy were within normal limits.[48] The IgG concentration, in contrast, was distinctly reduced, with a mean of 7 mg/ml in these patients, compared with 12 mg/ml in controls. The survival of ^{125}I-labeled IgG was markedly shortened in the patients with myotonic dystrophy, with IgG half-lives averaging 11.4 days in patients, compared with 23 days in controls.[48] A mean of 14% of the circulating IgG was catabolized per day in the patients, compared with 6.8% in controls. The rate of IgG synthesis was normal; thus, the reduction in IgG concentration was due solely to hypercatabolism.

   To characterize the nature of the defect better, IgG was prepared from the serum of a patient with myotonic dystrophy, labeled, and injected into a normal subject and into the patient from whom it was obtained. The IgG was catabolized normally in the control. But in the patient with myotonic dystrophy, it was catabolized at a higher rate, comparable with that of IgG from a normal donor. Thus, host factors appear to be responsible for the accelerated breakdown of IgG, rather than an abnormality of the IgG synthesized by the patient. Patients with myotonic dystrophy thus have an interesting but unexplained immunoglobulin abnormality characterized by isolated hypercatabolism of IgG.

Abnormal Immunoglobulin Interactions   Hypogammaglobulinemia and reduced immunoglobulin survival may be secondary to immunoglobulin interactions with other circulating immunoglobulins, presumably result-

ing from the development of antibodies to one of the immunoglobulin
classes. The development of IgG antibodies to IgA in patients with an
absence of only IgA has been discussed earlier. Another example of
hypercatabolism of an immunoglobulin (IgG) due to immunoglobulin
interaction has been noted in a patient with Sjögren's syndrome, with
an increase in monoclonal IgM and a marked reduction in serum IgG.[46]
This patient's serum contained a cryogel consisting of IgG and IgM that
began to form at 36 C. Neither the isolated IgG nor the isolated IgM
would gel *in vitro*. The isolated IgM, however, would gel if any human
IgG was added to it. This patient had a normal survival of IgM, IgA, IgE,
and albumin. The survival of IgG, however, was markedly shortened,
with a half-life of 11 days and a fractional catabolic rate of over 16%.
The short survival of IgG in this patient could be explained if complexes
of IgG and the patient's IgM formed *in vivo* and were then rapidly
catabolized.

*Hypogammaglobulinemia Secondary to Excessive
Loss of Immunoglobulins*

A third major pathophysiologic mechanism of hypogammaglobulinemia
is the loss of immunoglobulin into the urinary or gastrointestinal tract.
Patients with the nephrotic syndrome have a significant but selective
loss of immunoglobulins into the urine due to damage to the glomerulus.
In most of these patients, the sieving function of the glomerular mem-
brane is retained in part, and the relatively small immunoglobulins, such
as IgG, are lost into the urine much more rapidly than IgM.[6,19] When the
defect in the kidney is limited to the proximal convoluted tubule, as in
patients with the Fanconi syndrome, the pattern of proteins lost into
the urine is quite different from that seen in nephrosis. In tubular proteinuria, small proteins (molecular weight, 20,000–40,000), including
L chains of immunoglobulins, and such enzymes as lysozyme and ribo-
nuclease are lost into the urine, rather than large proteins, such as intact
immunoglobulins.[18,45] We have previously shown that the kidney plays
a major role in the catabolism of L chains.[30,49] It would appear that
small proteins, including L chains, are normally filtered by the glomerulus and taken up and catabolized by the proximal convoluted tubule.
In patients with abnormalities of the proximal convoluted tubule, this
catabolic process is markedly impaired, and increased quantities of these
proteins appear in the urine. In patients with uremia and nephron loss,

L-chain survival is prolonged by 4–10 times, with increased serum concentrations of this protein and small enzymes, such as lysozyme.

One of the significant contributions derived through the use of turnover studies of labeled plasma proteins has been the demonstration that
excessive gastrointestinal protein loss is a major pathophysiologic disorder leading to hypoproteinemia and hypogammaglobulinemia. Excessive loss of serum proteins into the gastrointestinal tract is a common
disorder that has been noted in association with over 70 diseases.[39]
This loss may be secondary to a variety of pathophysiologic mechanisms.
One such mechanism is an abnormality of the gastrointestinal lymphatics
that leads to loss of lymph into the gastrointestinal lumen in patients
with such disorders as intestinal lymphangiectasia,[44] Whipple's disease,[20]
lymphatic fistulas into the bowel,[26] and cardiac disease with right-sided
heart failure.[11,33] The hallmark morphologic lesion of this type of disorder is the dilated lymphatic channel of the small bowel.

We have studied the metabolism of immunoglobulins in patients with
intestinal lymphangiectasia.[35] The serum concentrations of all major
classes of immunoglobulins in 19 such patients were low. The total circulating and total body pools of each of these immunoglobulins were
reduced. The catabolic rate of the intravascular pool was increased to
34% per day for IgG, 59% per day for IgA, and 66% per day for IgM.
The excessive catabolism—i.e., the fraction by which the catabolism of
the intravascular pool of protein per day exceeded the normal amount—
was about the same for all three immunoglobulins. This apparent hypercatabolism was shown by ^{51}Cr–albumin[38] and [67]Cu–ceruloplasmin[42]
tests to be due to loss of proteins into the gastrointestinal tract. There
was apparent bulk loss of all serum proteins into the gastrointestinal
tract, with selection according to size. The rates of immunoglobulin synthesis in patients with intestinal lymphangiectasia were normal or slightly
increased. Patients with intestinal lymphangiectasia, as well as patients
with other disorders of the gastrointestinal lymphatics, have marked
lymphocytopenia and a reduction in serum immunoglobulin concentration; both lymphocytes and serum proteins are lost into the gastrointestinal tract. The lymphocyte depletion may lead to skin anergy and impaired homograft rejection. Our patients, for instance, could not be
sensitized to dinitrochlorobenzene, and skin grafts from unrelated donors
were not rejected during the 2-year period of observation in four patients
in whom this study was carried out. In two of them, a second skin graft
from the donors of the first graft showed no evidence of rejection during

the following year. Thus, patients with intestinal lymphatic disorders may lose both immunoglobulins and lymphocytes into the bowel and may develop anergy secondary to the lymphocytopenia.

SUMMARY

The five classes of immunoglobulins differ in man in their rates of synthesis, patterns of distribution, and rates of catabolism. These differences in metabolic behavior are determined by the Fc fragment. The catabolic pathways of the different immunoglobulins appear to be unique, and physiologic or pathophysiologic factors may affect the catabolism of one immunoglobulin without affecting that of the others.

Hypogammaglobulinemia may be secondary to a variety of pathophysiologic conditions. There is decreased synthesis of all classes of immunoglobulins in patients with sex-linked agammaglobulinemia, idiopathic acquired hypogammaglobulinemia, and hypogammaglobulinemia associated with thymic tumors. There is decreased synthesis of one immunoglobulin, IgA, in patients with ataxia-telangiectasia or isolated IgA deficiency; decreased synthesis is sometimes accompanied by accelerated catabolism of IgA when antibodies to IgA develop.

There is generalized hypercatabolism of many serum proteins in patients with familial idiopathic hypercatabolic hypoproteinemia or with the Wiskott-Aldrich syndrome. Isolated hypercatabolism of one immunoglobulin is noted in patients with myotonic dystrophy and in some patients with abnormal immunoglobulin–immunoglobulin interactions, as in those with mixed cryogels.

There is selective loss of immunoglobulins into the urine in most patients with the nephrotic syndrome and a generalized nonselective loss of proteins into the gastrointestinal tract in patients with protein-losing enteropathy.

REFERENCES

1. Bachmann, R. Studies on the serum γA-globulin level. III. The frequency of A-γA-globulinemia. Scand. J. Clin. Lab. Invest. 17:316–320, 1965.
2. Barandun, S. von, J. Aebersold, R. Bianchi, R. Kluthe, G. von Muralt, G. Poretti, and G. Riva. Proteindiarrhöe. Zugleich ein Beitrag zur Frage der sogenannten essentiellen Hypoproteinämie. Schweiz. Med. Wschr. 90:1458–1467, 1960.

3. Barth, W. F., R. D. Wochner, T. A. Waldmann, and J. L. Fahey. Metabolism of human gamma macroglobulins. J. Clin. Invest. 43:1036–1048, 1964.
4. Blaese, R. M., W. Strober, R. S. Brown, and T. A. Waldmann. The Wiskott-Aldrich syndrome. A disorder with a possible defect in antigen processing or recognition. Lancet 1:1056–1061, 1968.
5. Blaese, R. M., W. Strober, and T. A. Waldmann. Hypercatabolism of several serum proteins in the Wiskott Aldrich syndrome. J. Clin. Invest. 48:8a, 1969. (abstract)
6. Blainey, J. D., D. B. Brewer, J. Hardwicke, and J. F. Soothill. The nephrotic syndrome. Diagnosis by renal biopsy and biochemical and immunological analyses related to the response to steroid therapy. Quart. J. Med. 29:235–256, 1960.
7. Borsos, T., and H. J. Rapp. Hemolysin titration based on fixation of the activated first component of complement: Evidence that one molecule of hemolysin suffices to sensitize an erythrocyte. J. Immun. 95:559–566, 1965.
8. Brambell, F. W., W. A. Hemmings, and I. G. Morris. A theoretical model of γ-globulin catabolism. Nature 203:1352–1354, 1964.
9. Cooper, M. D., H. P. Chase, J. T. Lowman, W. Krivit, and R. A. Good. Wiskott-Aldrich syndrome. An immunologic deficiency disease involving the afferent limb of immunity. Amer. J. Med. 44:499–513, 1968.
10. Cooper, M. D., D. A. Raymond, R. D. Peterson, M. A. South, and R. A. Good. The functions of the thymus system and the bursa system in the chicken. J. Exp. Med. 123: 75–102, 1966.
11. Davidson, J. D., T. A. Waldmann, D. S. Goodman, and R. S. Gordon, Jr. Protein-losing gastroenteropathy in congestive heart-failure. Lancet 1:899–902, 1961.
12. Deichmiller, M. P., and F. J. Dixon. The metabolism of serum proteins in neonatal rabbits. J. Gen. Physiol. 43:1047–1059, 1960.
13. Ein, D., and T. A. Waldmann. Metabolic studies of a heavy chain disease protein. J. Immun. 103:345–348, 1969.
14. Fahey, J. L., and A. G. Robinson. Factors controlling serum γ-globulin concentration. J. Exp. Med. 118:845–868, 1963.
15. Fahey, J. L., and S. Sell. The immunoglobulins of mice. V. The metabolic (catabolic) properties of five immunoglobulin classes. J. Exp. Med. 122:41–58, 1965.
16. Farthing, C. P., J. Gerwing, and J. Shewell. The catabolism of ^{131}I-labelled homologous γ-globulin in normal, hyperthyroid and hypothyroid rats. J. Endocr. 21:83–89, 1960.
17. Freeman, T. Gamma globulin metabolism in normal humans and in patients. Series Hemat. 4:76–86, 1965.
18. Harrison, J. F., and J. D. Blainey. Low molecular weight proteinuria in chronic renal disease. Clin. Sci. 33:381–390, 1967.
19. Joachim, G. R., J. S. Cameron, M. Schwartz, and E. L. Becker. Selectivity of protein excretion in patients with the nephrotic syndrome. J. Clin. Invest. 43:2332–2346, 1964.
20. Laster, L., T. A. Waldmann, L. F. Fenster, and J. W. Singleton. Albumin metabolism in patients with Whipple's disease. J. Clin. Invest. 45:637–644, 1966.
21. Lippincott, S. W., S. Korman, C. Fong, E. Stickley, W. Wolins, and W. L. Hughes. Turnover of labeled normal gamma globulin in multiple myeloma. J. Clin. Invest. 39:565–572, 1960.
22. Matthews, C. M. The theory of tracer experiments with ^{131}I-labelled plasma proteins. Phys. Med. Biol. 2:36–53, 1957.
23. McFarlane, A. S. Effective trace-labelling of proteins with iodine. Nature 182:53, 1958.
24. Morell, A., W. Terry, and T. Waldmann. Relation between metabolic properties and serum concentration of IgG-subclasses in man. Clin. Res. 17:356, 1969. (abstract)
25. Peterson, R. D., M. D. Cooper, and R. A. Good. Lymphoid tissue abnormalities associated with ataxia-telangiectasia. Amer. J. Med. 41:342–359, 1966.

26. Riva, G., S. Barandun, H. Koblet, D. Nussle, and H. P. Witschi. Proteinverlierende Gastro-enteropathien: Klinik und Pathophysiologie, pp. 168–192. In H. Peeters, Ed. Protides of the Biological Fluids. Proceedings of the 11th Colloquium. Amsterdam: Elsevier Publishing Co., 1963. (Engl. summary)

27. Rogentine, G. N., Jr., D. S. Rowe, J. Bradley, T. A. Waldmann, and J. L. Fahey. Metabolism of human immunoglobulin D (IgD). J. Clin. Invest. 45:1467–1478, 1966.

28. Sell, S., and J. L. Fahey. Relationship between γ-globulin metabolism and low serum γ-globulin in germfree mice. J. Immun. 93:81–87, 1964.

29. Solomon, A., T. A. Waldmann, and J. Fahey. Clinical and experimental metabolism of normal 6.6S γ-globulin in normal subjects and in patients with macroglobulinemia and multiple myeloma. J. Lab. Clin. Med. 62:1–17, 1963.

30. Solomon, A., T. A. Waldmann, J. L. Fahey, and A. S. McFarlane. Metabolism of Bence Jones proteins. J. Clin. Invest. 43:103–117, 1964.

31. Spiegelberg, H., B. Fiskkin, and H. Grey. Catabolism of γG myeloma proteins of different subclasses in man. Fed. Proc. 27:731, 1968. (abstract)

32. Spiegelberg, H. L., and W. O. Weigle. The catabolism of homologous and heterologous 7S gamma globulin fragments. J. Exp. Med. 121:323–338, 1965.

33. Strober, W., L. S. Cohen, T. A. Waldmann, and E. Braunwald. Tricuspid regurgitation. A newly recognized cause of protein-losing enteropathy, lymphocytopenia and immunologic deficiency. Amer. J. Med. 44:842–850, 1968.

34. Strober, W., R. D. Wochner, M. H. Barlow, D. E. McFarlin, and T. A. Waldmann. Immunoglobulin metabolism in ataxia telangiectasia. J. Clin. Invest. 47:1905–1915, 1968.

35. Strober, W., R. D. Wochner, P. P. Carbone, and T. A. Waldmann. Intestinal lymphangiectasia: a protein-losing enteropathy with hypogammaglobulinemia, lymphocytopenia and impaired homograft rejection. J. Clin. Invest. 46:1643–1656, 1967.

36. Thieffry, S., M. Arthuis, J. Aicardi, and G. Lyon. L'ataxie-télangiectasie (7 observations personnelles). Rev. Neurol. 105:390–405, 1961.

37. Uhr, J. W., and G. Möller. Regulatory effect of antibody on the immune response. Advances Immun. 8:81–127, 1968.

38. Waldmann, T. A. Gastrointestinal protein loss demonstrated by 51_{Cr}-labelled albumin. Lancet 2:121–123, 1961.

39. Waldmann, T. A. Protein-losing enteropathy. Gastroenterology 50:422–443, 1966.

40. Waldmann, T. A., and L. Laster. Abnormalities of albumin metabolism in patients with hypogammaglobulinemia. J. Clin. Invest. 43:1025–1035, 1964.

41. Waldmann, T. A., E. J. Miller, and W. D. Terry. Hypercatabolism of IgG and albumin: A new familial disorder. Clin. Res. 16:45, 1968.

42. Waldmann, T. A., A. G. Morell, R. D. Wochner, W. Strober, and I. Sternlieb. Measurement of gastrointestinal protein loss using ceruloplasmin labeled with ^{67}copper. J. Clin. Invest. 46:10–20, 1967.

43. Waldmann, T. A., and P. J. Schwab. IgG (7S gamma globulin) metabolism in hypogammaglobulinemia: Studies in patients with defective gamma globulin synthesis, gastrointestinal protein loss, or both. J. Clin. Invest. 44:1523–1533, 1965.

44. Waldmann, T. A., J. L. Steinfeld, T. F. Dutcher, J. D. Davidson, and R. S. Gordon, Jr. The role of the gastrointestinal system in "idiopathic hypoproteinemia." Gastroenterology 41:197–207, 1961.

45. Waldmann, T. A., and W. Strober. Kinetic studies of immunoglobulin metabolism in immunologic deficiency. Birth Defects, Orig. Articl. Ser. 4:388–395, 1968.

46. Waldmann, T. A., and W. Strober. Metabolism of immunoglobulins. Progr. Allerg. 13:1–110, 1969.

47. Waldmann, T. A., W. Strober, R. M. Blaese, and A. J. Strauss. Thymoma, hypogamma-globulinemia, and absence of eosinophils. J. Clin. Invest. 46:1127–1128, 1967. (abstract)
48. Wochner, R. D., G. Drews, W. Strober, and T. A. Waldmann. Accelerated breakdown of immunoglobulin G (IgG) in myotonic dystrophy: A hereditary error of immunoglobulin catabolism. J. Clin. Invest. 45:321–329, 1966.
49. Wochner, R. D., W. Strober, and T. A. Waldmann. The role of the kidney in the catabolism of Bence Jones proteins and immunoglobulin fragments. J. Exp. Med. 126:207–221, 1967.
50. Young, R. R., K. F. Austen, and H. W. Moser. Abnormalities of serum gamma-1A globulin and ataxia telangiectasia. Medicine 43:423–433, 1964.

DISCUSSION

DR. SOOTHILL: I am anxious to place the data on ataxia-telangiectasia in their statistical context. In this series, every patient was grossly deficient in IgA, but that is not true of all patients with ataxia-telangiectasia. I wonder to what extent this series has been selected by the known interests of the group in Bethesda. Also, you cannot say that there is a disease, the sex-linked Bruton agammaglobu-linemia, in which all the immunoglobulins are deficient. Some members of such families may have deficiencies of only some of the immunoglobulins. There may be two brothers who show all the characteristic features of the antibody-deficiency syndrome, one with gross deficiency of all immunoglobulins, and the other with normal levels of IgM.

DR. WALDMANN: We have now seen 21 patients with ataxia-telangiectasia, of whom 14 have no detectable IgA; the other 7 have IgA in their serum. It appears that some patients with ataxia-telangiectasia lack IgE. In addition, most of the patients who are IgA-deficient have great quantities of low-molecular-weight IgM in their serum. The only families that we have seen with sex-linked hypo-gammaglobulinemia have reductions in all the immunoglobulins. I agree that other circumstances may exist.

DR. ALEXANDER: You mentioned with regard to the Wiskott-Aldrich syndrome that there was thrombocytopenia, and you had data regarding the metabolic turnover of albumin—I gather as a reference standard for metabolic turnover of other plasma proteins in relation to the immunoglobulins. Have you any infor-mation on the turnover of fibrinogen?

DR. WALDMANN: We have given some of the patients precursor amino acids, particularly guanido-labeled arginine, to study the survival of fibrinogen. We do not have the results of these studies yet. Nor do we know the survival of autolo-gous platelets in these patients. I know that the survival of other people's plate-lets is normal in these patients. They are on the platelet program and only rarely develop antibodies to platelets.

DR. ROBBINS: Their own and other platelets survive normally.

DR. ALEXANDER: I am interested in your patient with gelation of the plasma. How does the patient live?

DR. WALDMANN: The gelling occurred very close to body temperature. The patient's serum begins to gel at 36 C, when the viscosity of the serum changes drastically. And 22S complexes have been shown to form at this temperature. The patient, amazingly, does not have necrosis of the nose or fingers or Raynaud's phenomenon. She stays inside at all times when it is cold and has done quite well. Previously, whenever she went out in the winter, she would develop fever to 41 C and parotitis.

DR. BUCKLEY: Past approaches to the problem of compensating immunologically crippled patients have relied on the passive administration of antibiotics and human gamma globulin. Recently, we have experimentally evaluated the same problem in adults with a different approach. Specifically, we have tried to diminish their exposure to antigen. We have used a chemically defined diet to lessen the exposure of the immunologically compromised patient to bowel microflora. These patients have high rates of serum immunoglobulin catabolism. For example, we have observed a significant decrease in endogenous creatinine production in one patient after the use of a chemically defined and assimilable diet. The high cost of this experimental diet, currently about $7 a day, has limited the number of patients studied. Nonetheless, exploratory studies in six patients have been completed. Reversal of the symptoms and signs of chronic unexplained inflammatory disease have been observed in two of these patients. Experimental diet treatment of some of these patients has been associated with the return of the ability to maintain approximately normal quantities of immunoglobulins and circulating lymphocytes. Reduction of endogenous creatinine by one third suggests that a normal quantity of bowel flora may contribute to excessive tissue attrition in some patients. Is the metabolic attrition of immunoglobulin in immunologically crippled patients associated with similar catabolic changes involving other tissues? And can significant changes in nitrogen metabolism be demonstrated in these same patients?

DR. WALDMANN: We have studied one group of patients on a chemically defined diet; these patients, suffering from what we call "allergic gastroenteropathy," have extreme gastrointestinal protein loss, eosinophilia, asthma, and eczema. They have diarrhea and vomit on the ingestion of some foods. When placed on a completely defined diet, they had cessation of their gastrointestinal protein loss, eczema, asthma, and gastrointestinal symptoms. The introduction of the offending material, usually milk or one of the milk proteins, will immediately precipitate gastrointestinal protein loss, eosinophilia, Charcot-Leyden crystals in the stools, wheezing, diarrhea, and vomiting. We felt that an abnormal response to milk, whether immunologically mediated or not, was the background in these patients, and that they could be handled either by removing them from the offending material or by placing them on steroids. Immunoglobulins rose markedly when they were placed on therapy, because, although the rate of synthesis was the same, survival was increased fivefold or sixfold as the excessive gastrointestinal protein loss was eliminated. I know of no other metabolic characteristics in the hypercatabolic groups we discussed, which may involve other tissues.

DR. FAHEY: Have you ever found a gamma globulin that was defective in its catabolic properties?

DR. WALDMANN: Not since we have recognized that IgG3 is catabolized differently from other IgG immunoglobulins. At one time, it was thought that IgG3 was defective.

DR. FAHEY: Have you ever measured the turnover of a commercial gamma globulin preparation?

DR. WALDMANN: One cannot extrapolate from materials carefully prepared by gel filtration and DEAE cellulose chromatography and assume that commercial Cohn's fraction II, stored in various conditions, is going to behave in the same fashion. Frequently, there is 20–50% early-degradable material in commercial preparations. The half-lives of the commercial preparations that we tried were about 10 days, instead of 23 days. One can evaluate the quality of commercial gamma globulin preparations by studying their metabolism in experimental animals.

DR. FAHEY: Then you think increased catabolism of a preparation reflects something that happened to it after it came out of the body, inasmuch as no one has reported any abnormality of any gamma globulin preparation that has been carefully prepared? A rapid catabolism is due to something that happens afterwards?

DR. WALDMANN: Yes, especially in those preparations which are commercially radiolabeled.

DR. FAHEY: Would anybody have any objections to that comment? Dr. Clarke from Lederle Laboratories and Dr. Palmer from Hyland: both of you are involved in gamma globulin preparation. Do you test your preparations for turnover?

DR. PALMER: There is no routine testing in our process.

DR. CLARKE: We have studied our commercial preparations of gamma globulin from placental sources for a number of years by ultracentrifugation and have found small amounts of breakdown.

DR. FAHEY: Dr. Waldmann, do you want to comment on the use of the ultracentrifuge to predict turnover?

DR. WALDMANN: I have never found a test other than a turnover study that will adequately predict a good preparation in an animal or man. There are lots of things that can predict a terrible one.

DR. ELLIS: Is there any evidence that parenterally administered IgA goes into
secretions?

DR. WALDMANN: In studies using radioiodinated IgA, we showed that 90–97%
of the IgA of external secretions of man is locally produced. In addition, studies
of the relative rates of clearance of albumin and IgA from the serum to saliva
were performed using intravenously administered ^{131}I albumin and ^{125}I IgA. The
proteins had the same rate of appearance in the saliva. That is, there was no selective transport of IgA molecules. IgA does not readily enter the secretions following parenteral administration.

JOSEPH F. HEREMANS

Biochemical Features and Biologic Significance of Immunoglobulin A

Immunoglobulin A, or IgA, has been known since 1954 as one of the human serum proteins[113] (under the name of β_x- or β_2 A-globulin[21]) and since 1958 as one of the immune globulins.[52] Although earlier publications were concerned mainly with IgA as a serum protein and with its representation among the myeloma globulins,[53] there has in recent years been a shift of interest toward the significance of IgA in the immunologic defense of mucosal and glandular surfaces.

SERUM IMMUNOGLOBULIN A

Sera of animals as diverse as primates, mice, and insectivora contain immunoglobulins related to human serum IgA.[10, 38, 39, 75, 80, 81, 83, 108, 110] In several instances, however, proteins from different animal species originally believed to be IgA have turned out merely to represent subclasses of IgG. The horse's "T-globulin," for instance, is commonly mistaken for IgA.[111] Judging from amino acid sequence data on its a chains, IgA seems to be related more closely to IgM than to IgG.[1] Both IgM and IgA are richer in carbohydrate than IgG.

52

Normal human serum IgA has (in a ratio of 9:1) at least two subclasses differing in the structure of their a chains.[63,107] These subclasses are found in the same proportions among IgA myeloma proteins. The minor subclass (IgA2) of human IgA resembles mouse IgA,[2] in that both have a chains that are not linked to the L chains by disulfide bridges, as they are in the major subclass (IgA1).[47]

IgA is remarkable for its tendency to polymerize[52] by forming intermolecular disulfide bonds involving a cysteine residue of the a chain.[2] Unlike IgM, for which the pentamer is the stable form, the preferred form of IgA in normal human serum is the monomer. In the dog and mouse, and in many human IgA myeloma proteins, however, the dimer is the stable form. Even a 17S IgA myeloma protein, multiply aggregated, has been described.[105] IgA tends to form complexes with many other proteins, particularly albumin.[50,67]

IgA is catabolized much more rapidly than IgG, both in man[109] and in the mouse.[37] Combined with a lower rate of synthesis, this finding explains why IgA in human serum has a concentration between 200 and 250 mg/ml, compared with about 1,200 mg/ml for IgG. In most species of mammals, except primates, IgA is even less abundant than in man, often being reduced to the status of a trace component (e.g., in the cow and dog). Almost half the total body pool of human IgA is intravascular.[109] This proportion may be higher in animals whose serum IgA is of larger molecular weight than it is in man.

Ever since Schultze's first report on the subject,[92] a great variety of antibody activities have been demonstrated in human serum IgA (Table 1). Impressive though the list may be, it is nevertheless clear that serum IgA compares unfavorably with other serum immunoglobulins in its quantitative importance as a producer of antibodies. This must a priori be true in animal species that possess only traces of IgA in their serum. Antibodies of the IgA type have some distinct properties. There is, for instance, general agreement that they resist heating to 56 C. They have exhibited poor precipitating capacity with diphtheria toxoid[54] and blood group A substance.[58] Their agglutinating capacity is evident only with the polymer form and is largely lost on reductive cleavage with mercaptoethanol,[58] a procedure that also decreases their binding capacity sharply.[57] IgA antibodies have consistently been found not to be hemolytic and not to fix complement—with one curious exception, in which the concomitant presence of lysozyme was found to be required for

TABLE 1 Antibody Activities in Human Serum IgM, IgA, and IgG

Antigens	Distribution			References
	IgM	IgA	IgG	
Erythrocytes				
A (precipitins)	7/8	6/8	8/8	64
	(+)	(+)	(+++)	
A, B (hemagglutinins)	3/3	4/4	3/3	84
		11/11		
D		15/15	14/14	82
		3/32	32/32	4
	14/22	2/22	22/22	73
G	1/2	1/2	2/2	84
	(±)	(+)	(++)	
	1/1		1/1	73
c		2/3	3/3	82
		(+)	(+++)	
		0/2	2/2	4
			(+++)	
	6/8	1/8	8/8	73
C		0/2	2/2	82
			(±)	
E		0/3	3/3	82
			(+)	
K, k, Fy, Kp, Jk, P, s, U	–	– to ±	++	4, 82, 84
Le		1/1		84
	2/3	0/3	1/3	4
	5/5	0/5	1/5	73
Bacteria				
Brucella abortus (convalescence)	2/2	2/2	2/2	54
Corynebacterium diphtheriae toxoid (vaccination)	1/1	1/1	1/1[a]	54
Salmonella typhi (vaccination)				
H	1/1	1/1	1/1 }	104
O	1/1	1/1	0/1 }	
Escherichia coli (natural)	2/2	0/2	0/2	3
	+	++	+++	101
Vibrio cholerae (convalescence)				
Precipitin test	{ 240[b]	182[b]	210[b] }	39
	{ 160[b]	145[b]	183[b] }	
Neutralizing activity	–	–	+++	
Francisella tularensis				
Aerosol challenge	+++	++	+	15
Cardiolipin–lecithin test	14/20[c]	6/20[c]	19/20[c]	72

TABLE 1   (Continued)

Antigens	Distribution IgM	IgA	IgG	References
Viruses				
Poliovirus (natural)	1/17	16/17	16/17	5
Influenza A2				
Parainfluenza 3				
Polio 1	+[d]	+[e]	f	14
Coxsackie A9 (natural)				
Parainfluenza 1				
Infection	−	+	++	93
Vaccination	+	+	+++	
Parasites				
Trichinella spiralis (rabbit)	−	−	+++	34
Autoantigens				
Thyroglobulin	3/4	1/4	4/4	46
	1/11	0/11	11/11	73
Nuclear antigens				
Systemic lupus	16/17	13/17	17/17	13
	(++)	(+)	(+++)	
	12/20	5/20	20/20	73
Rheumatoid arthritis	18/18	16/18	16/18	13
	(+++)	(+)	(++)	
Parietal gastric cells (pernicious anemia)	0/72	g	62/72	59
	?	3/4	4/4	43
		(±)	(+++)	
Foreign proteins				
Insulin	0/11	0/11	11/11	74
	1/15	2/15	15/15	114
Milk proteins				
Casein; pool of sera	?	256[b]	256[b]	28
β-lactoglobulin; pool of sera	?	16[b]	64[b]	
Ragweed				
Untreated allergic patients	4/42	26/42	27/42	85
Treated allergic patients	14/48	34/48	46/46	
Horse serum albumin				
Allergic patient	0/1	1/1	1/1	42
Nonallergic subject	0/1	0/1	0/1	

[a]Precipitin.
[b]Titer.
[c]Secondary syphilis.
[d]Rarely.

[e]Possibly.
[f]Predominant in all cases.
[g]Minor amounts.

cell lysis.[4] Serum IgA does not become anticomplementary after heating,[11,94,106] and this property is not changed by removal of the sialic acid moiety.[106]

It has not been possible to allocate to serum IgA any precise place in the immunization sequence. IgA antibodies often appear only in antisera after other antibody classes have risen to high titers. This may be, however, because nearly all investigators of this subject have concentrated on immunization by the parenteral route. Recent studies in our laboratory have shown that mice given horse-spleen ferritin in their drinking water will develop circulating antibodies that are virtually restricted to the IgA class. It would be uncautious to generalize, inasmuch as Coombs *et al.*[28] have noted that, in the serum of infants, IgG antimilk antibodies nearly always predominated over antibodies of the IgA class. Similarly, among rabbits orally immunized with bovine serum albumin, Rothberg *et al.*[91] found IgA antibodies only in the animals that exhibited the strongest IgG serum antibody response.

The skin-sensitizing activity once tentatively attributed to IgA has been shown decisively by Ishizaka *et al.*[56] to belong to a different protein that tends to accompany IgA during its isolation—a finding that formed the basis for the discovery of immunoglobulin E.

EXOCRINE IMMUNOGLOBULIN A

Current thought concerning the biologic significance of IgA has been initiated by the discovery, by Tomasi and Zigelbaum,[99] that this protein is the predominant immunoglobulin in external secretions. In man, this has been demonstrated for milk and colostrum,[99] saliva,[99] tears,[27,61] nasal fluid,[8,86] bronchial fluid,[35,69,71] gastrointestinal secretions,[27,29,70] bile,[27] and secretions from the urinary passages.[97,102] Similar findings have been made in rabbits,[24,38] mice,[9] and dogs.[108] However, the temptation to label as IgA any immunoglobulin that predominates in secretions must be resisted; in cow's milk, for instance, the major immune component is not IgA, but a subclass of IgG (IgG1).

Exocrine IgA differs chemically from serum IgA in its higher sedimentation rate, which is about 11S, and in the presence of an additional polypeptide moiety, called the "secretory piece," in its molecule.[48,77,97,99] These properties have also been demonstrated (separately or together) in exocrine IgA from the rabbit,[25] dog,[60] and mouse[9] and are assumed to exist in several other mammalian species. The most plausible model for exocrine IgA is a dimer formed by two 7S serum IgA units with a possibly double-chained "secretory piece" whose molecular weight is about 50,000–76,000, bringing the total molecular weight to about 390,000.[25,77,97] Exocrine IgA has a particularly high resistance to destruction by proteolysis[26,97] (serum IgA has it to a lesser degree) and to reductive cleavage.[98]

That IgA from the blood gains access to external secretions to any large extent is considered very improbable on the basis of experiments with ^{131}I-labeled 7S IgA molecules,[22,98] although there is some evidence of selective excretion from the circulation.[94] There does seem to be general agreement that most of the IgA in external secretions has its origin in the rich plasma-cell population that infiltrates the stroma of mucosae and glandular structures. Not only are these cells extremely numerous (about 400,000/mm^3 in the lamina propria of the human duodenum[30]), but almost all of them can be shown to contain IgA.[33,34,68,101] In spite of one discordant report,[89] it has generally been found that mucosal and glandular plasma cells do not synthesize the "secretory piece" moiety of exocrine IgA and that this part of the molecule is produced by epithelial or glandular cells.[51,68,98,100] Whether the "secretory piece" is joined to 7S IgA by the epithelial cells or by a spontaneous process, whether IgA seeps out into the lumen of the glands through intercellular junctions or by transfer through epithelial cytoplasm, and whether the "secretory piece" plays a role in this process of excretion (as believed by some writers, who have called it a "transport piece"[94]) are all unsolved questions. The third question will probably have to receive a negative answer.[51]

Secretory IgA has been found to possess antibody activity against a great variety of antigens, as shown in Table 2, but in this regard two differences from serum IgA are immediately apparent. First, exocrine IgA is vastly more important than IgG or IgM as the carrier of antibody activities in secretions, whereas the reverse is true in serum. Second, not all antigens are equally capable of eliciting a response in the IgA of external secretions. For example, although blood group A and B substances readily give rise to exocrine IgA antibodies, rhesus antigens do not. Autoantibodies against epithelial components, when found in external secretions, usually belong to the IgG class, rather than the IgA

TABLE 2   Antibody Activities in IgM, IgA, and IgG Found in Human Secretions

Antigens	Secretions	Distribution			References
		IgM	IgA	IgG	
Erythrocytes					
A, B, AB	Saliva ⎱ Colostrum ⎰	?	++++	?	⎰ 98 ⎱ 4
Rh	Saliva ⎱ Colostrum ⎰	*a*	*a*	*a*	4
Bacteria					
Escherichia coli					
Lysis, agglutination	Colostrum	⎰ +? 2/7 (±)	+++ 7/7 (+++)	+? 0/7	⎱ 3
Fluorescence	⎰ Urine ⎱ Saliva	5/5 5/5	5/5 5/5	1/5 5/5	⎰ 101
Vibrio cholerae Neutralization (Cer-copithecus)	Jejunal fluid		+++	+++	40
Francisella tularensis hemagglutination	Nasal fluid	0/14	14/14 (+++)	0/14	15
Salmonella typhi					
Agglutination	Urine		++	++	104
Bentonite agglutination	Nasal fluid		+++	+	90
Cl. tetani toxoid: hemag-glutination	Urine	−	++	++	103
Viruses					
Poliovirus					
Neutralization	Nasal fluid	−	+++	±	14
Neutralization	Feces	?	+++	?	62
Radioprecipitin test	Colostrum and milk	−	++++	−	55
Radioprecipitin test	⎰ Saliva Duodenal fluid ⎱ Urine	0/10 0/22 ?	10/10 5/22 5/5	0/10 0/22 5/6	16
Rhinovirus					
Neutralization	Nasal fluid	±?	++++	±	88
Neutralization	Tears, saliva, and nasal fluid		+++	+?	36
Influenza, parainfluenza, polio, coxsackie, echo, adeno: neutralization	Nasal fluid	−	++++	?	8
Parainfluenza 1: neutra-lization	Nasal fluid	−	++++	±	93
Influenza:					
Neutralization	Nasal fluid, sputum, and saliva	?	++++	?	66

TABLE 2 (Continued)

Antigens	Secretions	Distribution			References
		IgM	IgA	IgG	
Neutralization, hemagglutination-inhibition	Nasal fluid		++++	+?	6
Autoantigens					
Parietal gastric cells					
Immunofluorescence	Gastric fluid	?	3/4 (+)	4/4 (+++)	43
Immunofluorescence	Gastric fluid	?	0/6	6/6	59
Intrinsic factor:					
Radioprecipitin test	Saliva	?	1/2	1/2	23
Radioprecipitin test	Gastric fluid	–	+	–	45

*a*Usually no antibody activity.

(Table 2). The first of these features is obviously a reflection of the quantitative predominance of IgA in secretions and need not be commented on further. The second feature might be largely explained by assuming that IgA antibodies arise preferentially after local, not systemic, antigenic stimulation of mucosal and glandular lymphoid tissues. It may be recalled that many oligosaccharides of bacterial or vegetal origin are structurally related to blood group AB substances and are probably present in food, as well as in the bacterial flora of the intestinal tract.

Exocrine IgA has thus been cast in the role of what earlier immunologists called "mucoantibodies" or, in the case of the feces, "copro-antibodies."[20] Arguments in favor of this approach have been discussed in a recent review.[49] Such antibodies are known to be produced by local contact of the mucosae with antigen, to appear in the corresponding secretion before detectable antibody is present in the serum, to exist in titers independent of those measured in the serum, and, frequently, to vanish while serum antibody is still present. Many of the exocrine IgA antibodies listed in Table 2 have been reported to exhibit similar characteristics. The superior protective value of such "mucoantibodies" has been demonstrated repeatedly.[49]

Succumbing to teleologic temptation, I once suggested that the tendency of IgA to form complexes with other macromolecules would endow it with precisely the adhesive properties that would make it an excellent "antiseptic paint," to use a term coined by Burnet.[19] In the same vein, he has speculated further that the particular resistance of IgA to proteolytic digestion would be another reason for nature to entrust this immunoglobulin with the exposed role of a sentry.[49] To close this digression, it may be noted that the inability to fix complement should be of no consequence in external secretions, because in such an environment phagocytosis of antigens would have little biologic significance.

CLINICAL ASPECTS OF IMMUNOGLOBULIN A DEFICIENCY

Deficiencies of serum or secretory IgA may occur in association with deficiencies of other immunoglobulins—e.g., as one element of combined hypogammaglobulinemia or agammaglobulinemia of any cause, in combination with decreased IgG and increased IgM, and in combination with decreased IgM and decreased IgG (the Giedion-Scheidegger syndrome). In addition, selective deficiency of serum or secretory IgA is found in some clinically healthy persons and in association with disease. Among the healthy persons with selective IgA deficiency are those rare subjects who enjoy perfect health despite an apparently complete lack of IgA,[87] and some relatives of patients with hypogammaglobulinemia or agammaglobulinemia.[49,50] In the clinically affected group are many patients with ataxia-telangiectasia; occasional patients, pediatric or adult, with recurrent but usually mild infections, particularly of the respiratory passages[44,96,112]; patients with "IgA-deficient sprue"[31,32]; and a few patients with such oddities as IgA deficiency associated with systemic lupus erythematosus[12] or various allergies.[112] It has been shown by Waldmann and Strober[109] that the lack of IgA in ataxia-telangiectasia is due not only to deficient synthesis but also to the presence of autoantibodies against IgA. It is possible, although not demonstrated, that the deficiency of IgA in the cases referred to as "oddities" is also of autoimmune origin. There is some evidence[95] that localized defects of exocrine IgA production, not associated with systemic IgA deficiency, may be responsible for some cases of chronic sinorespiratory infection.

One cannot fail to notice a serious discrepancy between this short clinical survey and the preceding discussion from which IgA emerged as the star figure of mucosal defenses. With the exception of the patients with IgA deficiency and recurrent mild infections, and disregarding the as yet poorly documented local deficiency of IgA, there is no evidence that patients with isolated IgA deficiency should find it difficult to mount an adequate defense against bacterial invaders attacking mucous surfaces. This paradox is lifted, however, by the observation[18,32] that in cases of isolated IgA deficiency the lacking immune globulin may be replaced by IgM, which appears in increased amounts in all secretions, while a corresponding increase occurs in the numbers of mucosal and glandular plasma cells of the IgM type. It is interesting that this "secretory IgM" should not be combined to "secretory piece,"[18] a finding that casts considerable doubt on the postulated significance of this "piece" in the process of transepithelial transfer of IgA.

One of the syndromes mentioned above interests me particularly: the rare disorder called "IgA-deficient sprue," in which intestinal malabsorption is combined with an almost complete lack of IgA in the serum and in all secretions.[31,32] It is remarkable that a gluten-free diet, although capable of improving the clinical manifestations of the disease, should so far have failed to restore the immunologic status to normal. This finding and the systemic nature of the lack of IgA have been taken to indicate that the immune defect was the primary abnormality and the steatorrhea either an independent disorder or a consequence of the immune defect. The latter hypothesis is strengthened by the knowledge that specific infestations of the gut may cause intestinal malabsorption.[79] However, as will be discussed later, the alternative hypothesis, placing emphasis on the epithelial abnormality itself, should not be discarded too lightly.

Because the intestinal malabsorption syndrome in IgA-deficient sprue may remain latent for many decades, one must seriously consider the possibility that it is not an obligatory facet of the disorder and that persons with good health and almost complete lack of IgA have an incompletely expressed form of IgA-deficient sprue. In a family recently discovered, the propositus had the full-blown form of IgA-deficient sprue, and several siblings exhibited an almost total lack of IgA without evidence of malabsorption.

SPECIAL RELATIONSHIPS BETWEEN
IMMUNOGLOBULIN A AND THE INTESTINE

The observations on IgA-deficient sprue emphasize one of the relationships of IgA to the intestinal mucosa. There are, however, still more fundamental connections between the gut and IgA that remain to be explored.

Origin of the IgA Type of Antibody Response of the Intestine

Recent work by our group has been aimed at answering the following questions: Do intestinal plasma cells synthesize antibody only in response to local (enteric) stimulation, or do they also participate in a systemic response to parenteral antigen? If the latter is true, will their response be of the IgA type? What class of antibodies, if any, is made by extraintestinal plasma cells in response to antigenic stimulation by the enteric route?

Germ-free mice (chosen because they had fewer plasma cells than animals reared conventionally) were immunized with horse-spleen ferritin by subcutaneous or intraperitoneal injection or orally (by taking ferritin in their drinking water for 30 days). Cells that had produced antibodies against ferritin were identified in tissue sections by the indirect method of immunohistochemical analysis, which involved exposure to fluoresceinated rabbit antiserum against ferritin after preliminary incubation with ferritin. In addition, such cells were typed according to the class of immunoglobulins that they contained by a sequential immunofluorescence technique.[76] After parenteral immunization, most of the antibody-producing cells were localized in the lymph nodes and spleen and contained antibody of the IgG1 and IgG2 classes; small numbers of the cells were also found in the lamina propria of the gut, and all the antibody produced by the latter cells was IgA. After oral immunization, however, most of the antibody-producing cells were confined to the lamina propria of the gut (Figure 1), and IgA was still almost the only type of antibody synthesized by these cells. The most curious finding, however, was that the few cells from extraintestinal lymphoid tissues that produced antibody in response to ingested antigen belonged exclusively to the IgA type.

These findings, while stressing the commitment of the gut to the syn-

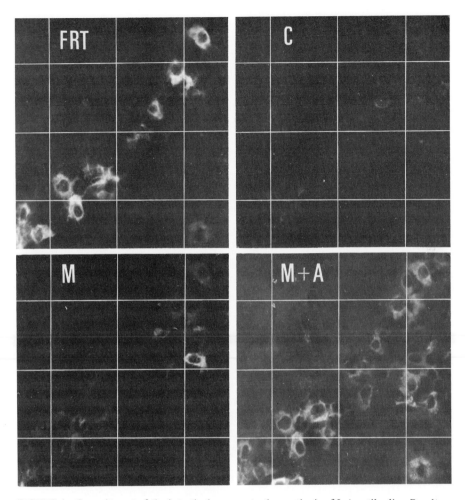

FIGURE 1   Commitment of the intestinal mucosa to the synthesis of IgA antibodies. Results
of sequential immunofluorescence analysis of a section of intestinal mucosa from a mouse that
had received horse-spleen ferritin in its drinking water for 30 days. FRT, plasma cells that contain antibodies to ferritin, revealed by the indirect immunohistochemical method (slide first
exposed to ferritin and then to fluorescein-labeled rabbit antiserum specific for ferritin). C, control; same field as in FRT, after destruction of the fluorochrome by strong ultraviolet radiation.
M, same field; after extinction of the fluorescence, as shown in C, the section was exposed to
fluorescein-labeled rabbit antimouse IgM; only one plasma cell is revealed to contain IgM, and
it does not belong to the population of ferritin-antibody producers (compare with FRT).
M + A, same field, after additional incubation with fluorescein-labeled antiserum to mouse IgA;
many plasma cells are revealed, including all the cells that were previously shown to contain
antibodies against ferritin.

thesis of IgA antibodies in response to oral and parenteral antigen, suggest two alternative hypotheses: (1) antigen coming from the intestinal lumen is processed during its resorption by the mucosa in such a way as to become "IgA-genic," i.e., to give rise to the IgA type of antibody response wherever it meets immunologically competent cells; or (2) the antigen is of indifferent nature but the lymphoid cells of the lamina propria are predifferentiated toward the synthesis of IgA antibodies. Intimate physical relationships have been shown to exist between epithelial cells and small lymphocytes—in this connection called "theliolymphocytes."[41] If the first hypothesis proves true, it may be speculated that epithelial cells are processers of antigen. Antigen would be made "IgA-genic" by them before being passed on to lymphoid cells, which, on being primed by such material, would be polarized into making IgA antibodies. Small amounts of "IgA-genic" antigen might gain access to the circulation (it has been convincingly demonstrated that soluble antigens are absorbed from the gut[17]), and, on reaching distant lymphoid tissues, these antigens would set up a weak antibody response, which would also be exclusively of the IgA type. If the second hypothesis is confirmed, it could mean that lymphoid cells differentiated for the synthesis of IgA antibodies would remain confined to the immediate vicinity of their place of birth, there to build a large population of IgA-producing plasma cells, which is typical of the lamina propria. Small numbers of IgA-predifferentiated cells would emigrate to other lymphoid tissues, setting up the weak extraintestinal IgA response noted in our experiments.

Contribution of the Gut to Plasma IgA

Kinetic studies of immunoglobulin metabolism by Waldmann and Strober[109] have indicated that, in man, IgA is synthesized at the rate of 24 mg/kg of body weight per day, and IgG at 34 mg/kg per day. If one assumes that the output of immunoglobulin per cell is the same for both immunoglobulins, it seems strange that there should be so few IgA plasma cells, compared with IgG cells, in the lymph nodes, spleen, and bone marrow. This discrepancy would vanish, however, if it were assumed that the rich IgA-cell population in mucosal and glandular tissues did not limit its function to providing IgA for the external secretions,

but also contributed significantly to the IgA pool of the blood and interstitial fluid. Here again, the gut, which constitutes the largest body store
of IgA-producing plasma cells, might have a special role to play.

Recent work in our laboratory has shown that the intestinal mucosa
may contribute large amounts of IgA to the bloodstream. This was
shown by comparing the concentrations of various proteins of different
molecular weights—orosomucoid, albumin, transferrin, a_2-macroglobulin
—and of the immunoglobulins IgG1, $IgG2_{ab}$, $IgG2_c$, IgM, and IgA, in the
serum and mesenteric lymph of normal adult dogs. Mesenteric lymph
may be considered a good sample of interstitial fluid from the lamina
propria of the intestine. If the IgA-producing cells from the latter tissue
contributed IgA into the blood, they would do so by first secreting this
protein into the intercellular fluid bathing them, thereby raising the
ratio of mesenteric lymph concentration to serum concentration above
the level expected from the molecular weight of IgA if this transfer did
not depend on an active system. The results indicated that 60–95% of
the IgA present in mesenteric lymph originated in the intestinal mucosa,
the remaining 5–40% being derived from the intestinal blood vessels.
Mesenteric lymph, at least in the dog, is known to contribute about half
the lymph flow of the thoracic duct,[78] so it should cause no wonder
that Mandel and Asofsky[65] found the IgA:IgG ratio in mouse thoracic
duct lymph to exceed the corresponding ratio in the serum considerably.
The flow of intestinal lymph in the anesthetized dog was found by Nix
et al.[78] to average 12.2 ml/hr, i.e., 293 ml/day. Considering that this
fluid has an IgA concentration of about 0.59 mg/ml, and assuming that
80% of this IgA is synthesized by the intestine, the gut's daily contribution to the plasma pool of IgA in the dog would amount to about
138 mg. The intravascular pool of IgA in the average dog being about
123 mg, this would mean that the intestine alone produces more IgA
per day than is present in the plasma at a given time.

The rate of catabolism of IgA in the dog has not been measured, but
an estimation, based on the data of Andersen et al.[7] for the fractional
rate of catabolism of IgG in the dog and on those of Waldmann and
Strober[109] for the catabolism of IgA and IgG in man, indicates that
some 75% of the intravascular pool of IgA may be lost daily in the dog.
It will be appreciated that the gut alone is sufficient to make good such
losses.

SUMMARY

IgA is a relatively unimportant component of the immune system in human blood and may have still less significance in many other species of mammals. In contrast, it is the main component of the immune system in external secretions. Exocrine IgA differs from serum IgA in its molecular constitution in that it contains a special polypeptide chain not found in serum IgA. Most or all of the exocrine IgA seems to be produced by the rich population of IgA-containing plasma cells in the stroma of glands and mucosae.

Isolated deficiency of IgA, known to occur in several different clinical syndromes, in particular in "IgA-deficient sprue," is not often associated with particular susceptibility of mucosal surfaces to infection, presumably because in many such cases its role is taken over by IgM, whose output into external secretions may be increased.

Animals (germfree mice) immunized with ferritin produce antibodies almost only of the IgA type. This antibody production is almost restricted to the gut, when the antigen is introduced orally. In such cases, the extraintestinal antibody response is weak and is remarkably restricted to IgA.

Analyses of the IgA content of mesenteric lymph indicate that the intestine contributes large amounts of IgA to the circulation, in addition to the IgA that is excreted into the lumen of the digestive tract.

The original data presented here are derived in part from work supported by grants 1026 and 1130 from the Fonds de la Recherche Scientifique Médicale, Brussels, Belgium.

REFERENCES

1. Abel, C. A., and H. M. Grey. Carboxy-terminal amino acids of gamma-A and gamma-M heavy chains. Science 156:1609–1610, 1967.
2. Abel, C. A., and H. M. Grey. Studies on the structure of mouse gamma-A myeloma proteins. Biochemistry 7:2682–2688, 1968.
3. Adinolfi, M., A. A. Glynn, M. Lindsay, and C. M. Milne. Serological properties of γA antibodies to *Escherichia coli* present in human colostrum. Immunology 10:517–526, 1966.
4. Adinolfi, M., P. L. Mollison, M. J. Polley, and J. M. Rose. γA-blood group antibodies. J. Exp. Med. 123:951–967, 1966.

5. Ainbender, E., R. Berger, M. M. Hevizy, H. D. Zepp, and H. L. Hodes. Radioautographic studies of poliovirus binding by human immunoglobulins. Proc. Soc. Exp. Biol. Med. 119:1166–1169, 1965.

6. Alford, R. H., R. D. Rossen, W. T. Butler, and J. A. Kasel. Neutralizing and hemagglutination-inhibiting activity of nasal secretions following experimental human infection with A2 influenza virus. J. Immun. 98:724–731, 1967.

7. Andersen, S. B., J. Glenert, and K. Wallevik. Gamma globulin turnover and intestinal degradation of gamma globulin in the dog. J. Clin. Invest. 42:1873–1881, 1963.

8. Artenstein, M. S., J. A. Bellanti, and E. L. Buescher. Identification of the antiviral substances in nasal secretions. Proc. Soc. Exp. Biol. Med. 117:558–564, 1964.

9. Asofsky, R., and M. B. Hylton. Secretory IgA synthesis in germfree and conventionally reared mice. Fed. Proc. 27:617, 1968. (abstract)

10. Audibert, F., and G. Sandor. Nature de la fraction antitoxine des immunsérums de cheval. C. R. Acad. Sci. 267:457–458, 1968.

11. Audran, R., and M. Steinbuch. Etude de l'activité anticomplémentaire des protéines sériques humaines: action "in vitro" de la globuline gamma-A. Path. Biol. 14:838–840, 1966.

12. Bachmann, R., C.-B. Laurell, and E. Svenonius. Studies on the serum gamma 1A-globulin level. II. Gamma 1A-deficiency in a case of systemic lupus erythematosus. Scand. J. Clin. Lab. Invest. 17:46–50, 1965.

13. Barnett, E. V., R. F. Bakemeier, J. P. Leddy, and J. H. Vaughan. Heterogeneity of antinuclear factors in lupus erythematosus and rheumatoid arthritis. Proc. Soc. Exp. Biol. Med. 118:803–806, 1965.

14. Bellanti, J. A., M. S. Artenstein, and E. L. Buescher. Characterization of virus neutralizing antibodies in human serum and nasal secretions. J. Immun. 94:344–351, 1965.

15. Bellanti, J. A., E. L. Buescher, W. E. Brandt, H. G. Dangerfield, and D. Crozier. Characterization of human serum and nasal hemagglutinating antibody to Francisella tularensis. J. Immun. 98:171–178, 1967.

16. Berger, R., E. Ainbender, H. L. Hodes, H. D. Zepp, and M. M. Hevizy. Demonstration of IgA polioantibody in saliva, duodenal fluid and urine. Nature 214:420–422, 1967.

17. Bernstein, I. D., and Z. Ovary. Absorption of antigens from the gastrointestinal tract. Int. Arch. Allerg. 33:521–527, 1968.

18. Brandtzaeg, P., I. Fjellanger, and S. T. Gjeruldsen. Immunoglobulin M: local synthesis and selective secretion in patients with immunoglobulin A deficiency. Science 160:789–791, 1968.

19. Burnet, F. M. The Clonal Selection Theory of Acquired Immunity, pp. 83–86. Nashville, Tenn.: Vanderbilt University Press, 1959.

20. Burrows, W., M. E. Elliott, and I. Havens. Studies on immunity to Asiatic cholera. IV. The excretion of coproantibody in experimental enteric cholera in the guinea pig. J. Infect. Dis. 81:261–281, 1947.

21. Burtin, P., L. Hartmann, J. Heremans, J. J. Scheidegger, F. Westendorp-Boerma, R. Wieme, C. Wunderly, R. Fauvert, and P. Grabar. Études immunochimiques et immunoélectrophorétiques des macroglobulinémies. Rev. Franc. Etud. Clin. Biol. 2:161–177, 1957.

22. Butler, W. T., R. D. Rossen, and T. A. Waldmann. The mechanism of appearance of immunoglobulin A in nasal secretions in man. J. Clin. Invest. 46:1883–1893, 1967.

23. Carmel, R., and V. Herbert. Intrinsic-factor antibody in the saliva of a patient with pernicious anaemia. Lancet 1:80–81, 1967.

24. Cebra, J. J., and J. B. Robbins. γA-immunoglobulin from rabbit colostrum. J. Immun. 97:12-24, 1966.
25. Cebra, J. J., and P. A. Small, Jr. Polypeptide chain structure of rabbit immunoglobulins. 3. Secretory gamma-A-immunoglobulin from colostrum. Biochemistry 6:503-512, 1967.
26. Cederblad, G., B. G. Johansson, and L. Rymo. Reduction and proteolytic degradation of immunoglobulin A from human colostrum. Acta Chem. Scand. 20:2349-2357, 1966.
27. Chodirker, W. B., and T. B. Tomasi, Jr. Gamma-globulins: quantitative relationships in human serum and nonvascular fluids. Science 142:1080-1081, 1963.
28. Coombs, R. R., W. E. Jonas, P. J. Lachmann, and A. Feinstein. Detection of IgA antibodies by the red cell linked antigen-antiglobulin reaction: Antibodies in the sera of infants to milk proteins. Int. Arch. Allerg. 27:321-337, 1965.
29. Crabbé, P. A. Le tissu lymphoide des muqueuses gastro-intestinales humaines. I. Caractéristiques sécrétoires. Presse Méd. 76:1734-1737, 1968.
30. Crabbé, P. A., A. O. Carbonara, and J. F. Heremans. The normal human intestinal mucosa as a major source of plasma cells containing gamma-A-immunoglobulin. Lab. Invest. 14:235-248, 1965.
31. Crabbé, P. A., and J. F. Heremans. Lack of gamma A-immunoglobulin in serum of patients with steatorrhoea. Gut 7:119-127, 1966.
32. Crabbé, P. A., and J. F. Heremans. Selective IgA deficiency with steatorrhea. A new syndrome. Amer. J. Med. 42:319-326, 1967.
33. Crabbé, P. A., and J. F. Heremans. The distribution of immunoglobulin-containing cells along the human gastrointestinal tract. Gastroenterology 51:305-316, 1966.
34. Crandall, R. B., J. J. Cebra, and C. A. Crandall. The relative proportions of IgG-, IgA- and IgM-containing cells in rabbit tissues during experimental trichinosis. Immunology 12: 147-158, 1967.
35. Dennis, E. G., M. M. Hornbrook, and K. Ishizaka. Serum proteins in sputum of patients with asthma. J. Allerg. 35:464-471, 1964.
36. Douglas, R. G., Jr., R. D. Rossen, W. T. Butler, and R. B. Couch. Rhinovirus neutralizing antibody in tears, parotid saliva, nasal secretions and serum. J. Immun. 99:297-303, 1967.
37. Fahey, J. L., and S. Sell. The immunoglobulins of mice. V. The metabolic (catabolic) properties of five immunoglobulin classes. J. Exp. Med. 122:41-58, 1965.
38. Feinstein, A. Character and allotypy of an immune globulin in rabbit colostrum. Nature 199:1197-1199, 1963.
39. Felsenfeld, O., A. D. Felsenfeld, W. E. Greer, and C. W. Hill. Relationship of some vibrio antibodies to serum immune globulins in man and in *Cercopithecus aethiops*. J. Infect. Dis. 116:329-334, 1966.
40. Felsenfeld, O., W. E. Greer, and A. D. Felsenfeld. Cholera toxin neutralization and some cellular sites of immune globulin formation in *Cercopithecus aethiops*. Nature 213: 1249-1251, 1967.
41. Fichtelius, K. E. The gut epithelium—a first level lymphoid organ? Exp. Cell Res. 49: 87-104, 1968.
42. Fink, J. N., R. Patterson, and J. J. Pruzansky. The characterization of human antibody to heterologous serum protein. J. Allerg. 38:84-92, 1966.
43. Fisher, J. M., C. Rees, and K. B. Taylor. Antibodies in gastric juice. Science 150:1467-1469, 1965.
44. François, R., D. Rosenberg, R. Creyssel, and Y. Manuel. Syndrome d'infections à répétition par carence en bêta-2-A-globulines. Arch. Franc. Pediat. 22:913-927, 1965.

45. Goldberg, L. S., J. Shuster, M. Stuckey, and H. H. Fudenberg. Secretory immunoglobulin A: autoantibody activity in gastric juice. Science 160:1240–1241, 1968.

46. Goodman, H. C., E. D. Exum, and J. Robbins. Radioimmunoelectrophoresis of thyroid antigens and anti-thyroglobulin antibodies in clinical and experimental thyroiditis. J. Immun. 92:843–853, 1964.

47. Grey, H. M., C. A. Abel, W. J. Yount, and H. G. Kunkel. A subclass of human γA-globulins (γA2) which lacks the disulfide bonds linking heavy and light chains. J. Exp. Med. 128:1223–1236, 1968.

48. Hanson, L. A., and B. G. Johansson. Studies on secretory IgA, pp. 141–151. In J. Killander, Ed. Gamma Globulins. Structure and Control of Biosynthesis. Nobel Symposium 3. New York: John Wiley & Sons, Inc., 1967.

49. Heremans, J. F. Immunoglobulin formation and function in different tissues. Curr. Top. Microbiol. Immun. 45:131–203, 1968.

50. Heremans, J. F. Les globulines sériques du système gamma. Leur nature et leur pathologie. Arscia, Brussels, and Masson, Paris, 1960.

51. Heremans, J. F., and P. A. Crabbé. Immunohistochemical studies on exocrine IgA, pp. 129–139. In J. Killander, Ed. Gamma Globulins. Structure and Control of Biosynthesis. Nobel Symposium 3. New York: John Wiley & Sons, Inc., 1967.

52. Heremans, J. F., M. T. Heremans, and H. E. Schultze. Isolation and description of a few properties of the β_{2A}-globulin of human serum. Protides Biol. Fluids 6:166–172, 1958.

53. Heremans, J. F., J.-P. Vaerman, A. O. Carbonara, J. A. Rodhain, and M. T. Heremans. Gamma-1A-globulin (β_{2A}-globulin): its isolation, properties, functions and pathology. Protides Biol. Fluids 10:108–121, 1962.

54. Heremans, J. F., J.-P. Vaerman, and C. Vaerman. Studies on the immune globulins of human serum. II. A study of the distribution of anti-Brucella and anti-diphtheria antibody activities among γ_{ss}-, γ_{IM}- and γ_{1A}-globulin fractions. J. Immun. 91:11–17, 1963.

55. Hodes, H. L., R. Berger, E. Ainbender, M. M. Hevizy, H. D. Zepp, and S. Kochwa. Proof that colostrum polio antibody is different from serum antibody. J. Pediat. 65:1017, 1964. (abstract)

56. Ishizaka, K., T. Ishizaka, and M. M. Hornbrook. Physico-chemical properties of human reaginic antibody. IV. Presence of a unique immunoglobulin as a carrier of reaginic activity. J. Immun. 97:75–85, 1966.

57. Ishizaka, K., T. Ishizaka, and E. H. Lee. Immunochemical properties of human gamma A isoagglutinin. II. The effect of reduction and alkylation. J. Immun. 95:771–780, 1965.

58. Ishizaka, K., T. Ishizaka, E. H. Lee, and H. Fudenberg. Immunochemical properties of human gamma-A isohemagglutinin. I. Comparisons with gamma-G and gamma-M globulin antibodies. J. Immun. 95:197–208, 1965.

59. Jeffries, G. H., and M. H. Sleisenger. Studies of parietal cell antibody in pernicious anemia. J. Clin. Invest. 44:2021–2028, 1965.

60. Johnson, J. S., and J. V. Vaughan. Canine immunoglobulins. I. Evidence for six immunoglobulin classes. J. Immun. 98:923–934, 1967.

61. Josephson, A. S., and D. W. Lockwood. Immunoelectrophoretic studies of the protein components of normal tears. J. Immun. 93:532–539, 1964.

62. Keller, R., and J. E. Dwyer. Neutralization of poliovirus by IgA coproantibodies. J. Immun. 101:192–202, 1968.

63. Kunkel, H. G., and R. A. Prendergast. Subgroups of gamma-A immune globulins. Proc. Soc. Exp. Biol. Med. 122:910–913, 1966.

64. Kunkel, H. G., and J. H. Rockey. β_{2A} and other immunoglobulins in isolated anti-A antibodies. Proc. Soc. Exp. Biol. Med. 113:278–281, 1963.

70 Immunoglobulin Classes

65. Mandel, M. A., and R. Asofsky. Studies of thoracic duct lymphocytes of mice. I. Immunoglobulin synthesis in vitro. J. Immun. 100:363–370, 1968.
66. Mann, J. J., W. R. Waldman, Y. Togo, G. G. Heiner, A. T. Dawkins, and J. A. Kasel. Antibody response in respiratory secretions of volunteers given live and dead influenza virus. J. Immun. 100:726–735, 1968.
67. Mannik, M. Binding of albumin to γA-myeloma proteins and Waldenström macroglobulins by disulfide bonds. J. Immun. 99:899–906, 1967.
68. Martinez-Tello, F. J., D. G. Braun, and W. A. Blanc. Immunoglobulin production in bronchial mucosa and bronchial lymph nodes, particularly in cystic fibrosis of the pancreas. J. Immun. 101:989–1003, 1968.
69. Masson, P. L., and J. F. Heremans. Molecular size of gamma-A-immunoglobulin from bronchial secretions. Biochim. Biophys. Acta 120:172–173, 1966.
70. Masson, P. L., J. F. Heremans, and C. Dive. Studies of the proteins of secretions from two villous tumours of the rectum. Gastroenterologia 105:270–282, 1966.
71. Masson, P. L., J. F. Heremans, and J. Prignot. Studies on the proteins of human bronchial secretions. Biochim. Biophys. Acta 111:466–478, 1965.
72. Matuhasi, T., K. Mizuoka, and M. Usui. Studies on the fluorescent treponemal antibody test using fluorescent anti-gamma, anti-alpha, anti-mu, anti-lambda, anti-kappa chains and beta-ICA, E globulin reagents. Bull. WHO 34:466–472, 1966.
73. Matuhasi, T., and M. Usui. Immunoglobulin class and light chain type of human antibodies. Studies with anti-gammaG, -gammaM, -gammaA-globulin, -beta ICA, E-globulins and anti-kappa, -lambda chains reagents. Jap. J. Exp. Med. 36:407–421, 1966.
74. Morse, J. H., and J. F. Heremans. Immunoelectrophoretic analysis of human insulin-binding antibody and its papain-produced fragments. J. Lab. Clin. Med. 59:891–897, 1962.
75. Murphy, F. A., O. Aalund, J. W. Osebold, and E. J. Carroll. Gamma globulins of bovine lacteal secretions. Arch. Biochem. 108:230–239, 1964.
76. Nash, D. R., P. A. Crabbé, and J. F. Heremans. Sequential immunofluorescent staining: a simple and useful technique. Immunology 16:785–790, 1969.
77. Newcomb, R. W., D. Normansell, and D. R. Stanworth. A structural study of human exocrine IgA globulin. J. Immun. 101:905–914, 1968.
78. Nix, J. T., F. C. Mann, J. L. Bollman, J. H. Grindlay, and E. V. Flock. Alterations of protein constituents of lymph by specific injury to the liver. Amer. J. Physiol. 164:119–122, 1951.
79. Olson, L. J., and J. A. Richardson. Intestinal malabsorption of D-glucose in mice infected with *Trichinella spiralis*. J. Parasit. 54:445–451, 1968.
80. Picard, J., J. Heremans, and G. Vandebroek. Serum proteins found in primates. I. Proteins of man, *Macaccus irus* and *Lemur mongoz*. Vox Sang. 7:190–213, 1962.
81. Picard, J., J. Heremans, and G. Vandebroek. Serum proteins found in primates. II. Serum proteins of some other primate species. Vox Sang. 7:425–448, 1962.
82. Prager, M. D., and J. Bearden. Blood group antibody activity among γ_{1A}-globulins. J. Immun. 93:481–488, 1964.
83. Rask-Nielsen, R., J. F. Heremans, H. E. Christensen, and R. Djurtoft. Beta-2A (= beta-3-II=gamma-1A) mouse leukemia with "flame cells" in leukemic infiltrations and degenerative lesions in muscles. Proc. Soc. Exp. Biol. Med. 107:632–636, 1961.
84. Rawson, A. J., and N. M. Abelson. Studies of blood group antibodies. VI. The blood group isoantibody activity of γ_{1A}-globulin. J. Immun. 93:192–198, 1964.
85. Reisman, R. E., C. E. Arbesman, and Y. Yagi. Radioimmunoelectrophoretic studies of ragweed-binding antibodies in allergic sera. J. Allerg. 36:362–373, 1965.

86. Remington, J. S., K. L. Vosti, A. Lietze, and A. L. Zimmerman. Serum proteins and antibody activity in human nasal secretions. J. Clin. Invest. 43:1613–1624, 1964.

87. Rockey, J. H., L. A. Hanson, J. F. Heremans, and H. G. Kunkel. Beta-2A-aglobulinemia in two healthy men. J. Lab. Clin. Med. 63:205–212, 1964.

88. Rossen, R. D., R. G. Douglas, Jr., T. R. Cate, R. B. Couch, and W. T. Butler. The sedimentation behavior of rhinovirus neutralizing activity in nasal secretion and serum following the rhinovirus common cold. J. Immun. 97:532–538, 1966.

89. Rossen, R. D., C. Morgan, K. C. Hsu, W. T. Butler, and H. M. Rose. Localization of 11 S external secretory IgA by immunofluorescence in tissues lining the oral and respiratory passages in man. J. Immun. 100:706–717, 1968.

90. Rossen, R. D., S. M. Wolff, and W. T. Butler. The antibody response in nasal washings and serum to S. typhosa endotoxin administered intravenously. J. Immun. 99:246–254, 1967.

91. Rothberg, R. M., S. C. Kraft, and R. S. Farr. Similarities between rabbit antibodies produced following ingestion of bovine serum albumin and following parenteral immunization. J. Immun. 98:386–395, 1967.

92. Schultze, H. E. The synthesis of antibodies and proteins. Clin. Chim. Acta 4:610–626, 1959.

93. Smith, C. B., J. A. Bellanti, and R. M. Chanock. Immunoglobulins in serum and nasal secretions following infection with type 1 parainfluenza virus and injection of inactivated vaccines. J. Immun. 99:133–141, 1967.

94. South, M.-A., M. D. Copper, F. A. Wollheim, R. Hong, and R. A. Good. The IgA system. I. Studies of the transport and immunochemistry of IgA in the saliva. J. Exp. Med. 123:615–627, 1966.

95. South, M.-A., W. J. Warwick, F. A. Wollheim, and R. A. Good. The IgA system. III. IgA levels in the serum and saliva of pediatric patients—evidence for a local immunological system. J. Pediat. 71:645–653, 1967.

96. Stoelinga, G. B. Dysimmunoglobulinaemie bij kinderen, pp. 78–81. Centrale Drukkerij N.V. Nijmegen, 1966.

97. Tomasi, T. B., Jr., and D. S. Czerwinski. The secretory IgA system. Birth Defects, Orig. Artic. Series 4:270–275, 1968.

98. Tomasi, T. B., Jr., E. M. Tan, A. Solomon, and R. A. Prendergast. Characteristics of an immune system common to certain external secretions. J. Exp. Med. 121:101–124, 1965.

99. Tomasi, T. B., Jr., and S. Zigelbaum. The selective occurrence of gamma-1A globulins in certain body fluids. J. Clin. Invest. 42:1552–1560, 1963.

100. Tourville, D. R., R. H. Adler, J. Bienenstock, and T. B. Tomasi, Jr. The human secretory immunoglobulin system: Immunohistological localization of gamma A, secretory "piece," and lactoferrin in normal human tissues. J. Exp. Med. 129:441–429, 1969.

101. Tourville, D., J. Bienenstock, and T. B. Tomasi, Jr. Natural antibodies of human serum, saliva, and urine reactive with Escherichia coli. Proc. Soc. Exp. Biol. Med. 128:722–727, 1968.

102. Turner, M. W. Characterization of antibodies in normal human urine by gel-filtration and antigenic analysis. Protides Biol. Fluids 12:453–456, 1964.

103. Turner, M. W., and D. S. Rowe. Antibodies of IgA and IgG classes in normal human urine. Immunology 12:689–699, 1967.

104. Turner, M. W., and D. S. Rowe. Characterization of human antibodies to Salmonella typhi by gel-filtration and antigenic analysis. Immunology 7:639–656, 1964.

105. Vaerman, J.-P., H. H. Fudenberg, C. Vaerman, and W. J. Mandy. On the significance of the heterogeneity in molecular size of human serum γA-globulins. Immunochemistry 2:263–272, 1965.

106. Vaerman, J.-P., and J. F. Heremans. Effect of neuraminidase and acidification on complement-fixing properties of human IgA and IgG. Int. Arch. Allerg. 34:49–52, 1968.
107. Vaerman, J.-P., and J. F. Heremans. Subclasses of human immunoglobulin A based on differences in the alpha polypeptide chains. Science 153:647–649, 1966.
108. Vaerman, J.-P., and J. F. Heremans. The immunoglobulins of the dog–I. Identification of canine immunoglobulins homologous to human IgA and IgM. Immunochemistry 5: 425–432, 1968.
109. Waldmann, T. A., and W. Strober. Kinetic studies of immunoglobulin metabolism in immunologic deficiency. Birth Defects, Orig. Artic. Series 4:388–392, 1968.
110. Wang, A. C., J. Shuster, A. Epstein, and H. H. Fudenberg. Evolution of antigenic determinants of transferrin and other serum proteins in primates. Biochem. Genet. 1:347–358, 1968.
111. Weir, R. C., R. R. Porter, and D. Givol. Comparison of the C-terminal amino-acid sequence of two horse immunoglobulins IgG and IgG(T). Nature 212:205–206, 1966.
112. West, C. D., R. Hong, and N. H. Holland. Immunoglobulin levels from the newborn period to adulthood and in immunoglobulin deficiency states. J. Clin. Invest. 41:2054–2064, 1962.
113. Williams, C. A. Immuno-electrophoresis: a new method for the analysis of complex antigen and antibody mixtures. Applications to human serum antigens and hyperimmune horse serum. Thesis. New Brunswick, N.J.: Rutgers University Press, 1954.
114. Yagi, Y., P. Maier, D. Pressman, C. E. Arbesman, R. E. Reisman, and A. R. Lenzner. Multiplicity of insulin binding antibodies in human sera. Presence of antibody activity in γ-, β_{2A}-, and β_{2M}-globulins. J. Immun. 90:760–769, 1963.

DISCUSSION

DR. MILLS: Some patients with IgA deficiency malabsorption syndrome are improved by broad-spectrum antibiotics. Do you have any information on the role of alterations in the bacterial flora in the gut in the malabsorption syndrome?

DR. HEREMANS: There is plenty of clinical evidence of the favorable effect of broad-spectrum antibiotic therapy on the malabsorption syndrome in patients with sprue in general, and the same seems to apply to patients with IgA-deficient sprue, but the results are not really very clear-cut. Recently, a study of experimental infection of the mouse with *Trichinella spiralis* has shown that intestinal absorption became pathologic as soon as the infection set in. There is a clear possibility that the digestive disturbance in these patients is a consequence of the unchecked development of an abnormal bacterial flora in the gut.

We have tried to do some bacterial studies on that, but it is very difficult. My only excuse for not having succeeded in demonstrating anything is that it has been reported by several authors in the literature that no one can really describe the normal bacterial flora of the human small intestine, so that we do not know what a pathologic flora would look like.

DR. EDWARDS: Does the mesenteric- or the gut-synthesized IgA contribute to the other secretory levels of IgA, such as in the parotid solution, saliva, and the naso-pharyngeal area?

DR. HEREMANS: We have no direct evidence on that. The only comment I can make is that in patients with IgA-deficient sprue, where something obviously is wrong with the gut and nothing is demonstrably wrong with other mucosae (such patients have absolutely no symptoms in relation to the nose, the throat, or the eyes), there is no IgA in other external secretions. But I do not know whether the gut is responsible for providing IgA to other mucosae or whether any other relationship of that kind exists.

DR. FUDENBERG: Has anyone found an absence of secretory IgA in the presence of normal serum IgA? If so, have such patients had unusually high frequencies of respiratory or gastrointestinal infection?

DR. HEREMANS: As far as I can remember, patients described by Mary-Ann South and co-workers had normal or high serum IgA, with deficient IgA in their parotid saliva and possibly in respiratory secretions. These patients were stated to have a high incidence of local infections.

JOHN MILLS, ROBERT M. CHANOCK, JOHN VAN KIRK,
JOSEPH A. BELLANTI, *and* JOHN C. PERKINS

Biology of Antibodies to Infectious Agents in Respiratory Secretions

Progress in the biologic sciences occurs during periods of heightened
interest in particular fields. These periods are often initiated by advances in investigative techniques. That nasal secretions, saliva, and tears
contained substances that would react with infectious agents was first
observed early in this century,[2, 84, 100] shortly after the demonstration of
similar substances in blood and peritoneal fluid by Buchner, Bordet,
Pfeiffer, Gruber, Widal, and Ehrlich. Interest in respiratory secretory
antibody increased markedly between 1941 and 1951, when a number
of studies of respiratory antibody to influenza virus were published.
Little further work was done until the mid-1960's; then rapid advances
in the techniques of respiratory virology and immunochemistry resulted
in the present burgeoning of publications related to local antibody. The
purpose of this paper is to discuss work on the presence and development of local antibody in the respiratory tract and associated structures
(such as the parotid and lacrimal glands) and to review its possible role
in protection against infection. Some recent data from our laboratory
concerning the role of local antibody in immunity to respiratory syncytial viral and rhinoviral infection in adults also will be presented. The

discussion will be oriented primarily toward viral infections, because most of the recent studies have dealt with viruses, rather than bacteria or other microorganisms.

First, we should mention the methods used to obtain respiratory secretions. "Nasal washes" refers usually to material collected by instilling saline (or other innocuous salt solution, usually iso-osmolar) into the nares of humans and having them expel the saline and accompanying mucus into a container. In infants, the saline–mucus mixture is removed by suction. Nasal washes are often concentrated by lyophilization, even though it causes a reduction in the apparent concentration of immunoglobulins, probably by inducing aggregation.[91] In our experience, such loss is usually less than 30%. Collected by this method, the protein concentration of nasal washes from a single person can vary as much as fourfold from day to day, and the variation between persons can be as great as 20-fold.[94] Although protein and IgA concentrations tend to be related, the proportion may vary widely from time to time, making protein concentration unreliable as an index of IgA concentration (for examples, see the data presented by Rossen *et al.*[91,94] and Smith *et al.*[97]). The presence of occult blood in nasal washes (detected by guaiac or benzidine test) does not appear to influence the immunoglobulin composition markedly.[94]

"Sputum" refers to material collected by having volunteers cough into a container, usually soon after arising. Although partially contaminated by saliva, it is probably representative of tracheobronchial secretions. Because most of the volunteers used in experiments to study local antibody have been prisoners (men who are almost invariably heavy smokers), sputum collected from them may differ significantly both qualitatively and quantitatively from that of the normal population, particularly the pediatric population. Such possible differences have, to our knowledge, not been studied. In experimental animals, tracheobronchial secretions have been obtained by washing the airways with saline immediately post mortem.[35, 38]

Saliva is usually obtained from adults by stimulating secretion with paraffin wax or lemon, and special devices are often used to collect parotid secretions directly from Stensen's duct. Immunologic differences between whole-mouth saliva and parotid secretions have not been looked for but may exist, in view of pronounced differences in the other constituents of the secretions of the various salivary glands.

In the older literature, techniques of immunoglobulin characterization have included ammonium sulfate fractionation, heat resistance (56 C for 30 min) and sensitivity (70 C), and specific absorption by antigen; more recently, gel filtration, gradient centrifugation, immunoelectrophoresis, immunodiffusion, absorption with immunoglobulin-specific antisera, and radioimmunobinding have also been used. Unless otherwise noted, the inhibitory substances cited in this paper have been characterized as immunoglobulins.

ANTIBODIES IN RESPIRATORY SECRETIONS

Antibodies to a wide variety of viruses and bacteria have been demonstrated in respiratory secretions (see, for example, references 3, 71, 72, 88, and 96). The earlier work, which largely concerned salivary antibodies to bacteria and bacterial toxins, has been reviewed by Kraus and Konno,[71] Pierce,[83] and Gay.[53,54] In general, appreciable levels of agglutinins, precipitins, and hemagglutinins to a number of bacteria could be found in saliva, although no attempt was made to characterize them as immunoglobulins other than by showing the specificity of the reaction. Quantitatively, it was found that low or undetectable serum titers to a given bacterium were associated with an absence of salivary "antibodies"; however, in subjects with higher serum titers, there was only a general correlation between these levels and those in saliva. The findings with regard to tears have been similar.[59,96]

Five groups of investigators have attempted to demonstrate the antibody nature of antibacterial substances in respiratory secretions: Kraus and Konno,[71,72] antibacterial antibodies in saliva; Remington et al.,[88] antibodies to tetanus and diphtheria toxoids in nasal washes; Brandtzaeg et al.,[14] antibacterial antibodies in saliva; Tourville et al.,[104] antibodies to *Escherichia coli* in urine and saliva; and Buescher, Bellanti, and co-workers,[8,16] antibodies to *Francisella tularensis* in respiratory secretions. Brandtzaeg et al.[14] and Tourville et al.[104] were able to show adsorption of IgA from saliva onto various bacteria by means of immunofluorescence; Tourville et al. were also able to demonstrate adsorption of IgG and IgM, although the levels of IgM in saliva were too low to detect by the Ouchterlony technique. Unfortunately, in neither instance were tests done to demonstrate that the binding of the immunoglobulins to the bacteria was immunologically specific; therefore, a nonspecific adsorption of the antibodies to the bacteria cannot be excluded.

Bellanti, Buescher, and co-workers[8, 16] found hemagglutinating antibodies to *F. tularensis* in nasal washes. The specificity of the reaction was indicated by two observations: normal subjects had no detectable antibody to this bacterium in serum or nasal washes, and antibodies developed only after infection or percutaneous vaccination. These antibodies behaved like secretory IgA on gel filtration. Similar findings were reported by Remington *et al.*[88] for tetanus and diphtheria toxoids: only subjects with high serum titers to these antigens due to repeated vaccination had detectable nasal antibodies.

Neutralizing antibodies to many viruses have been found in respiratory secretions since 1917, when Amoss and Taylor[2] reported neutralization of poliovirus by nasal mucus. The viruses studied have been primarily those which infect via the respiratory passages, including influenza viruses A, B, and C, parainfluenza viruses 1, 2, and 3, respiratory syncytial virus, adenoviruses, enteroviruses, rhinoviruses, and measles virus.[3, 5, 7, 9, 19, 46, 64, 68, 98, 105, 108] As is the case with antibacterial antibodies, there is a general correlation of neutralizing antibody levels between serum and secretions.[3, 5, 24, 25] The principal antibody activity found is in IgA, with variable but usually smaller amounts of activity in IgG. Polio and measles viruses have been studied by radioimmunodiffusion, which allows specific identification of the immunoglobulins that bind to the virus. In the case of poliovirus, only IgA binding activity was found in respiratory and intestinal secretions; but with measles virus, some IgG binding activity was also detected in occasional nasal washes.[9, 10, 81]

We have determined nasal-wash titers of neutralizing antibodies to respiratory syncytial virus in 103 prison volunteers. The titers ranged from 1 : 8 to 1 : 2,000 when corrected to an IgA concentration of 20 mg/ 100 ml. All the men had detectable antibody, as might be expected from the fact that all adults have experienced repeated respiratory syncytial viral infections and have moderate amounts of serum neutralizing antibodies. Although there was a significant correlation between the serum and nasal-wash titers, the predictive value of the correlation was low.

Nasal secretions also contain various other, nonantibody substances, including lysozyme, transferrin, interferon, and some mucoproteins, all of which may be important in preventing or controlling respiratory infections.[58, 89, 90, 94]

STIMULATION OF ANTIBODY FORMATION IN SECRETIONS

Infection with Live Bacteria and Viruses

A specific increase in the antibody titer of secretions was described by
Francis and Brightman,[48] who observed rises in nasal titers of neutralizing antibodies in nine of 10 persons ill with influenza due to the A_o
subtype. The rises were demonstrated by comparing nasal washes taken
during the acute phase of illness and 3 weeks thereafter. Francis later
showed that these nasal neutralizing substances had the properties of
antibodies.[45,47]

More recently, rises in nasal titer of neutralizing antibodies were demonstrated after rhinovirus type 1 infections[86] and, less regularly, after
respiratory syncytial and parainfluenza type 3 infections in infants.[70]
Kim *et al.*[70] studied antibody in serum and nasal secretions from 17 infants and children aged 2–40 months. The nasal washes were taken during the acute illness and 3 weeks thereafter. Seven of these children
developed a fourfold or greater rise in level of neutralizing antibodies;
a fourfold or greater fall in titer occurred in seven; and in three children
the levels were unchanged. Interestingly, two of the youngest patients,
aged 2 and 4 months, had high nasal titers of neutralizing antibodies
initially, and these levels did not change after 3 weeks.

Studies on secretory antibody formation during experimental viral
infection were done by Fazekas de St. Groth and Donnelley on influenza infection in mice.[36,38-40] Hemagglutination-inhibiting antibodies
were shown to develop in bronchial washings and serum of mice infected intranasally with influenza virus. The antibodies appeared 7 days
after inoculation (at a time when viral replication had apparently already
terminated) and reached maximal titers within approximately 2 weeks
in both serum and bronchial washings. Much lower bronchial titers were
obtained if live virus was administered by a nonrespiratory route. Serum
and bronchial titers decreased approximately tenfold in 12 weeks.[36]
Similar kinetics of pulmonary antibody formation in the mouse have
been observed by other workers.[65]

In adult volunteers, nasal neutralizing antibodies are formed after experimental influenza infection. Alford *et al.*[1] gave approximately 10^5
$TCID_{50}$ (median tissue-culture infective dose) of influenza A2/Beth/
10/63 to eight men who lacked detectable nasal and serum antibodies

or who had low levels of serum antibodies; each became infected. Neutralizing-antibody activity was first detected in nasal secretions 10–14 days after inoculation and was primarily associated with 11S IgA. Serum and nasal titers rose simultaneously, but after 3 weeks the nasal titers fell, despite the persistence of high serum titers. Variations in antibody titers did not correlate with severity of illness, recovery of virus, or the magnitude of the serum-antibody response. The nasal washes used in this study were not concentrated, and the titers were uncorrected for differences in IgA concentration; thus, an early rise in nasal antibody could have been missed.

Mann, Waldman, and co-workers[75,108] administered $10^{5.5}$ $TCID_{50}$ of live influenza A2/Rockville/1/65 to 12 prison volunteers and studied the neutralizing-antibody response to the infecting virus and to a heterologous strain, A2/Beth/10/63, in whole saliva, sputum, and nasal washings. Nasal washings were not concentrated, and titers were not corrected for differences in protein or IgA concentration. All became infected, as indicated by a fourfold or greater rise in serum or secretory titer. One week after challenge, an increase in titer was noted in both serum and secretions. In sera, the geometric mean titer increased 16-fold by 1½ weeks and 32-fold by 4 weeks. In sputum, an eightfold rise developed by 1 week, which increased to 16-fold by 2 weeks and fell to eightfold at 4 weeks. The development of nasal antibodies was more gradual, increasing slowly to a mean peak fourfold rise by 3 weeks. The maximal response in saliva, a mean 1.5-fold rise, occurred at 1 week and did not change thereafter. It is of interest that three volunteers did not develop illness or a significant serum-antibody response but developed a significant rise in secretory antibody titer. The antibody in secretions was shown, by absorption with immunoglobulin-specific antiserum, to be primarily IgA.

Togo *et al.* (unpublished data) have shown that infection with a strain of influenza A2/Ann Arbor/6/60, presumably attenuated by growth at suboptimal temperature (25 C), also produced rises in serum and secretory antibody. An apparent increase in antibody titer was seen in some persons 3 days after inoculation, although most exhibited a response by the seventh day. Antibodies in both sera and secretions appeared to persist for at least 2½ months.

The nasal-antibody response to experimental infection with parainfluenza type 1 virus was studied by Smith *et al.*[97] in experiments

TABLE 1 Serologic Response and Subsequent Resistance to Live-Virus Challenge of Volunteers Who Were Infected Intranasally with Parainfluenza Virus Type 1 or Who Received Inactivated Vaccine Intramuscularly[a]

Group	Treatment	Initial Antigenicity Trial (Phase 1)						Subsequent Challenge Trial (Phase 2)	
		Serum Antibodies				Nasal Antibodies			
		No. Men	% with ≥4-fold Rise	Reciprocal Geometric Mean Titer		% Who Developed Antibodies	Reciprocal Geometric Mean at 5 Weeks	No. Men Challenged with $10^{4.5}$ TCID$_{50}$	No. Men Infected
				Before	5 Weeks After Infection or Vaccination				
1	Intranasal infection with parainfluenza type 1 virus	35	51	35	48	83	5.2	20[b]	0[c]
2	2 IM injections of inactivated parainfluenza type 1 vaccine	25	80	37	90	12	<1	9[d]	6[c]

[a] Adapted from Chanock et al.[28]
[b] Each of these men developed antibodies in nasal secretions after infection in phase 1.
[c] Difference in infection rates between infected and vaccinated men was significant ($p \leq 0.02$, chi square with Yates correction, df = 1).
[d] Each of these men developed a fourfold or greater rise in serum antibodies after administration of vaccine.

performed in our laboratory. Seven volunteers lacking detectable nasal antibodies were challenged with $10^{4.5}$ $TCID_{50}$ of a strain of parainfluenza type 1 virus that had been passed twice in kidney tissue culture of African green monkey. A rise in the geometric mean nasal titer of neutralizing antibodies to parainfluenza type 1 was detected 1 week after challenge. The peak mean titer was reached at 2 weeks and was maintained until at least the fifth week. Between 5 and 24 weeks after inoculation, there was a fourfold fall in mean nasal titer. IgA levels were determined for four of the volunteers, and significant secretory-antibody responses were evident if the serologic data were corrected to a constant IgA concentration. In this study, data on serum antibodies were not obtained until 3 weeks after infection, so that it was not possible to compare the rate of antibody increase in nasal washes and in serum. Additional data from this study are summarized in Table 1 (group 1); of interest was the finding that a significant proportion of the men developed a rise in nasal antibodies without an accompanying serum-antibody response.

Douglas *et al.*[30] studied the serum and secretory neutralizing-antibody response to rhinoviral infection. They challenged 13 prison volunteers with 0.1 or 15 $TCID_{50}$ of rhinovirus 15 in a fine-particle aerosol. Nasal washes (unconcentrated), tears, and parotid saliva were studied; antibody titers were not corrected for variations in IgA concentration. All the men became infected after challenge. Specimens were obtained every 2–3 days for 24 days from four men who were given the 15-$TCID_{50}$ challenge. None of these men had detectable neutralizing antibodies (at a 1 : 2 dilution) in serum or secretions before challenge. Neutralizing activity was first detected in serum between 14 and 17 days after inoculation and rose to a geometric mean titer of 1 : 32 by 24 days. Antibody activity could not be detected in secretions until after 21 days; by 24 days after challenge, 10 of the 13 men who were infected had developed detectable neutralizing antibodies in their nasal secretions. The concentration of IgA in the nasal washes was 10–30 mg/100 ml, suggesting that excessive dilution of the nasal washes by the collecting fluid did not cause the apparent delay in appearance of antibodies. The major secretory-antibody activity was shown to be associated with 11S IgA,[92] with a variable proportion of activity associated with IgG; the rises in titer were specific for rhinovirus 15. Despite the antibody rise in blood, nasal washes, tears, and saliva, the infecting rhinovirus could be isolated only from nasal washes. However, the fact that volunteers in this study could be infected with 0.1 $TCID_{50}$ of rhinovirus type 15 raises some doubt about the sensitivity of the tissue-culture isolation method.

Slightly different results were obtained in a similar study by Cate *et al.*[24,25] with the same virus. In this experiment, a fourfold or greater rise in nasal and serum antibodies was detected as early as 1 week after challenge in one of ten men who lacked detectable antibodies initially. Three of ten men exhibited rises by 2 weeks. In this group, the geometric mean titers in serum and nasal washes tended to rise in parallel, in contrast with the earlier rise in serum titer found by Douglas *et al.*[30] This parallel rise was also noted in another eight men with initially detectable antibodies in secretions who became infected. Transient fourfold rises in nasal-wash titer were seen in three of six men with preexisting serum and secretory antibodies who did not shed detectable virus. The rises were specific to rhinovirus 15, and the secretory antibodies were largely IgA. The discrepancy between these two studies of the kinetics of secretory-antibody formation during rhinoviral infection is not readily apparent; the only methodologic difference between the studies involves the size of the viral challenge, which was slightly smaller in the investigation of Douglas *et al.*[30]

Two members of the enterovirus group have been studied for evidence of stimulation of formation of respiratory antibodies. Rossen *et al.*[91] successfully challenged 12 prison volunteers with 32–676 $TCID_{50}$ of Coxsackie A-21 virus; shedding of virus began 1–3 days after challenge and lasted for over 17 days. All except one of the volunteers were seronegative at the start of the investigation; 50% developed a fourfold or greater serum-antibody rise by 17 days, and all did so by 4 weeks. Nasal washes were obtained until 16–17 days after inoculation, and at that time all specimens were free of antibody activity, as were the preinoculation washings. Later nasal washes were not collected.

Ogra *et al.*[81] studied the antibody response in serum, nasal washes, and intestinal secretions of infants immunized with oral live poliovirus vaccine. Nasal washes and intestinal secretions were collected and concentrated to a uniform protein concentration, and immunoglobulin-specific poliovirus antibody was measured by radioimmunoassay. The sera and secretions were free of antibodies before immunization. After 16–21 days, an increase in IgA poliovirus-specific antibody could be demonstrated in both nasal and duodenal secretions. The increased titers were maintained at or near the maximal level for several months to a year. The serum titers rose within several days after vaccination, but, because nasal-wash or duodenal specimens were not taken before 16 days, the temporal response in the three systems could not be compared.

In another study, by Ogra and Karzon,[79] intracolonic instillation of live poliovirus vaccine induced virus multiplication in the colon (but not in the duodenum or nasopharynx), and the antibody response was confined to lower intestinal secretions and serum. In this instance, a rise in the level of serum antibodies was detected at 1 week in most cases, but the rise in colonic antibodies appeared slightly later, between 1 and 3 weeks after inoculation. Studies to determine whether viremia had occurred after intracolonic immunization were not done.

Bellanti *et al.*[9] studied the immune response in secretions of nine children vaccinated parenterally with live measles vaccine. Radioimmuno-diffusion was used in conjunction with gradient centrifugation to characterize the immunoglobulins responsible for the antibody response. Two weeks after inoculation, each of the nine children had developed a fourfold or greater rise in serum antibodies (the mean rise was eightfold), but only three had developed detectable nasal antibodies. Transient rises occurred later in another five, but in no instance did the level of antibodies appear to be well maintained. The nasal washes used in this study were not concentrated, but contained moderate amounts of IgA, so that the explanation for the delayed, often weak, and transient nasal-antibody response probably lies in the diminished level of multiplication in the nasopharynx of the vaccine measles virus given parenterally.[33]

We have studied the nasal- and serum-antibody response in adult volunteers challenged with live respiratory syncytial virus; the results are presented later in this paper.

Bellanti, Buescher, and co-workers[8, 16] studied the nasal secretory response to infection with *Francisella tularensis*. Aerosol administration of this organism in seronegative subjects produced rises in nasal and serum titers beginning 4–7 days after challenge, peaking at 3 weeks, and being fairly well maintained for several months. There were some unusual features of this system: the serum-antibody response was confined almost exclusively to IgM, and an IgA antibody was also induced by percutaneous live vaccination. However, the level of nasal antibody did seem to be higher after aerosol immunization.

Immunization with Inactivated Bacteria and Viruses

Many attempts to immunize the respiratory tract locally with dead antigens have been made since Cecil and Steffen[26] showed that intratracheal administration of formalinized pneumococci in monkeys prevented pneumonia on challenge with virulent pneumococci, even though detectable levels of serum antibodies were not induced. Other early animal investigations that demonstrated the development of respiratory antibodies after immunization with inactivated bacterial antigens include those of Turró and Domingo,[106] Bull and McKee,[17,18] and Walsh, Cannon, and Sullivan.[22,110-112] Fazekas de St. Groth and Donnelley[38,39] showed that intranasal administration of inactivated influenza virus in mice stimulated levels of tracheobronchial antibodies that were nearly as high as those seen after intranasal infection. In this study, a significant serum-antibody response also occurred after intranasal vaccination.

Perhaps the earliest attempt to vaccinate humans by the respiratory route was that of Quilligan and Francis,[87] who in 1943 administered inactivated influenza vaccine intranasally to children. Serum-antibody titers rose substantially after intranasal vaccination, but not as high as after subcutaneous administration. However, despite Francis's prior interest in nasal antibodies, secretions were not examined in these experiments, and information regarding protection was not obtained.

Similar studies have been performed more recently by Waldman *et al.*,[107] Kasel *et al.*,[69] and Fulk *et al.*[52] with simultaneous study of nasal- and serum-antibody responses. Intranasal or subcutaneous immunization resulted in nearly comparable serum titers, but appreciable levels of nasal or sputum neutralizing antibodies tended to develop more often, to be higher, and to persist longer after intranasal administration of vaccine.

In contrast, Ogra and Karzon[80] have recently shown that intranasal administration of inactivated poliovirus vaccine produced an increase of nasal antibodies within 4–7 days without a rise in serum antibodies. Revaccination after the antibody had disappeared produced a primary type of secretory-antibody response without evidence of an anamnestic reaction. The nasal-antibody response to dead virus differed from the response to live virus, in that the antibody activity was lost rather quickly— within 2–3 months—whereas, after live poliovirus vaccine, it appeared to persist for a year or more.[80,81]

Perkins and colleagues[82] were successful in stimulating both nasal- and serum-antibody formation with an inactivated rhinovirus vaccine administered intranasally, and Fulk and co-workers (unpublished data) have shown that inactivated parainfluenza virus type 3 administered intranasally will stimulate nasal-antibody production in some volunteers.

Several investigators have observed the appearance of antibodies in respiratory secretions after parenteral immunization with inactivated influenza, parainfluenza, and measles virus antigens.[9,38,49,52,69,75,97,107] Parenteral immunization with inactivated poliovirus vaccine, however, did not produce detectable levels of nasal or duodenal secretory antibodies.[81] Freund[50] and Rossen *et al.*[95] observed the development of nasal antibodies to *Salmonella typhosa* after parenteral administration, and Walsh and Cannon[110] described a similar finding with pneumococci.

Parenteral immunization produced lower and more transient antibody titers than local immunization, and only in a small fraction of the subjects studied. However, serum-antibody levels tended to be comparable after local and parenteral immunization.[9,28,38,52,69,81]

One example of these differences is shown in Table 1. Parenteral immunization with inactivated parainfluenza type 1 virus induced detectable levels of nasal antibodies in only 12% of those vaccinated, as opposed to 83% of men infected intranasally with the virus; furthermore, the nasal titers induced by parenteral inoculation were uniformly lower than those seen after viral infection. Although viral infection did not produce as marked a serum-antibody response as parenteral immunization, the differences between the two groups were not large.[28]

Systemic immunization with inactivated influenza virus produced a respiratory tract antibody response predominantly of the IgA type, but parenteral inactivated measles vaccine resulted in nasal antibodies with activity in both IgG and IgA.[9,75]

In mice, Fazekas de St. Groth, Donnelley, and Graham[37,40-42] found that the low level of bronchial secretory antibody induced by parenteral immunization with inactivated influenza vaccine could be raised (with a concomitant increase in resistance to infection) by intrabronchial instillation of agents that induce mild inflammation—so-called pathotopic vaccination. Such a procedure has yet to be tried in man.

In summary, secretory-antibody production may occur after local or systemic immunization with either live or inactivated organisms. The most pronounced secretory-antibody response appears to develop after local administration of a live organism capable of multiplying in the respiratory tract.

Several questions and problems concerning secretory-antibody production remain. (1) Are there wide variations in the apparent persistence of secretory antibodies after infection with different agents? (2) Differences among viruses (and bacteria) in ability to stimulate secretory-antibody formation need to be explored. (3) A more thorough study of the kinetics of secretory- and serum-antibody response after infection needs to be undertaken. When do levels of serum and secretory antibody first increase? Are these antibody systems synchronous in their time course? Does the IgA system have an efficient immunologic memory? The apparent lack of immunologic memory for IgA has been partially demonstrated in the case of poliovirus.[80, 81] (4) The relationship between the location of antigen and the site of antibody synthesis needs to be resolved. Although the available evidence now supports the local (submucosal) synthesis of secretory antibody in the respiratory tract,[21, 93] parenteral vaccination at a distant site can result in the appearance of antibodies in respiratory secretions, and local immunization often results in serum-antibody production and, in at least one instance, in secretory-antibody production at other sites.

Several examples will illustrate the apparent divergent behavior of different viruses in the latter regard. Douglas *et al.*[30] showed that, during rhinovirus type 15 infection, live virus could be demonstrated only in the nasopharynx, but antibody levels rose in serum, saliva, and tears, as well as in nasal secretions. In contrast, Ogra and Karzon[79] found that intracolonic administration of live poliovirus vaccine resulted in an antibody response restricted to the area of viral multiplication and serum. Kraus and Volk[73] found that infection of one cornea of a rabbit with smallpox produced resistance to subsequent smallpox challenge only in the previously infected cornea. Inactivated poliovirus administered intranasally did not induce a serum-antibody response,[80] but intranasal instillation of an inactivated rhinovirus vaccine often produced an antibody response in serum that was apparently greater than that in nasal secretions.[82] It seems reasonable to suppose that migration of antigen may occur after immunization, but this remains to be established.

ROLE OF LOCAL RESPIRATORY ANTIBODIES IN PROTECTION AGAINST INFECTION AND DISEASE

It has been known for many years that immunity to influenza virus is not always related to the level of serum antibodies, and Francis suggested as early as 1940 that this might be due to the relative importance of secretory antibodies, whose concentration varied independently of that of serum antibody.[43-47] The observation that resistance is not strictly proportional to serum-antibody level has since been extended to some other respiratory pathogens, the rhinoviruses and paramyxoviruses.[23-25,66,98] Although high levels of serum antibodies are associated with protection against infection with some respiratory viruses, it has not been determined whether this is due to coincident high titers of secretory antibodies.[13,76]

In one unusual ecologic circumstance, it has been possible to dissociate the effect of serum antibody from that of local respiratory antibody. Young infants, although possessing high levels of maternally derived serum antibody to respiratory syncytial virus (RSV), nevertheless develop severe bronchiolitis or pneumonia as a result of RSV infection.[27,28] Indeed, the highest incidence of serious RSV lower respiratory tract disease is seen during the first 4 months of life, when maternally derived serum-antibody levels are moderately high.

Furthermore, induction of higher titers of serum antibody by parenteral injection of an inactivated RSV vaccine did not prevent infection; in fact, when recipients of the vaccine became infected, they developed more serious disease than their unvaccinated cohorts.[27] In these circumstances, it is clear that serum neutralizing antibody itself does not provide significant protection. We have suggested that serum antibody, in addition to not conferring resistance, may actually participate in the production of pulmonary damage when it interacts with RSV in the lungs of young infants.[27] Inasmuch as reinfection of older persons usually leads to a less severe illness than that seen in early infancy, there must be a mechanism for providing partial resistance to the effects of the virus. It is reasonable to postulate that local respiratory tract antibody may be responsible for such resistance by preventing or suppressing virus replication. A recent study testing this hypothesis will be described later in this presentation.

Evidence that the presence of secretory antibodies plays an important role in protecting against respiratory infection comes from cases of isolated IgA deficiencies such as ataxia-telangiectasia. Some persons with such a deficiency are susceptible to an increased incidence of upper respiratory infections, often with chronic bacterial complications.[6,20,62,99] They often have problems of malabsorption, which may also be related to the role of IgA in preventing local multiplication of micro-organisms.[12,56]

Persons with low or absent IgA who escape recurrent respiratory infections may compensate by an increased secretion of IgM or IgG antibodies onto the respiratory epithelium.[6,15,101]

The importance of secretory antibodies in protection has been experimentally demonstrated by passive intranasal immunization against influenza virus and *Hemophilus pertussis* with antibody derived from serum or nasal washes.[34,42,45,60,77,102] Sniffing of lyophilized hyperimmune horse serum has been used for many years in the Soviet Union and is claimed to be an effective prophylactic against epidemic influenza.[113]

Fazekas de St. Groth and Donnelley[39] demonstrated that protection of mice against influenza A virus was a function of secretory antibodies, rather than serum antibodies. In man, the role of secretory, rather than serum, antibodies in protection against respiratory infection was first demonstrated by Smith and associates.[98] They showed that nasal antibodies exerted a marked protective effect against infection with parainfluenza type 1 virus (Table 2). When given type 1 virus, 13 of 17 men with a nasal-antibody titer less than 1:3 became infected, whereas only one of 17 men with a nasal-antibody titer greater than 1:3 was infected. The difference in illness rates was comparable. In both groups, the presence of a low (i.e., less than 48) or high (i.e., greater than 48) serum titer of antibodies did not influence the occurrence of infection; hence, resistance was not related to serum antibodies *per se*.

Ogra and Karzon have shown a definite protective effect of local anti-

TABLE 2   Comparison of Protective Effect of Serum and Local Antibodies Against Challenge with $10^{4.5}$ $TCID_{50}$ of Parainfluenza Type 1 Virus[a]

Nasal-Antibody Titer	Serum-Antibody Titer		Value of p[b] for Serum-Antibody Differences
	$<$48 (Infected/Total)	$<$48 (Infected/Total)	
$<$1:3	10/13	3/4	$>$0.3
$>$1:3	1/9	0/8	$>$0.3
Value of p[b] for nasal-antibody differences	$<$0.01	$<$0.05	

[a]Adapted from Smith *et al.*[98]
[b]Fisher Exact test.

bodies in poliovirus infection.[79] Children immunized with poliovirus via
the colon developed an unmodified nasopharyngeal infection when challenged orally with poliovirus vaccine, despite the presence of a high level
of serum antibodies. Replication of virus in the colon was suppressed,
and this was attributed to the previously induced coproantibodies. In a
parallel study,[80] they stimulated nasal antibodies, without altering the
level of serum antibodies, by administering inactivated vaccine intranasally and showed that the presence of nasal antibodies was associated
with a marked reduction in virus multiplication in the nasopharynx after
challenge with live poliovirus vaccine.

Four independent studies, by Waldman, Kasel, Fulk, and their associates,[52,69,107,109] support the hypothesis that the level of local respiratory antibodies is correlated with the resistance of man to influenzal
infection. Waldman *et al.*[109] demonstrated that aerosol administration
of inactivated influenza vaccine provided greater protection against
natural infection than did subcutaneous vaccination, although comparable levels of serum antibodies were induced by the two methods of
administration; titers of nasal antibodies were not determined. Waldman
et al.,[107] Fulk *et al.*,[52] and Kasel *et al.*[69] immunized volunteers by intranasal administration of antigen and showed that this route of application
was superior to the parenteral route in inducing high levels of nasal antibodies, but was only slightly less effective than parenteral immunization
in stimulating serum-antibody formation; protection studies were not
done. Joosting and collaborators[68] were not able to detect a protective
effect of nasal antibodies on illness resulting from infection with influenza C virus, but the number of men studied was small.

Some preliminary data from a recent volunteer study by Perkins and
his collaborators in our laboratory suggest that nasal antibodies may
also be the primary determinant of resistance to rhinoviral infection.[82]
They immunized seronegative volunteers either intranasally or intramuscularly with an inactivated rhinovirus type 13 vaccine that had previously been shown to induce serum antibodies when given intramuscularly and both serum and nasal antibodies when given intranasally. The
vaccinated volunteers were then challenged with 10^2 $TCID_{50}$ of the
homologous rhinovirus, as were seronegative volunteers who served as a
control group. Only the intranasal route of immunization offered significant protection against illness, despite the fact that the serum-
antibody titers of those vaccinated intranasally were lower than those

TABLE 3 Comparison of Protective Effect of Inactivated Rhinovirus Type 13 Vaccine Administered Intranasally or Intramuscularly to Seronegative Volunteers

Route of Administration	No. Volunteers	Reciprocal Geometric Mean Serum-Antibody Titer after Vaccine	Response to Subsequent Challenge with Approximately 10^2 $TCID_{50}$ of Rhinovirus Type 13[a]	
			Upper Respiratory Tract Illness	No Illness
(A) Intranasal[b]	28	53.8	10	18
(B) Intramuscular[c]	11	72.5	9	2
(C) Not given	23	< 4	18	5

[a] p (chi square with Yates correction)
 A versus C < 0.01
 A versus B   0.02
 A versus B + C   0.01
 B versus C   0.5

[b] 2 ml given four times at 1- to 2-week intervals; 26 of 28 volunteers developed a fourfold or greater increase in serum antibodies.
[c] 1 ml given twice, 4 weeks apart; 10 of the 11 volunteers given this vaccine developed a fourfold or greater increase in serum antibodies.

of the parenterally vaccinated group (Table 3). Secretory antibody developed in most of the intranasal vaccinees, whereas this type of response was infrequent after intramuscular vaccination.[82] Cate *et al.*[24] have also shown a correlation between level of nasal secretory antibody and protection against infection with another rhinovirus (type 15), but they were unable to distinguish clearly between the protective effects of serum and secretory antibodies.

Other studies in which a possible role of respiratory antibodies in protection against infection has been suggested, but not proved, have been done by Tremonti *et al.*,[105] with parainfluenza type 2 viral infection in man; Ehrenkranz,[32] with nasal colonization of humans by *Staphylococcus aureus*; Bull and McKee[17,18] and Walsh, Cannon, and Sullivan,[22,110-112] with pneumococcal infection in rabbits; Cecil and Steffen,[26] with pneumococcal infection in monkeys; Dow,[31] North and Anderson,[78] Gray,[57] and Cooper,[29] with *Hemophilus pertussis* infection in mice; and Hornick, Buescher, Bellanti, and their associates,[8,16,63] with *Francisella tularensis* infection in man.

We have studied the role of secretory antibodies in resistance of adults to RSV infection. As mentioned previously, this virus is a common cause of bronchiolitis and pneumonia in infants, but causes only upper respiratory illness in adults.[11,66,67,74] It has been assumed that the presence of pre-existing local antibodies in adults confers resistance to lower respiratory tract involvement during reinfection with this virus.[27] We undertook this study as one step in the investigation of this hypothesis.

The nasal washes from 103 men were concentrated, adjusted to an IgA level of 20 mg/100 ml, and then titrated for RSV neutralizing antibodies by a plaque-reduction technique. Sixteen men were selected for inclusion in the study: eight with low nasal-antibody titer (1 : 5.7 to 1:16.4), and eight with high nasal titer (1:80 to 1:1,295). The nasal- and serum-antibody titers of these men are illustrated in Figure 1. There was a 27-fold difference between the geometric mean nasal titers of the

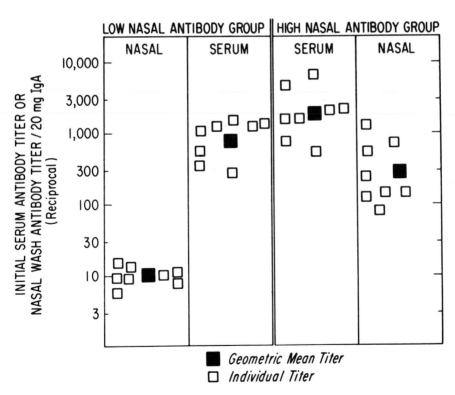

FIGURE 1   Initial serum and nasal titers of antibodies in 16 men later challenged with respiratory syncytial virus.

two groups, with no overlap of the individual titers. Although there was only a 2½-fold difference between the geometric mean serum titers of the two groups, with great overlapping of individual titers, the difference was statistically significant (t test; $p = 0.035$). The men were challenged with a suspension of the A2 strain of RSV prepared after 21 passages in calf kidney culture.[51] In a previous study, 10^4–10^5 $TCID_{50}$ of this virus suspension produced a common cold illness in volunteers.[51]

Administration of about $10^{2.9}$ $TCID_{50}$ of virus—500 plaque-forming units (pfu)—resulted in upper respiratory symptoms in a few of the men, but not definite colds. Each of the men became infected, as indicated by recovery of virus from freshly collected unfrozen throat washings, and there were no important differences between the two groups, either in mean day of onset of virus excretion or in mean duration of virus excretion. The shortest duration of virus excretion by a volunteer was 2 days, and the longest, 7; both men were in the low-nasal-titer group.

To detect possible quantitative differences in virus excretion, the throat washings collected on the sixth and seventh days following ad-

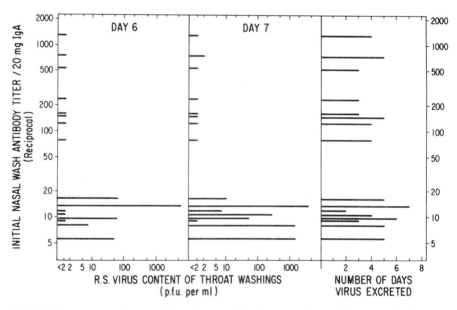

FIGURE 2   Correlation between titer of nasal antibodies and pattern of virus excretion in 16 men infected with respiratory syncytial virus.

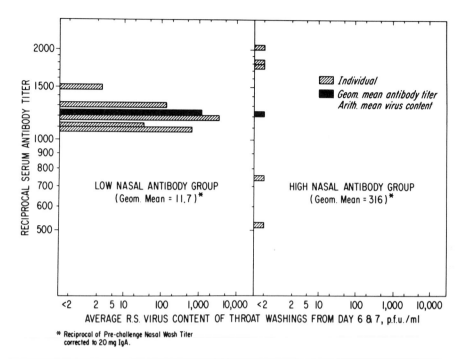

FIGURE 3   Lack of effect of serum antibodies on respiratory syncytial virus excretion, as shown by matching five men from the low-nasal-antibody group and five from the high-nasal-antibody group for geometric mean serum-antibody titer.

ministration of virus were titered by the plaque technique in HEp-II cells; the results are summarized in Figures 2 and 3. In Figure 2, the amount and duration of virus excretion are related to the initial nasal antibody titers. The amount of virus excreted was influenced by the antibody titer, but infection *per se* and duration of virus excretion were not. Because there was a small but significant difference between the serum titers of these two groups, we analyzed a subgroup consisting of five men from each group matched for geometric mean serum-antibody titer. Virus excretion data for these two matched groups are presented in Figure 3. The prechallenge geometric mean serum titers of these two groups were nearly identical, but there was a 27-fold difference between the geometric mean nasal titers. None of the specimens from the high-nasal-titer men yielded virus; in contrast, specimens from all the men in the low-nasal-titer group were positive, with an average virus content of

TABLE 4 Summary of Serologic and Virologic Studies of Men Inoculated with 500 pfu of Respiratory Syncytial Virus

Group	No. Volunteers	No. with ≥4-fold Rise in Indicated Antibody Titer			No. with ≥4-fold Rise in Any Antibody Titer	Duration of Virus Excretion, Range, Days	Peak Virus Content of Throat Washings, $\log_{10}$ pfu/ml	
		Serum Neutralizing	Serum Complement-Fixing	Nasal Neutralizing			Range	Geometric Mean
Low nasal-antibody titer	8	2	4	5	6	2-7	<0.3-5.0	2.4
High nasal-antibody titer	8	0	0	0	0	3-5	<0.3	<0.3

94

1,000 pfu/ml of throat washing. Indeed, of 19 previously virus-positive throat washings from the high-titer group that were retitered, only two yielded virus, whereas 21 of 25 were positive in the low-titer group. Virus titers were never higher than 2 pfu/ml in the high-titer group but ranged from 2 to 100,000 pfu/ml in the low-titer group (see Table 4). Evaluation of the effect of one cycle of freezing and thawing indicated that this manipulation effected a twofold to tenfold decrease in titer of virus in throat washings.

The neutralizing-antibody response in serum and nasal secretions and the complement-fixing (CF) antibody response in serum were studied in the 16 men, and the data are summarized in Table 4. Of the eight men with low initial nasal-antibody titers, only two had a fourfold or greater rise in serum neutralizing antibodies, whereas four developed significant levels of serum CF antibodies. In addition, five of the men developed a fourfold or greater rise in level of nasal-neutralizing antibodies. The two men who exhibited a serum neutralizing-antibody response also developed both nasal-antibody and serum-CF-antibody responses. In fact, these two men had the largest increases in nasal-antibody titer of the group and excreted the most virus in their throat washings. Virus excretion and antibody data on one of these men are illustrated in Figure 4. Of the four men with a serum-CF-antibody response, three had a significant rise in nasal neutralizing-antibody titer. The two men who had no change in serum- or nasal-antibody levels excreted virus for a short time (2 and 3 days), and the virus content of their throat washings was rela-

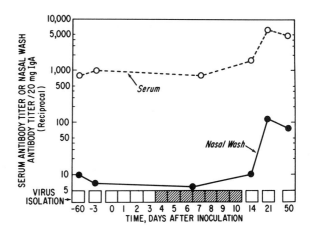

FIGURE 4   Rises in both serum and nasal titers of antibodies in a volunteer after infection.

tively low. None with a high initial nasal-antibody titer developed an increase in either nasal or serum antibodies, despite virus excretion for as long as 5 days.

It is clear that high titers of secretory antibodies to RSV did not prevent infection after challenge with 500 pfu of virus, but did markedly decrease the excretion of virus. Why did high titers of secretory neutralizing antibodies fail to prevent infection? It is possible that the inoculum was too large, overwhelming even high levels of local antibodies, and that protection would have been demonstrated if the challenge dose had been smaller. In the case of the biophysically similar parainfluenza type 1 virus, secretory-antibody titers of $1:3$ or greater apparently afforded complete protection against a much larger challenge dose, $10^{4.5}$ $TCID_{50}$, in most subjects.

It seems likely that RSV is relatively insensitive to secretory antibodies and is able to initiate infection in the presence of such antibodies. This interpretation is consistent with the frequent occurrence of natural reinfection in normal adults, all of whom apparently possess secretory antibodies. The interpretation does not deny an effect of secretory antibodies. In part, the insensitivity of RSV to secretory antibodies may arise from the ability of RSV infection to spread by recruitment of uninfected cells into an infected syncytium, in this manner evading the effects of antibodies. In addition, failure of IgA to fix complement may contribute to its relative inability to act against RSV, inasmuch as neutralization of the virus is in part complement-dependent.[4,61,85,103]

The observed effect of local antibodies on RSV excretion might be produced either (1) by decreasing virus replication through limiting the extent of initial infection or its subsequent spread or (2) by simply neutralizing the virus produced during infection. The latter seems less likely as a primary mode of action, in that immunologic responses were not detected in the high-nasal-titer group, although infection occurred. In our view, it is more likely that the primary effect of secretory antibodies is to decrease virus replication. A similar effect of secretory antibodies on poliovirus infection was noted by Ogra and Karzon.[80] The phenomenon of reduced virus multiplication after immunization has also been observed in parainfluenza type 3 viral infection of sheep.[55]

The antibody response to RSV infection in our volunteers was not particularly rapid; the most significant increase in secretory-antibody titers occurred between 2 and 3 weeks after inoculation, some time after virus excretion had ceased. In children, the secretory-antibody response may occur somewhat more rapidly, explaining the presence of neutralizing activity in the nasal secretions of infants and children at the time of admission to the hospital for RSV lower respiratory tract disease.[70]

SUMMARY AND CONCLUSIONS

1. Antibodies to viruses and bacteria are found in various secretions: sputum, saliva, tears, and nasal mucus. These antibodies, in man, are primarily 11S IgA.

2. Development of secretory antibodies has been shown to occur after natural or experimental infection with a number of myxoviruses, picornaviruses, and a few bacteria. In addition, secretory antibodies can be stimulated by local application of inactivated viral and bacterial antigens. Either infection or local vaccination can induce a significant change in secretory antibodies, apparently without necessarily affecting serum antibodies. Antibodies may appear in respiratory secretions after parenteral immunization; however, this type of response occurs irregularly and is generally of a lesser magnitude and more transient than the response evoked by local immunization.

3. In a few instances—such as influenza in mice and parainfluenza virus, respiratory syncytial virus, and poliovirus in man—secretory antibodies (as distinct from serum antibodies) have been shown to have a definite protective effect, either by apparently preventing infection altogether or by markedly limiting virus production.

4. If later work confirms the critical role of secretory antibodies in resistance to other viral and bacterial respiratory infections, then it will be clear that efforts to increase secretory-antibody levels will be effective in preventing disease. This selective stimulation of secretory antibodies could most logically be accomplished by immunization with live attenuated viruses, but dead vaccines given locally and perhaps the technique of pathotopic vaccination, as described by Fazekas de St. Groth, Donnelley, and Graham,[37,40,41] may also prove useful.

5. More information about the secretory-antibody response and its significance are needed before the final strategy of immunization via the respiratory tract can be developed. For example, we lack an understand-

ing of the pattern of development (and decline) of secretory antibodies after infection with the major respiratory tract pathogens. Attempts at immunization would be facilitated if we knew the level of secretory antibodies that provide protection against respiratory agents.

6. Knowledge of the level of secretory antibodies that permits reinfection in the absence of symptoms might hasten development of effective immunoprophylaxis.

7. The magnitude, duration, and immunologic memory of the secretory-antibody response induced by attenuated organisms and inactivated antigens must be defined and compared before a choice between these techniques can be made.

We should like to acknowledge the invaluable technical assistance of Mr. Walter James, Mr. Ike Fishburne, Mr. H. C. Turner, Miss Ena Camargo, and Mrs. Barbara Walls. We are indebted to Dr. Julius Kasel for several helpful discussions. The personnel and inmates of the Lorton Reformatory, District of Columbia Department of Corrections, Lorton, Virginia, are to be thanked for their cooperation in the volunteer studies.

REFERENCES

1. Alford, R. H., R. D. Rossen, W. T. Butler, and J. A. Kasel. Neutralizing and hemagglutination-inhibiting activity of nasal secretions following experimental human infection with A2 influenza virus. J. Immun. 98:724–731, 1967.
2. Amoss, H. L., and E. Taylor. Neutralization of the virus of poliomyelitis by nasal washings. J. Exp. Med. 25:507–523, 1917.
3. Artenstein, M. S., J. A. Bellanti, and E. L. Buescher. Identification of the antiviral substances in nasal secretions. Proc. Soc. Exp. Biol. Med. 117:558–564, 1964.
4. Baughman, R. H., J. D. Fenters, G. S. Marquis, Jr., and J. C. Holper. Effect of complement and viral filtration on the neutralization of respiratory syncytial virus. Appl. Microbiol. 16:1076–1080, 1968.
5. Bell, E. J. The relationship between the antipoliomyelitic properties of human nasopharyngeal secretions and blood serums. Amer. J. Hyg. 47:351–369, 1948.
6. Bellanti, J. A., M. S. Artenstein, and E. L. Buescher. Ataxia-telangiectasia: Immunologic and virologic studies of serum and respiratory secretions. Pediatrics 37:924–933, 1966.
7. Bellanti, J. A., M. S. Artenstein, and E. L. Buescher. Characterization of virus neutralizing antibodies in human serum and nasal secretions. J. Immun. 94:344–351, 1965.
8. Bellanti, J. A., E. L. Buescher, W. E. Brandt, H. G. Dangerfield, and D. Crozier. Characterization of human serum and nasal hemagglutinating antibody to *Francisella tularensis*. J. Immun. 98:171–178, 1967.
9. Bellanti, J. A., R. L. Sanga, B. Klutinis, B. Brandt, and M. S. Artenstein. Antibody responses in serum and nasal secretions of children immunized with inactivated and attenuated measles-virus vaccines. New Eng. J. Med. 280:628–633, 1969.

10. Berger, R., E. Ainbender, H. L. Hodes, H. D. Zepp, and M. M. Hevizy. Demonstration of IgA polioantibody in saliva, duodenal fluid and urine. Nature 214:420–422, 1967.
11. Berglund, B. Respiratory syncytial virus infections in families. A study of family members of children hospitalized for acute respiratory disease. Acta Paediat. Scand. 56:395–404, 1967.
12. Bird, D. C., J. B. Jacobs, M. Silbiger, and S. M. Wolff. Hypogammaglobulinemia with nodular lymphoid hyperplasia of the intestine. Report of a case with rectosigmoid involvement. Radiology 92:1535–1536, 1969.
13. Bloom, H. H., K. M. Johnson, R. Jacobsen, and R. M. Chanock. Recovery of parainfluenza viruses from adults with upper respiratory illnesses. Amer. J. Hyg. 74:50–59, 1961.
14. Brandtzaeg, P., I. Fjellanger, and S. T. Gjeruldsen. Adsorption of immunoglobulin A onto oral bacteria in vivo. J. Bact. 96:242–249, 1968.
15. Brandtzaeg, P., I. Fjellanger, and S. T. Gjeruldsen. Immunoglobulin M: local synthesis and selective secretion in patients with immunoglobulin A deficiency. Science 160:789–791, 1968.
16. Buescher, E. L., and J. A. Bellanti. Respiratory antibody to *Francisella tularensis* in man. Bact. Rev. 30:539–541, 1966.
17. Bull, C. G., and C. M. McKee. Respiratory immunity in rabbits. VI. The effects of immunity on the carrier state of the pneumococcus and *Bacillus bronchisepticus*. Amer. J. Hyg. 8:723–729, 1928.
18. Bull, C. G., and C. M. McKee. Respiratory immunity in rabbits. VII. Resistance to intranasal infection in the absence of demonstrable antibodies. Amer. J. Hyg. 9:490–499, 1929.
19. Burnet, F. M., D. Lush, and A. V. Jackson. A virus-inactivating agent from human nasal secretion. Brit. J. Exp. Path. 20:377–385, 1939.
20. Buser, F., R. Bütler, and R. M. Du Pan. Susceptibility to infection and IgA deficiency in the infant. J. Pediat. 72:29–33, 1968.
21. Butler, W. T., R. D. Rossen, and T. A. Waldmann. The mechanism of appearance of immunoglobulin A in nasal secretions in man. J. Clin. Invest. 46:1883–1893, 1967.
22. Cannon, P. R., and T. E. Walsh. Studies on the fate of living bacteria introduced into the upper respiratory tract of normal and intranasally vaccinated rabbits. J. Immun. 32:49–62, 1937.
23. Cate, T. R., R. B. Couch, and K. M. Johnson. Studies with rhinoviruses in volunteers: Production of illness, effect of naturally acquired antibody, and demonstration of a protective effect not associated with serum antibody. J. Clin. Invest. 43:56–67, 1964.
24. Cate, T. R., R. D. Rossen, R. G. Douglas, Jr., W. T. Butler, and R. B. Couch. The role of nasal secretion and serum antibody in the rhinovirus common cold. Amer. J. Epidem. 84:352-363, 1966.
25. Cate, T. R., R. D. Rossen, R. G. Douglas, and R. B. Couch. Nasal secretion antibody in the rhinovirus common cold. Clin. Res. 13:293, 1965. (abstract)
26. Cecil, R. L., and G. I. Steffen. Vaccination of monkeys against pneumococcus type I pneumonia by means of intratracheal injection of pneumococcus type I vaccine. Public Health Rep. 37:2735-2744, 1922.
27. Chanock, R. M., R. H. Parrott, A. Z. Kapikian, H. W. Kim, and C. D. Brandt. Possible role of immunologic factors in pathogenesis of RS virus lower respiratory tract disease, p. 125. In M. Pollard, Ed. Perspectives in Virology. (6th ed.) New York: Harper & Row Publishers, Inc., 1968.
28. Chanock, R. M., C. B. Smith, W. T. Friedewald, R. H. Parrott, B. R. Forsyth, H. V. Coates, A. Z. Kapikian, and M. A. Gharpure. Resistance to parainfluenza and respiratory syncytial virus infection—implications for effective immunization and preliminary study of an

attenuated strain of respiratory syncytial virus, pp. 53–61. In First International Conference on Vaccines Against Viral and Rickettsial Diseases of Man. Scientific Publ. No. 147. Washington, D.C.: Pan American Health Organization, World Health Organization, 1967.

29. Cooper, G. N. Active immunity in mice following the intranasal injection of sub-lethal doses of living *Haemophilus pertussis*. J. Path. Bact. 64:65–74, 1952.

30. Douglas, R. G., Jr., R. D. Rossen, W. T. Butler, and R. B. Couch. Rhinovirus neutralizing antibody in tears, parotid saliva, nasal secretions and serum. J. Immun. 99:297–303, 1967.

31. Dow, R. P. Active immunization by the intranasal route: A comparison of various *H. pertussis* antigens. Canad. Public Health J. 31:370–375, 1940.

32. Ehrenkranz, N. J. Nasal rejection of experimentally inoculated *Staphylococcus aureus*: Evidence for an immune reaction in man. J. Immun. 96:509–517, 1966.

33. Enders, J. F., and S. L. Katz. Present status of live rubeola vaccines in the United States, pp. 295–300. In First International Conference on Vaccines Against Viral and Rickettsial Diseases of Man. Scientific Publ. No. 147. Washington, D.C.: Pan American Health Organization, World Health Organization, 1967.

34. Evans, D. G. The protective properties of pertussis antisera in experimental infection. J. Path. Bact. 56:49–54, 1944.

35. Fazekas de St. Groth, S. Influenza: A study in mice. Lancet 1:1101–1105, 1950.

36. Fazekas de St. Groth, S. Studies in experimental immunology of influenza. VI. The duration of induced immunity. Aust. J. Exp. Biol. Med. Sci. 28:559–568, 1950.

37. Fazekas de St. Groth, S. Studies in experimental immunology of influenza. IX. The mode of action of pathotopic adjuvants. Aust. J. Exp. Biol. Med. Sci. 29:339–352, 1951.

38. Fazekas de St. Groth, S., and M. Donnelley. Studies in experimental immunology of influenza. III. The antibody response. Aust. J. Exp. Biol. Med. Sci. 28:45–60, 1950.

39. Fazekas de St. Groth, S., and M. Donnelley. Studies in experimental immunology of influenza. IV. The protective value of active immunization. Aust. J. Exp. Biol. Med. Sci. 28:61–75, 1950.

40. Fazekas de St. Groth, S., and M. Donnelley. Studies in experimental immunology of influenza. V. Enhancement of immunity by pathotopic vaccination. Aust. J. Exp. Biol. Med. Sci. 28:77–85, 1950.

41. Fazekas de St. Groth, S., M. Donnelley, and D. M. Graham. Studies in experimental immunology of influenza. VIII. Pathotopic adjuvants. Aust. J. Exp. Biol. Med. Sci. 29:323–337, 1951.

42. Fazekas de St. Groth, S., and D. M. Graham. Studies in experimental immunology of influenza. X. Passive immunity and its enhancement. Aust. J. Exp. Biol. Med. Sci. 32:369–386, 1954.

43. Francis, T., Jr. A rationale for studies in the control of epidemic influenza. Science 97:229–235, 1943.

44. Francis, T., Jr. Epidemic influenza. Bull. N.Y. Acad. Med. 17:268–279, 1941.

45. Francis, T., Jr. Factors conditioning resistance to epidemic influenza. Harvey Lect. 37:69–99, 1941–42.

46. Francis, T., Jr. The inactivation of epidemic influenza virus by nasal secretions of human individuals. Science 91:198–199, 1940.

47. Francis, T., Jr. The significance of nasal factors in epidemic influenza, p. 41. In Problems and Trends in Virus Research. Philadelphia: University of Pennsylvania Press, 1941.

48. Francis, T., Jr., and I. J. Brightman. Virus-inactivating capacity of nasal secretions in the acute and convalescent stages of influenza. Proc. Soc. Exp. Biol. Med. 48:116–117, 1941.

49. Francis, T., Jr., H. E. Pearson, E. R. Sullivan, and P. M. Brown. The effect of subcutaneous vaccination with influenza virus upon the virus-inactivating capacity of nasal secretions. Amer. J. Hyg. 37:294–300, 1943.

50. Freund, J. Distribution of immune agglutinins in the serum and organs of rabbits. J. Immun. 14:101–110, 1927.
51. Friedewald, W. T., B. R. Forsyth, C. B. Smith, M. A. Gharpure, and R. M. Chanock. Low-temperature-grown RS virus in adult volunteers. JAMA 204:690–694, 1968.
52. Fulk, R. V., D. S. Fedson, M. A. Huber, J. R. Fitzpatrick, B. F. Howar, and J. A. Kasel. Antibody responses in children and elderly persons following local or parenteral administration of an inactivated influenza virus vaccine, A_2/Hong Kong/68 variant. J. Immun. 102:1102–1104, 1969.
53. Gay, F. P. Local or tissue immunity. Arch. Path. 1:590–604, 1926.
54. Gay, F. P. Local resistance and local immunity to bacteria. Physiol. Rev. 4:191–214, 1924.
55. Gilmour, N. J., A. Drysdale, R. G. Stevenson, D. E. Hore, and J. F. Brothersoon. Reaction of young adult sheep to vaccination and infection with myxovirus parainfluenza 3. J. Comp. Path. 78:463–468, 1968.
56. Gorback, S. L., J. G. Banwell, R. Mitra, B. D. Chatterjee, B. Jacobs, and D. N. Guha Mazumder. Bacterial contamination of the upper small bowel in tropical sprue. Lancet 1:74–77, 1969.
57. Gray, D. F. The influence of virulence on the immunising potency for mice of *Haemophilus pertussis*, phase 1. J. Path. Bact. 59:235–246, 1947.
58. Gresser, I., and H. B. Dull. A virus inhibitor in pharyngeal washings from patients with influenza. Proc. Soc. Exp. Biol. Med. 115:192–196, 1964.
59. Hegner, C. A. Ueber das Vorkommen von Agglutininen in der Tränenflüssigkeit. Klin. Mbl. Augenheilk. 57:48–50, 1916.
60. Henle, W., J. Stokes, Jr., and D. R. Shaw. Passive immunization of mice against human influenza virus by the intranasal route. J. Immun. 40:201–212, 1941.
61. Heremans, J. F., J.-P. Vaerman, and C. Vaerman. Studies on the immune globulins of human serum. II. A study of the distribution of anti-Brucella and anti-diphtheria antibody activities among γ_{ss}-, γ_{1M}- and γ_{1A}-globulin fractions. J. Immun. 91:11–17, 1963.
62. Hobbs, J. R. Immune imbalance in dysgammaglobulinaemia type IV. Lancet 1:110–114, 1968.
63. Hornick, R. B., and H. T. Eigelsbach. Aerogenic immunization of man with live Tularemia vaccine. Bact. Rev. 30:532–538, 1966.
64. Howitt, B. F. Relationship between nasal and humoral antipoliomyelitic substances. J. Infect. Dis. 60:113–121, 1937.
65. Isaacs, A., and G. Hitchcock. Role of interferon in recovery from virus infections. Lancet 2:69–71, 1960.
66. Johnson, K. M., H. H. Bloom, M. A. Mufson, and R. M. Chanock. Natural reinfection of adults by respiratory syncytial virus. Possible relation to mild upper respiratory disease. New Eng. J. Med. 267:68–72, 1962.
67. Johnson, K. M., R. M. Chanock, D. Rifkind, H. M. Kravetz, and V. Knight. Respiratory syncytial virus. IV. Correlation of virus shedding, serologic response, and illness in adult volunteers. JAMA 176:663–667, 1961.
68. Joosting, A. C., B. Head, M. L. Bynoe, and D. A. Tyrrell. Production of common colds in human volunteers by influenza C virus. Brit Med. J. 4:153–154, 1968.
69. Kasel, J. A., E. B. Hume, R. V. Fulk, Y. Togo, M. Huber, and R. B. Hornick. Antibody responses in nasal secretions and serum of elderly persons following local or parenteral administration of inactivated influenza virus vaccine. J. Immun. 102:555–562, 1969.
70. Kim, H. W., J. A. Bellanti, J. O. Arrobio, J. Mills, C. D. Brandt, R. M. Chanock, and R. H. Parrott. Respiratory syncytial virus neutralizing activity in nasal secretions following natural infection. Proc. Soc. Exp. Biol. Med. 131:658–661, 1969.
71. Kraus, F. W., and J. Konno. Antibodies in saliva. Ann. N.Y. Acad. Sci. 106:311–329, 1963.

72. Kraus, F. W., and J. Konno. The salivary secretion of antibody. Alabama J. Med. Sci. 2:15–22, 1965.

73. Kraus, R., and R. Volk. Weitere Studien über Immunität bei Syphilis und bei der Vakzination gegen Variola. Wien. Klin. Wschr. 19:620–621, 1906.

74. Kravetz, H. M., V. Knight, R. M. Chanock, J. A. Morris, K. M. Johnson, D. Rifkind, and J. P. Utz. Respiratory syncytial virus. III. Production of illness and clinical observations in adult volunteers. JAMA 176:657–663, 1961.

75. Mann, J. J., R. H. Waldman, Y. Togo, G. G. Heiner, A. T. Dawkins, and J. A. Kasel. Antibody response in respiratory secretions of volunteers given live and dead influenza virus. J. Immun. 100:726–735, 1968.

76. Morris, J. A., J. A. Kasel, M. Saglam, V. Knight, and F. A. Loda. Immunity to influenza to antibody levels. New Eng. J. Med. 274:527–535, 1966.

77. North, E. A. Passive immunization by the intranasal route in experimental pertussis. Aust. J. Exp. Biol. Med. Sci. 24:253–259, 1946.

78. North, E. A., and G. Anderson. Active immunization by the intranasal route in experimental pertussis. Med. J. Aust. 2:228–231, 1942.

79. Ogra, P. L., and D. T. Karzon. Distribution of poliovirus antibody in serum, nasopharynx and alimentary tract following segmental immunization of lower alimentary tract with polio-vaccine. J. Immun. 102:1423–1430, 1969.

80. Ogra, P. L., and D. T. Karzon. Poliovirus antibody response in serum and nasal secretions following intranasal inoculation with inactivated poliovaccine. J. Immun. 102:15–23, 1969.

81. Ogra, P. L., D. T. Karzon, F. Righthand, and M. MacGillivray. Immunoglobulin response in serum and secretions after immunization with live and inactivated poliovaccine and natural infection. New Eng. J. Med. 279:893–900, 1968.

82. Perkins, J. C., D. N. Tucker, K. L. S. Knopf, R. P. Wenzel, A. Z. Kapikian, and R. M. Chanock. Comparison of protective effect of neutralizing antibody in serum and nasal secretions in experimental rhinovirus type 13 illness. Amer. J. Epidem. 90:519, 1969.

83. Pierce, A. E. Specific antibodies at mucous surfaces. Vet. Rev. Annot. 5:17–36, 1959.

84. Pollaci, G., and S. Ceraulo. Das agglutinations vermögen eineger kör perflüssigkeiton beim Mediterranfeiber. Central. Bakteriol. 52:268, 1909.

85. Potash, L., R. S. Lees, and B. H. Sweet. Increased sensitivity for detection of respiratory syncytial virus neutralizing antibody by use of unheated sera. Bact. Rev. p. 122, 1966. (abstract)

86. Price, W. H., H. Emerson, I. Ibler, R. Lachaine, and A. Terrell. Studies of the JH and 2060 viruses and their relationship to mild upper respiratory disease in humans. Amer. J. Hyg. 69:224–249, 1959.

87. Quilligan, J. J., Jr., and T. Francis, Jr. Serological response to intranasal administration of inactive influenza virus in children. J. Clin. Invest. 26:1079–1087, 1947.

88. Remington, J. S., K. L. Vosti, A. Lietze, and A. L. Zimmerman. Serum proteins and antibody activity in human nasal secretions. J. Clin. Invest. 43:1613–1624, 1964.

89. Rose, H. M. Inhibitory and enhancing effects of secretions of human respiratory tract on influenza virus. Fed. Proc. 9:390, 1950. (abstract)

90. Rossen, R. D., R. H. Alford, W. T. Butler, and W. E. Vannier. The separation and characterization of proteins intrinsic to nasal secretion. J. Immun. 97:369–378, 1966.

91. Rossen, R. D., W. T. Butler, T. R. Cate, C. F. Szwed, and R. B. Couch. Protein composition of nasal secretion during respiratory virus infection. Proc. Soc. Exp. Biol. Med. 119:1169–1176, 1965.

92. Rossen, R. D., R. G. Douglas, Jr., T. R. Cate, R. B. Couch, and W. T. Butler. The sedimentation behavior of rhinovirus neutralizing activity in nasal secretion and serum following the rhinovirus common cold. J. Immun. 97:532–538, 1966.

93. Rossen, R. D., C. Morgan, K. C. Hsu, W. T. Butler, and H. M. Rose. Localization of 11 S external secretory IgA by immunofluorescence in tissues lining the oral and respiratory passages in man. J. Immun. 100:706–717, 1968.

94. Rossen, R. D., A. L. Schade, W. T. Butler, and J. A. Kasel. The proteins in nasal secretions: A longitudinal study of the γA-globulin, γG-globulin, albumin, siderophilin, and total protein concentrations in nasal washings from adult male volunteers. J. Clin. Invest. 45:768–776, 1966.

95. Rossen, R. D., S. M. Wolff, and W. T. Butler. The antibody response in nasal washings and serum to *S. typhosa* endotoxin administered intravenously. J. Immun. 99:246–254, 1967.

96. Sapse, A. T., J. Ivanyi, W. Stone, Jr., B. Bonavida, and E. E. Sercarz. Tears as carriers of antibodies. I. Presence of antibodies to diverse antigens in rabbit tears. Arch. Ophthal. 77:526–529, 1967.

97. Smith, C. B., J. A. Bellanti, and R. M. Chanock. Immunoglobulins in serum and nasal secretions following infection with type 1 parainfluenza virus and injection of inactivated vaccines. J. Immun. 99:133–141, 1967.

98. Smith, C. B., R. H. Purcell, J. A. Bellanti, and R. M. Chanock. Protective effect of antibody to parainfluenza type 1 virus. New Eng. J. Med. 275:1145–1152, 1966.

99. South, M. A., M. D. Copper, F. A. Wollheim, and R. A. Good. The IgA system. II. The clinical significance of IgA deficiency: Studies in patients with agammaglobulinemia and ataxia-telangiectasia. Amer. J. Med. 44:168–178, 1968.

100. Staubli, C. Experimentelle untersuchungen über die ausscheidung der typhus agglutinine. Central. Bakteriol. 33:375, 1903.

101. Stobo, J. D., and T. B. Tomasi. A low molecular weight immunoglobulin antigenically related to 19 S IgM. J. Clin. Invest. 46:1329–1337, 1967.

102. Stokes, J., Jr., and D. R. Shaw. Production of passive immunity against influenza virus by introducing immune serums into the respiratory tract. Amer. J. Dis. Child. 58:653, 1939.

103. Tomasi, T. B., Jr. Human immunoglobulin A. New Eng. J. Med. 279:1327–1330, 1968.

104. Tourville, D., J. Bienenstock, and T. B. Tomasi, Jr. Natural antibodies of human serum, saliva, and urine reactive with *Escherichia coli*. Proc. Soc. Exp. Biol. Med. 128:722–727, 1968.

105. Tremonti, L. P., J. S. Lin, and G. G. Jackson. Neutralizing activity in nasal secretions and serum in resistance of volunteers to parainfluenza virus type 2. J. Immun. 101:572–577, 1968.

106. Turró, R., and P. Domingo. Les anticorps locaux dans les immunités locales. C. R. Soc. Biol. 88:410–412, 1923.

107. Waldman, R. H., J. A. Kasel, R. V. Fulk, Y. Togo, R. B. Hornick, G. G. Heiner, A. T. Dawkins, Jr., and J. J. Mann. Influenza antibody in human respiratory secretions after subcutaneous or respiratory immunization with inactivated virus. Nature 218:594–595, 1968.

108. Waldman, R. H., J. J. Mann, and J. A. Kasel. Influenza virus neutralizing antibody in human respiratory secretions. J. Immun. 100:80–85, 1968.

109. Waldman, R. H., J. J. Mann, and P. A. Small. Immunization against influenza. Prevention of illness in man by aerosolized inactivated vaccine. JAMA 207:520–524, 1969.

110. Walsh, T. E., and P. R. Cannon. Immunization of the respiratory tract. A comparative study of the antibody content of the respiratory and other tissues following active, passive and regional immunization. J. Immun. 35:31–46, 1938.

111. Walsh, T. E., and P. R. Cannon. Studies on acquired immunity in rabbits to intranasal infection with type I pneumococcus. J. Immun. 31:331–346, 1936.

112. Walsh, T. E., F. L. Sullivan, and P. R. Cannon. Local formation of antibody by the nasal mucosa. Proc. Soc. Exp. Biol. Med. 29:675–676, 1932.

113. Zhdanov, V. M., and V. D. Soloviev. Some results of the study of Asian influenza. Amer. Rev. Resp. Dis. 83:178–192, 1961.

DISCUSSION

DR. FAHEY: If secretory antibodies can be a prime determinant of resistance to respiratory infections, can they be implicated in resistance to the common cold?

DR. CHANOCK: I can recapitulate Dr. Perkins's experience with regard to the rhinoviruses. These viruses, of which there are approximately 100, are responsible for most common colds in adults. He showed that vaccine given intramuscularly, which stimulated high levels of serum antibodies, did not protect volunteers when they were later challenged with a very small dose of virus. When the same vaccine was given intranasally, lower levels of serum antibodies were stimulated, but the vaccine provided protection.

There is evidence that the conventional approach to immunization against respiratory disease that has been used successfully for viruses that travel through the body and have a viremic phase and a tissue phase in the viscera would probably not work. The reason is that we are concerned primarily with infections that are localized in the surface areas of the respiratory tract. There is epidemiologic and clinical evidence that high levels of serum antibodies fail to protect against respiratory syncytial virus, which we now know to be the major respiratory tract pathogen early in life. This virus is unusual, in that, instead of avoiding the first few months of life, it selectively produces its effect then. The incidence of severe disease is greatest when antibodies derived from maternal sources are at the highest level. As the placentally transferred antibodies decrease, the incidence of severe disease caused by this virus also decreases. Experience with an inactivated vaccine indicated that the induction of high levels of serum antibodies in young infants did not provide protection. In fact, it induced a state of altered reactivity, so that when they were infected later in infancy or early childhood, at a time when respiratory syncytial virus does not normally produce severe disease, they became quite ill and experienced life-threatening types of disease.

Thus, we have evidence from many different sources that serum antibodies are not protective. The conventional approach of preparing an antigen, inoculating it under the skin, and stimulating serum antibody is not going to be very effective. I think this is the basis for the relative ineffectiveness of the influenza vaccine as it is presently compounded and used. Our major efforts are in the direction of developing an attenuated vaccine that can be given locally to stimulate the secretory antibodies that we feel are the major determinant of resistance. We are not going to give secretory antibodies. We are going to induce the development of secretory antibodies. That is an important distinction. The passive approach would be rather expensive and would not represent a permanent solution of the problem. What we have to do is induce the body to develop its own secretory antibodies. That is a much more efficient way of approaching disease control.

DR. HEREMANS: Old-time pediatricians have always insisted on the superiority of breastfeeding, not with regard to protection against *any* kind of infection, but with regard to protection against gastrointestinal infection in newborns. When one goes through the literature, one gets the impression that there must be some truth in the old belief. That may indeed have been the first and primordial application of the principle of local passive immunization.

DR. ROBBINS: The biologic role of IgA after it combines with antigen, whether it be a virus, bacterium, or other particle, is unclear. In collaboration with Martin Schulkind and David Eddy of the Universities of Florida and Leeds in England, we isolated in pure form IgG and secretory IgA anti-*Salmonella typhimurium* "O" antibodies from intestinal perfusate and from the colostrum of rabbits. Rabbits that received injections of dead bacteria developed no secretory antibody, but those that received live bacteria intraperitoneally or orally formed a sufficient amount of antibody that pure antibody could be isolated by absorption and elution from the bacteria. These purified antibodies, when mixed with live bacteria and precolostral calf serum, showed no bactericidal activity, whereas IgG isolated from intestinal perfusate and serum showed bactericidal activity. The addition of 1 μg of lysozyme to this reaction mixture, to ascertain whether lysozyme might potentiate the effect of IgA in the presence of complement, as reported by Adinolfi for human colostrum, did not have any effects. Preliminary experiments showed that IgA, when preincubated with bacteria, acts as a blocking agent for IgG and IgM isolated from the small intestine and serum. Live bacteria, preincubated with IgA isolated from the small intestine perfusate and given to pathogen-free mice intravenously, are not cleared from the blood in 1 hr. IgG from serum and intestinal perfusates gives essentially the same specific activities, whereas serum IgM, as previously reported, gives much higher values. In these experiments, the IgA may have been slightly contaminated by other proteins, but we could not detect contaminants by diffusion experiments or ultracentrifugation analysis.

IgA must do something as a secondary reaction to its combination with antigen. It does not kill bacteria in the presence of complement or permit organization, activities demonstrable for other immunoglobulins. We demonstrated one activity: incubation *in vitro* of 10^{15} dead bacteria with 100 μg of IgA or IgG followed by injection of the coated bacteria into rabbits that do not have detectable agglutinins in their serum will suppress the immune response to the antigen used. In another experiment, 10^8 live salmonellae were injected into

2-week-old rabbits that had no pre-existing agglutinins in their serum and whose mothers had no agglutinins. Both IgG and IgA have similar capacity to suppress the immune response, both in serum and in the fluid of the small intestine. The passively administered antibody suppressed the immune response, even after the biologically active parts of the molecules were cleaved by proteolysis. These experiments leave open the question of the role of IgG and IgA after they combine with the infective particles.

EZIO MERLER

Immunoglobulin M

Macroglobulins were recognized as a separate entity after the technique of ultracentrifugation was introduced to study the physical chemistry of serum proteins. Heidelberger and Pedersen[7] and Kabat[9] demonstrated that antibodies could be separated into light and heavy components and that the heavy components, having a sedimentation coefficient of 18.4S, were β-globulins. It was believed for a time that the light and heavy components were characteristic of various animal species and that man, rabbit, and monkey possessed only the light variety.[25] Waldenström,[26] however, showed that macroglobulins were present in a high concentration in the sera of some patients with myeloma, and it was recognized soon after that they were normal constituents of serum. In 1958 it was found that these proteins were made up of smaller, identical components. The complex could be reduced by thiol reagents into subunits that were prevented from reaggregating by alkylation of the sulfhydryl groups.[2] This classic experiment has provided the insight for a great deal of the structural work on all immunoglobulins that has been done in the last 10 years.

Macroglobulins appear in the centrifuge as a series of discrete, fast-sedimenting components; 65–85% of the protein has a sedimentation coefficient of approximately 19S. The remainder is composed of dimers and polymers of the 19S complex in an apparent state of equilibrium. The molecular weight of the 19S component has been reported as 870,000[10,15] or 970,000,[23] depending on the pH and ionic strength of the solvent used. This difference in molecular weight became significant when the numbers were used to help build structural models.

It is generally accepted that reduction of the 19S complex yields five subunits. But, although some studies suggested that each subunit had a molecular weight of 180,000 and was composed of chains (two L and two μ), another study indicated that the subunit had different composition. In this latter study, first, reduction of the macroglobulin by cysteine yielded a subunit of molecular weight 200,000, which was stable in the presence of acids and denaturing agents. Second, reduction of the macroglobulin by thiol and then alkylation of the sulfhydryl groups yielded a subunit of molecular weight 160,000; found with this subunit were materials of lower molecular weight, presumed to be L chains. Third, acidification or denaturation of reduced and alkylated subunits yielded two μ chains, each with a molecular weight of 67,000, and an L chain with a molecular weight of 22,000 (Table 1). On the basis of these experiments, it was suggested that each subunit was composed of two μ chains and three L chains; that is, the molecule was internally asymmetric. Unfortunately, these studies were done on small numbers of myeloma proteins, so that these two structures are not mutually exclusive but may represent two different subclasses of immunoglobulins. It would be conceptually pleasing if the three major classes of immunoglobulins shared a common architecture, as well as a common structural component—the L chain. Irrespective of the structure of each subunit,

TABLE 1   Molecular Weights and Chain Composition of IgM and its Subunits (IgM$_s$), Considering the Protein as Symmetric and Asymmetric

Composition of the Protein	Symmetric Protein			Asymmetric Protein		
	No. Chains			No. Chains		
	μ	L	Molecular Weight	μ	L	Molecular Weight
IgM	10	10	890,000	10	15	970,000
IgM$_s$	2	2	180,000	{ 2	3	200,000
				2	1	160,000

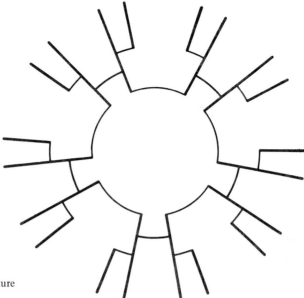

FIGURE 1   Tentative structure
of IgM.

the 19S complex is symmetric (Figure 1). The subunits are arranged in a
circle and are joined by a single disulfide bond,[18] which is presumably at
the C terminus of the μ chain. The electron microscope has revealed
molecules with "spider-like" structures with an electron-dense center
and five projections of various lengths, which are often looped.[24]
Antigen–antibody interaction of the macroglobulin appears to take
place through these projections.

Macroglobulins have been reported to contain 190 sulfhydryl groups
per molecule,[16] or 19 disulfide bonds per subunit. A knowledge of the
distribution of cysteines on the polypeptide chain and the number of
interchain disulfide bonds in each subunit would be helpful in defining
the structure of the molecule. This information, however, is not available; macroglobulins are variously labile to reductive cleavage and to
alkylation, owing to differing reactivities of disulfide bonds in individual
preparations, and it is not possible to distinguish between interchain and
intrachain bonds. It is not known whether intrachain loops similar to
those found in γ chains are also present in μ chains. Limited amino acid
sequences at both the N and C termini of the μ chain[1,27] seem to indicate homology between them and γ chains.

Limited proteolysis with papain, pepsin, and trypsin has been invaluable in studying the structure of IgG. Similar techniques and procedures have been applied to the study of IgM. The results obtained have, however, fallen short of expectations. IgM counterparts of F(ab')2, Fab, and Fc fragments were produced, but their yield is generally lower than expected and is sometimes so low as to be insignificant. Studies on the depolarization of fluorescence have indicated that the molecule has considerable internal freedom of rotation[13] like IgG, whereas studies of optical rotatory dispersion have indicated that there are significant differences in conformation between IgG and IgM.[3] The extensive amount of proteolysis favors the evidence that the polypeptide chains are loosely folded and extended structures, not only on the microscope grid but in solution.

The primary function of an antibody is to combine with its antigen. Given the complex structure of the macroglobulins, it became of some interest to define the number of combining sites per molecule. There have been three approaches to the problem:

1. By using a Waldenstrom macroglobulin with rheumatoid factor activity, it was shown that each mole of antibody bound five moles of IgG.[12] Each Fab fragment of the macroglobulin, however, combined with antigen. Not all rheumatoid factors exhibited this behavior, and in some only a portion of the Fab fragments combined with IgG. These experiments indicate that each subunit is potentially bivalent, but that, in the intact molecule, when the antigen is IgG, it is only monovalent.

2. By using rabbit IgM antibodies to sheep erythrocytes, reduced and alkylated subunits were prepared, only half of which could bind to antigen.[4] In these experiments, the subunits consisted apparently of one L and one μ chain; that is, they were half as big as the IgM_s subunits commonly obtained by reduction and alkylation of IgM. The reason for this difference is not clear; the authors attribute it to the low concentration of reactants in the reduction mixture. Whether this unusual structure contributed to the results of these experiments is not known. The results contrast with the previous one and indicate that subunits are monovalent whether they are dissociated or present in the intact molecule

3. By using a human IgM antibody to *Salmonella typhosa* and equilibrium dialysis, it was shown that the IgM antibody possessed 10 antigen-combining sites.[11] In this study, the ligand was a tetrasaccha-

ride, which is the antigenic determinant of the *S. typhosa* endotoxin.
Each subunit was therefore bivalent in the intact molecule. This last
study contrasts with both the previous ones. It has, however, the advantage over them that measurements were done in a state of thermo-
dynamic equilibrium. The Scatchard plot (Figure 2) was, within experimental error, a straight line, justifying the assumption that the antigen-
specific regions represented a set of equivalent and independent binding
sites, homogeneous in their ability to bind the ligand—a construction
that clearly would not be deduced for the previous experiments. Also,
through use of equilibrium dialysis, a study that had shown that a
rabbit IgM antibody obtained early in the immunologic response possessed one combining site per subunit[21] has recently been extended to

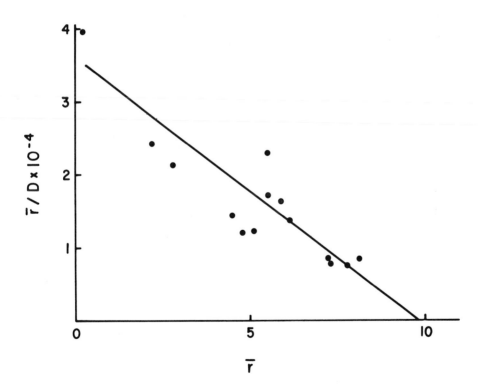

FIGURE 2   The binding of tetrasaccharide (haptene of *S. typhosa* endotoxin) by human IgM
antibody. $\bar{r}$/D (the number of moles of oligosaccharide bound per mole of antibody divided by
the molar concentration of free oligosaccharide in the antibody-containing compartment of the
dialysis cell) is plotted against $\bar{r}$. (Reprinted with permission from Merler *et al.*[11])

show that this antibody has two sets of antigen-combining sites of five sites each, one of low affinity for the haptene and one of high affinity.[20]

Unquestionably, the IgM antibody has 10 potential combining sites. In some instances, only five are expressed. Whether this is caused by IgM antibodies of different structure, by heterogeneity of the antibody molecule produced by variations of the polypeptide chains, or by heterogeneity produced by the assembly of different subunits is not known. Like IgG, macroglobulins are molecularly heterogeneous. The L chains, as in all immunoglobulins, are subdivided into κ and λ chains. At least two subclasses of μ chains with different serologic specificity not related to L chains have been described.[5] So have determinants that are expressed only when κ and μ chains are combined, but not when they are separate.[17] To date, no genetic subgroups of IgM have been described. By using a rabbit IgM antibody, fixation of complement was shown to be associated with only a small percentage of antigen–antibody complexes.[8] These experiments demonstrate that both the L and μ chains are heterogeneous in their serologic and biologic function and presumably in their amino acid sequence, but not in their overall structure. This heterogeneity is common to all immunoglobulins. It has no bearing, however, on the antibody activity of the molecule, particularly if assembly of the 19S complex is from identical subunits; that is, if one molecule contains all κ chains or all complement-fixing μ chains, the antibody activity of the complex should be indistinguishable from that of its subunits. There is no evidence that macroglobulins or other immunoglobulins are mosaics of various subunits bound to form a heterogeneous complex. Of course, it is possible that macroglobulins are not all structurally identical and that in the normal animal there are a small number of molecules that are asymmetric—the variety with three L chains—and that these molecules have been singled out in the studies with the myeloma proteins. In these sera, they may have become the only macroglobulin present. But if the IgM antibody of *S. typhosa* is at all indicative of the distribution of macroglobulins in normal sera, this asymmetric variety should not be too common.

A characteristic feature of all macroglobulins is their content of carbohydrate, which accounts for up to 10% of the molecule by weight.[19] About half this sugar is simple hexose, and the remaining half, fucose, hexosamine, and sialic acid. Almost all the carbohydrate is associated with the μ chain and is present on the Fc fragment.[14] Most of the human serum antibodies to the lipopolysaccharide antigens are IgM. These antibodies comprise the heterophile (Forssmann) and Wassermann antibodies, cold agglutinins, isohemagglutinins, and antibodies to the O antigens (endotoxins) of gram-negative bacteria.

Between 5% and 10% of the total serum antibody is found in the IgM. IgM antibodies are found in the circulation early, following primary antigenic stimulation. In many instances, these antibodies diminish in concentration and nearly disappear as immunization proceeds. These observations[22] prompted a flurry of investigations from which it was concluded that antigen stimulation provokes synthesis of IgM antibodies, primitive antibodies in the scheme of evolution, to be followed by synthesis of IgG antibodies, more specialized molecules, higher in the evolutionary development. Further investigation has shown that there is probably no sequence of antibody formation, but rather a sequence of antibody detectability,[6] inasmuch as fewer IgM molecules than IgG molecules can be detected in a system that measures antibody titers.

Although specific functions have been assigned to most IgG, IgA, and IgE immunoglobulins, IgM immunoglobulins are still unclassified. We know that they are complex and highly efficient antibodies, that they are synthesized early during the immunologic response, and that they are short-lived. They are present in lower vertebrates as the only antibody, and in mammals they are produced in response to antigenic stimulation with most carbohydrates. We do not know, however, why they are present at all. Many questions about the structure have been answered. We can expect in the near future to see extensive amino acid sequence data of the pathologic monoclonal macroglobulins and, presumably, increasing indication of the heterogeneity of the normal proteins. Many of the structural uncertainties will probably be cleared up. Elucidation of the biologic mechanism that determines the production of these molecules and their biosynthesis may, however, not be too readily available, and this, of course, constitutes the major challenge to future investigations in this field.

REFERENCES

1. Bennett, J. C. The amino-terminal sequence of the heavy chain of human immunoglobulin M. Biochemistry 7:3340–3344, 1968.
2. Deutsch, H. F., and J. I. Morton. Human serum macroglobulins and dissociation units. I. Physicochemical properties. J. Biol Chem. 231:1107–1118, 1958.

3. Dorrington, K. J., and C. Tanford. The optical rotatory dispersion of human γM-immunoglobulins and their subunits. J. Biol. Chem. 243:4745–4749, 1968.

4. Frank, M. M., and J. H. Humphrey. The subunits in rabbit anti-Forssmann IgM antibody. J. Exp. Med. 127:967–982, 1968.

5. Franklin, E. C., and B. Frangione. Two serologically distinguishable subclasses of μ-chains of human macroglobulins. J. Immun. 99:810–814, 1967.

6. Freeman, M. J., and A. B. Stavitsky. Radioimmunoelectrophoretic study of rabbit anti-protein antibodies during the primary response. J. Immun. 95:981–990, 1965.

7. Heidelberger, M., and K. O. Pedersen. The molecular weight of antibodies. J. Exp. Med. 65:393–414, 1937.

8. Hoyer, L. W., T. Borsos, H. J. Rapp, and W. E. Vannier. Heterogeneity of rabbit IgM antibody as detected by C′1a fixation. J. Exp. Med. 127:589–603, 1968.

9. Kabat, E. A. The molecular weight of antibodies. J. Exp. Med. 69:103–118, 1939.

10. Lamm, M. E., and P. A. Small, Jr. Polypeptide chain structure of rabbit immunoglobulins. II. Gamma-M-immunoglobulin. Biochemistry 5:267–276, 1966.

11. Merler, E., L. Karlin, and S. Matsumoto. The valency of human gamma-M immunoglobulin antibody. J. Biol. Chem. 243:386–390, 1968.

12. Metzger, H. Characterization of a human macroglobulin. V. A. Waldenström macroglobulin with antibody activity. Proc. Nat. Acad. Sci. USA 57:1490–1497, 1967.

13. Metzger, H., R. L. Perlman, and H. Edelhoch. Characterization of a human macroglobulin. IV. Studies of its conformation by fluorescence polarization. J. Biol. Chem. 241:1741–1744, 1966.

14. Mihaesco, C., and N. M. Seligmann. Papain digestion fragments of human IgM globulins. J. Exp. Med. 127:431–453, 1968.

15. Miller, F., and H. Metzger. Characterization of a human macroglobulin. I. The molecular weight of its subunit. J. Biol. Chem. 240:3325–3333, 1965.

16. Miller, F., and H. Metzger. Characterization of a human macroglobulin. II. Distribution of the disulfide bonds. J. Biol. Chem. 240:4740–4745, 1965.

17. Miller, E. J., and W. D. Terry. Antigenic determinants of human IgM requiring interaction of μ- and κ-chains. J. Immun. 101:1300–1307, 1968.

18. Morris, J. E., and F. P. Inman. Isolation of the monomeric subunit of immunoglobulin M with its interchain disulfide bonds intact. Biochemistry 7:2851–2857, 1968.

19. Müller-Eberhard, H. J., H. G. Kunkel, and E. C. Franklin. Two types of γ-globulin differing in carbohydrate content. Proc. Soc. Exp. Biol. Med. 93:146–150, 1956.

20. Onoue, K., A. L. Grossberg, Y. Yagi, and D. Pressman. Immunoglobulin M antibodies with ten combining sites. Science 162:574–576, 1968.

21. Onoue, K., Y. Yagi, A. L. Grossberg, and D. Pressman. Number of binding sites of rabbit macroglobulin antibody and its subunits. Immunochemistry 2:401–415, 1965.

22. Smith, R. T., and V. D. Eitzman. The development of the immune response. Characterization of the response of the human infant and adult to immunization with Salmonella vaccines. Pediatrics 33:163–183, 1964.

23. Suzuki, T., and H. F. Deutsch. Dissociation, reaggregation, and subunit structure studies of some human γ-M-globulins. J. Biol. Chem. 242:2725–2738, 1967.

24. Svehag, S. E., B. Chesebro, and B. Bloth. Ultrastructure of gamma-M immunoglobulin and alpha macroglobulin: electron-microscopic study. Science 158:933–936, 1967.

25. Tiselius, A., and E. A. Kabat. Electrophoretic study of immune sera and purified antibody preparations. J. Exp. Med. 69:119–131, 1939.

26. Waldenstrom, J. Abnormal proteins in myeloma. Advances Intern. Med. 5:398–440, 1952.

27. Wikler, M., H. Köhler, T. Shinoda, and F. W. Putnam. Macroglobulin structure: homology of mu and gamma heavy chains of human immunoglobulins. Science 163:75–78, 1969.

DISCUSSION

DR. DEUTSCH: Papain digestion of macroglobulins has been shown to give a rather large Fc fragment that contains almost all the carbohydrate present on IgM. The inference is that it is possible to remove a type of Fab fragment from the IgM molecule and to preserve a ring type of Fc structure that is linked by the inter-chain sulfhydryl groups of the μ chain. When one takes this papain-digested fraction, which sediments at 10S or 11S, and treats it with mercaptan, it is converted into smaller fragments. I think one of the reasons why one generally gets small fragments is that papain is a sulfhydryl enzyme and some splitting of the inter-subunit bonds occurs. The IgM subunits are very labile to papain digestion, but some of the Fc polymer, which then can be degraded further by mercaptan, is produced. I think this is a fairly reasonable picture, but it should be pointed out that the digestion of IgM is different from that of IgG.

H. G. SCHWICK, J. FISCHER, *and* H. GEIGER

Human Immunoglobulins A and M for Clinical Use

Human gamma globulin used nowadays for prophylaxis or therapy consists almost exclusively of IgG. In preparations of gamma globulin, specific antibodies against various pathogenic agents and toxins are concentrated about 20-fold, compared with the antibody content of the donor serum. All of them, whether obtained by fractionation with ethanol, neutral salts, or acridinium lactate, contain only traces of IgA and IgM.[5]

In measuring the antibody content of highly purified IgG, IgA, and IgM isolated from plasma of immunized blood donors, we were able to show that some antibodies can be demonstrated preferentially in one or the other of the three classes of immunoglobulins. Antibodies against protein antigens are found mainly in IgG, antibodies against carbohydrate antigens are found in IgM, and some virus antibodies occur equally in IgA and IgG.[10] In addition, it is known that antibodies contained in different immunoglobulins differ qualitatively. Thus, IgM antibodies are characterized by their high complement-binding activity.[9] Therefore, we found it necessary to develop a method for manufacturing gamma globulin preparations with increased contents of IgA and IgM for clinical investigation.

116

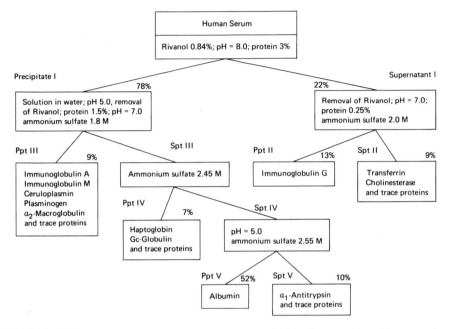

FIGURE 1   Serum fractionation by means of a combined Rivanol–ammonium sulfate procedure.

In our method for producing normal gamma globulin, the main portion of IgA and IgM is found in a fraction called precipitate III[2] (Figure 1). This fraction is the starting material for the purification of IgA and IgM. The principle of this method is shown in Figure 2. We have prepared several batches of gamma globulin for clinical tests. Their composition is shown in Table 1. The contents of IgA and IgM in the gamma globulin preparations were determined quantitatively by radial immunodiffusion.[1]

In the last few years, it has been shown by quantitative immunologic assays that the contents of IgG, IgA, and IgM in serum can differ in various diseases.[11] Therefore, several authors[6,7,13] have called for the manufacture of IgA and IgM preparations for clinical use. Hobbs[7] recently published data about isolated lack of IgA and IgM in a fairly large number of patients. The same author, together with Milner and Watt,[8] has demonstrated that IgM deficiency occurs with an increase in meningococcal meningitis and septicemia. However, infections of the lungs are frequently observed in cases of IgA deficiency.[14]

Our clinical tests, which have not yet been finished, involve prophylaxis against infections in newborn and premature infants. We hope that these investigations will answer the question of whether infections with *Escherichia coli*, salmonellae, and pyogenic organisms, which often cause death in premature infants, can be prevented.

Extensive clinical experiments are going on with regard to prophylaxis against infections in patients treated with cytostatics and postoperative prophylaxis against wound infections combined with disturbances of the wound-healing process in old people. The starting point of this study was our observation[4] of an increase of immunologically detectable immunoglobulins in old people with a decrease of antibody

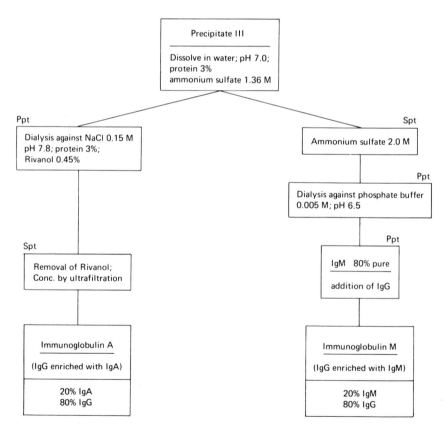

FIGURE 2   IgA and IgM preparations from precipitate III.

TABLE 1   Composition of Gamma Globulin Containing IgA and IgM for Clinical Testing

Lot	Content of Immunoglobulin %	Total Content of Immunoglobulins (electrophoresis), %
IgA-Enriched Gamma Globulins		
280967	28	94.5
271167	19	96
030168	24	95
080168	23	95
130568	25	95
IgM-Enriched Gamma Globulins		
100566	22	95
101067	19	99
070268	21	95
130368	22	95
210268	21	95

activities in their serum.[12] Gierhake[3] has demonstrated that an increase of wound infections in old people may depend on the antibody content of their serum. The gamma globulin preparations containing IgA and IgM are used in clinical cases in which deficiencies of IgA and IgM are manifest.

Summarizing the results of our clinical investigations, we can say that gamma globulin enriched in IgA and IgM is well tolerated after repeated intramuscular application.

REFERENCES

1. Becker, W. von, W. Rapp, H. G. Schwick, and K. Störiko. Methoden zur quantitativen Bestimmung von Plasmaproteinen durch Immunpräzipitation. Z. Klin. Chem. 6:113–122, 1968.
2. Dietzel, E., and H. Geiger. Gewinnung und Eigenschaften therapeutisch wichtiger Human-Plasma-proteine. Behringwerk-Mitteilungen 43:129–159, 1964.
3. Gierhake, F. W. Postoperative Wundheilungsstörungen und Staphylokokken-hospitalismus. Med. Welt 45:2444–2446, 1966.
4. Haferkamp, O., D. Schlettwein-Gsell, H. G. Schwick, and K. Störiko. Serum protein in an aging population with particular reference to evaluation of immune globulins and antibodies. Gerontologia 12:30–36, 1966.

5. Heiner, D. C., and L. Evans. Immunoglobulins and other proteins in commercial preparations of gamma globulin. J. Pediat. 70:820–827, 1967.
6. Hitzig, W. H. Therapie mit Immunglobulinen. Mschr. Kinderheilk 115:356–364, 1967.
7. Hobbs, J. R. Immune imbalance in dysgammaglobulinaemia type IV. Lancet 1:110–114,
   1968.
8. Hobbs, J. R., R. D. Milner, and P. J. Watt. Gamma-M deficiency predisposing to meningococcal septicaemia. Brit. Med. J. 4:583–586, 1967.
9. Humphry, J. H., and R. R. Dourmashkin. Electron microscope studies of immune cell
   lysis, pp. 175–186. In G. E. Wolstenholme and J. Knight, Eds. Complement. CIBA Foundation Symposium. Boston: Little, Brown and Co., 1965.
10. Schwick, H. G. Die Verteilung von Antikörpern in Human-Immunoglobulinen. G. Mal.
    Infett. 18 (Suppl.): 965–976, 1966.
11. Schwick, H. G. Immunological methods in clinical chemistry, p. 93. In Sixth International
    Congress on Clinical Chemistry, Munich, 1966. Vol. I. Clinical Protein Chemistry. Basel:
    S. Karger, 1968.
12. Schwick, H. G., and W. Becker. Humoral antibodies in older humans. In Bayer Symposium I:
    Current Problems in Immunology. Berlin, Heidelberg, New York: Springer, 1969. 253 pp.
13. Stiehm, E. R., J.-P. Vaerman, and H. H. Fudenberg. Plasma infusions in immunologic de-
    ficiency states: Metabolic and therapeutic studies. Blood 28:918–937, 1966.
14. Vesin, P. Les carences en immunoglobulines. Essai de classification bio-clinique. Protides
    Biol. Fluids 14:361–365, 1966.

DISCUSSION

DR. SOOTHILL: Dr. Schwick, what is your evidence for the assertion that the patients did better on the IgA- and IgM-containing material than on standard gamma globulin? It is extremely difficult to obtain evidence of this type, as the Medical Research Council working party found even with a twofold dose difference.

I should like to point out the statistical difficulties of the problem we are dealing with. Dr. Chandra, working with me now, noted in Indian infants a high incidence of disseminated nonprogressive vaccinia affecting about one in a thousand of two different populations who received the same lymph. This is presumably a hematogenous dissemination of the virus, and it represents a threshold test of an immunity function in these infants. He brought the serum of these patients to us. They are highly significantly deficient in IgM and IgA, compared with a control series from the same population. This suggests that clinically significant IgM deficiency may occur in 0.1% of the population.

DR. SCHWICK: I agree with you that it is difficult to test this preparation of immunoglobulins clinically and compare it with normal gamma globulin. In both cases in which the preparation was tested in Hamburg, children who for years had received gamma globulin every 4 weeks, and suffered repeated infections, remained free of infections when the gamma globulin was changed to this IgA- and IgM-enriched preparation. That is all I can say.

DR. BALLIEUX: With the IgA-enriched fraction, what are the dose and the frequency of treatment in patients with ataxia-telangiectasia?

DR. SCHWICK: In the studies in Hamburg, the IgA-enriched gamma globulin was given in 2 weeks. It is a 10% solution, and it was given in amounts of 0.2–0.5 ml/kg of body weight.

KIMISHIGE ISHIZAKA

Immunoglobulin E

Studies on the relationship between immunoglobulin structure and biologic function of antibodies revealed that the immunologic properties of antibodies depend on the immunoglobulin class to which the antibodies belong, which in turn depends on the structure of the heavy chains of the antibody molecules.[3,11] That suggested that human reaginic antibodies, having characteristic immunologic properties, may have a unique heavy-chain structure and may belong to a unique immunoglobulin class. Evidence existed that reagins were not immunoglobulins G, A, M, or D.[6,10] Radioimmunoelectrophoresis indicated the presence of a unique immunoglobulin in a reagin-rich fraction of atopic patients' sera.[8] In this experiment, rabbits were immunized with reagin-rich fractions, and the antisera obtained were absorbed with normal IgG, IgA, and IgD myeloma proteins. The absorbed antiserum gave a γ_1 precipitin band with a reagin-rich fraction from ragweed-sensitive serum, which combined with radioactive ragweed allergen in radioimmunoelectrophoresis. This finding indicated that the γ_1 globulin had a unique antigenic structure, different from that of the four immunoglobulins, and that it had reagin activity. We have called this protein γE globulin.[8]

CORRELATION BETWEEN γE AND REAGINIC ANTIBODIES

The relationship between γE and human reaginic antibodies has been studied. It was found by radioimmunodiffusion that the presence of reaginic antibody against ragweed allergen correlated with the presence of γE antibody against the allergen. Patients' sera containing antibodies against other allergens did not show the radioactive γE band when radioactive ragweed allergen was used to develop radioimmunodiffusion.[8,9]

It was found that the skin-sensitizing activity of the patients' sera was precipitated with the antibody specific for γE. To date, we have studied more than 20 reaginic sera that contained skin-sensitizing antibodies against ragweed, grass pollen, horse dandruff, egg white, house dust, and penicillin. In all cases, skin-sensitizing activity was precipitated by anti-γE. These findings indicate that association of reaginic activity with γE is not limited to the ragweed system but is also present in the other allergen–reagin systems.

The Prausnitz-Küstner (P-K) titer of sera from ragweed-sensitive patients quantitatively paralleled the concentration of γE antibody to the allergen, as measured by antigen-binding activity.[7] However, no correlation was obtained between the P-K titer and the IgG, IgA, or IgM antibody concentration in the patients' sera.

Physicochemical similarities were found between reaginic antibody and γE antibodies. When atopic patients' sera were fractionated by ion-exchange chromatography, gel filtration, sucrose density-gradient ultracentrifugation, and gel electrophoresis, distribution of reaginic activity paralleled that of γE antibody, as detected by radioimmunodiffusion.[9]

Finally, we have isolated γE from a reaginic serum. The preparation contained γE antibody, but not IgG, IgA, or IgM antibody, to ragweed allergen and had a very high P-K titer. All the reaginic activity in the preparation was precipitated by anti-γE.[4] This finding clearly showed that γE antibody has skin-sensitizing activity. In summarizing these observations, one can conclude that γE is the carrier of reaginic activity in atopic patients' sera.

ANTIGENIC STRUCTURE

To show that γE represents a distinct immunoglobulin class, we studied its antigenic structure.[13] It has been shown by radioimmunoelectrophoresis that γE has κ and λ L-chain determinants that are common to all immunoglobulins. γE also has antigenic determinants that are not shared by any of the other immunoglobulin classes; moreover, it does not have any of the major antigenic determinants present in the other four known immunoglobulin classes. This indicates that γE is not a subclass of the immunoglobulins. These pieces of information, together with the presence of antibody activity associated with γE, are sufficient for the conclusion that γE represents a distinct immunoglobulin class and should be called IgE. Furthermore, myeloma protein ND, described by Johansson and Bennich,[19] was proved to be an IgE myeloma protein.[1] In an experiment, an IgE fraction from a reaginic serum was placed in the center well of an Ouchterlony plate, and the peripheral wells were filled with the antisera specific for each immunoglobulin class and with a rabbit antiserum specific for the Fc portion of the ND protein. The anti-ND and anti-IgE sera gave a single precipitin band of identical specificity with the IgE fraction, and the precipitin band combined radioactive ragweed allergen in autoradiograms (Figure 1). It is apparent that both anti-ND and anti-IgE precipitated the same protein. Similarly, the ND protein and normal IgE gave a single precipitin band of identical specificity with the anti-IgE and anti-ND. These results clearly show that myeloma ND protein is an IgE myeloma protein and that the IgE antigenic determinants are present in the Fc portion of the IgE.

Recently, another patient (P.S.) afflicted with IgE myeloma was found, in Hanover, New Hampshire.[21] His bone marrow was infiltrated with plasma cells, and 60% of his peripheral leukocytes were plasma cells. The serum did not contain a detectable amount of IgA, IgM, or IgD, and the concentration of IgG was about 200 mg/100 ml. The serum gave a strong precipitin band with anti-IgE at a dilution of 1 : 100. Evidence was obtained that the plasma cells both in the bone marrow and

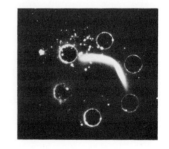

FIGURE 1 Radioimmunodiffusion showing the antigenic identity of myeloma ND protein with IgE. A reagin-rich fraction was placed in the center well, and antisera specific for each of the five immunoglobulins and for myeloma ND were placed in peripheral wells. Anti-IgE and anti-ND showed a precipitin band of identical specificity with the reagin-rich (γE) fraction. Autoradiography showed that the precipitin band combined radioactive antigen. Antisera from top in clockwise direction: anti-ND, anti-IgE, anti-IgD, anti-IgM, anti-IgA, and anti-IgG.

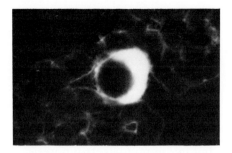
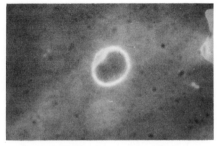

FIGURE 2 Fluorescent staining of a plasma cell in bone marrow (left) and a lymphoid cell in peripheral blood (right) of IgE myeloma patient P.S. The cells were stained by anti-IgE.

in the peripheral blood form IgE. Smears of bone marrow and buffy coats were treated with guinea pig anti-IgE antiserum and subsequently stained with a fluoresceinated antibody to guinea pig immunoglobulins. The plasma cells and peripheral lymphocytes were stained (Figure 2). Guinea pig antibodies specific for the other immunoglobulins did not stain any of the cells. The myeloma protein in the serum was isolated by DEAE cellulose-column chromatography and gel filtration through Sephadex G-200. PS myeloma protein and ND protein gave a single precipitin band of identical specificity against an anti-IgE raised to normal IgE (Figure 3, left). Both ND protein and PS protein belonged to

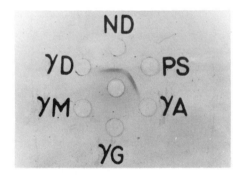
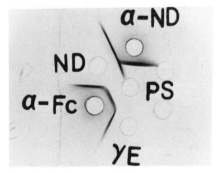

FIGURE 3   Left, antigenic identity of two IgE myeloma proteins (ND and PS). Antiserum specific for normal IgE (center well) gave a precipitin band of identical specificity with the myeloma proteins. Right, antigenic structure of IgE myeloma proteins. The precipitin band between ND protein and the antiserum specific for ND protein showed a spur over the precipitin band with PS protein. The antiserum specific for the Fc fragment of the ND protein (a-Fc) showed a precipitin band of identical specificity with ND protein, PS protein, and normal IgE.

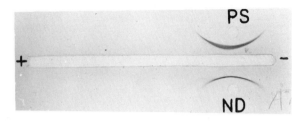

FIGURE 4   Immunoelectrophoresis of IgE myeloma proteins ND and PS, developed with an antiserum specific for IgE.

the λ type. When the proteins were tested by immunoelectrophoresis, they had identical γ_1 mobility (Figure 4). The only antigenic difference between the two myeloma proteins was the presence of idiotypic determinants. When the proteins were placed in peripheral wells against an antiserum specific for ND protein, the PS protein showed a reaction of bending and partial fusion with ND. Similarly, ND showed partial fusion with PS when anti-PS serum was used. The antigenic determinants accounting for these differences are not present in the Fc portion of the molecule. As shown in Figure 3 (right), the antiserum specific for the Fc fragment of the ND protein gave a single precipitin band of complete fusion with the ND protein, PS protein, and normal IgE isolated from an atopic patient's serum.

The normal concentration of IgE in serum is low. According to Johansson *et al.*,[20] it was in the range of 0.1–0.7 μg/ml, with an average of 0.3 μg/ml. The concentration of protein can be significantly higher in some atopic patients, although that is not necessarily the case.

PHYSICOCHEMICAL PROPERTIES AND STRUCTURE

The physicochemical properties of IgE are summarized in Table 1. There is too little IgE in serum to isolate it for structural studies. Therefore, all available information on its structure has been obtained from the two IgE myeloma proteins. Bennich and Johansson[2] have reduced the ND protein with mercaptoethanol, alkylated with iodoacetamide, and isolated two components that correspond to H and L chains. The yield of L chains was 20% of the total protein, and their molecular weight, calculated from the amino acid composition, was 22,500 (see Table 2). It was assumed that the molecule contains two L chains and two H chains. If the assumption is correct, the molecular weight of the H chain (ε)

TABLE 1 Physicochemical Properties of the Immunoglobulins

Property	IgG	IgM	IgA	IgD	IgE
Electrophoretic mobility	γ_1-γ_2	γ_1	γ_1	γ_1	γ_1
Sedimentation coefficient, $S^{\circ}_{20,W}$	6.6	18	6.6	7.0	8.2
DEAE cellulose chromatography (M/1)[a]	0.005	0.15	0.035	0.035	0.02
Molecular weight	150,000	900,000	180,000	?	200,000[b]
Carbohydrate, %	2.9	11.8	7.5	?	10.7[b]

[a]Molarity of salt at which protein is eluted.
[b]Determined for protein ND only.

should be approximately 75,000. Papain digestion of the myeloma protein produced two fragments that correspond to the Fc and Fab fragments of IgG. The IgE-antigenic determinants were present in Fc, but not in Fab fragments. The sedimentation coefficient of the Fc fragment was 5S, and its molecular weight was estimated to be 100,000. These data indicate that the Fc fragment of the IgE myeloma protein represents a portion of heavy (ϵ) chains. After pepsin digestion of the protein and then gel filtration, approximately 52% of the material was recovered as a 6S fragment. The fragment contained λ chains and corresponded to $(Fab')_2$. Both Fc and $(Fab')_2$ contained 11% carbohydrate, whereas λ chain did not. Distribution of cysteine and methionine residues in H and L chains was estimated from chemical analysis of the isolated H and L chains and $(Fab')_2$ fragment. From these findings, Bennich and Johansson[2] proposed a schematic model of the IgE myeloma pro-

TABLE 2 Properties of IgE Myeloma Protein ND

	Molecular Weight	Sedimentation Coefficient, $S^{\circ}_{20,W}$	Total Carbohydrate	Cysteine	Methionine
Myeloma protein ND	196,000	7.9	10.71	42	18
Light chain (λ), 214 aa	22,500	–	0	5	1
Heavy chain (ND)	75,500	–	14	16	8
$(Fab')_2$	104,000	6.1	10.76	18	10
Fd'	29,500	–	19	4	4
½ "Fc"=(Heavy-Fd')	46,000	–	11	12	4

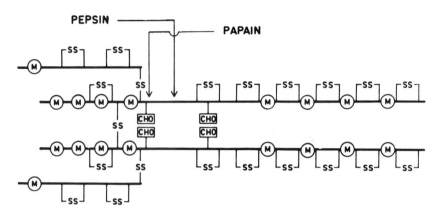

FIGURE 5   Schematic diagram of IgE myeloma protein. M, methionine. CHO, carbohydrate.

tein, as shown in Figure 5. Apparently, the large numbers of methionine residues per ϵ chain and of cysteine residues in the Fc portion of the molecules are characteristics of this immunoglobulin. As will be discussed later, this structure might be related to peculiar biologic properties of IgE antibodies.

IMMUNOLOGIC PROPERTIES

As already described, IgE antibodies give P-K reactions in normal persons. Assuming that IgE antibodies have avidity comparable with that of IgG antibodies, the minimal sensitizing dose of IgE antibody in the patients' sera was calculated from antigen-binding activity. This dose in six patients' sera studied was 2×10^{-6} μgN (micrograms of protein nitrogen).[7]

IgE antibodies are responsible for the passive cutaneous anaphylaxis (PCA) reaction in monkeys. With *Macaca irus*, about 30 times as much IgE antibody was required to sensitize the monkey skin as to sensitize human skin in the P-K reaction. Evidence was obtained in this experiment that neither IgG nor IgA antibodies sensitize monkey skin for PCA reactions. However, IgE antibody did not give a PCA reaction in the guinea pig, even when a reaginic fraction having a P-K titer of 1:10,000 was used for passive sensitization. Recently, we studied the possibility of sensitizing guinea pig skin for reversed PCA reactions with IgE myeloma protein. The IgE myeloma protein was injected intracutaneously into guinea pigs, which received intravenous injections of anti-IgE 3 hr later. The results showed that even 100 μgN/ml of IgE myeloma protein failed to sensitize guinea pig skin. It is clear that IgE can sensitize both human and monkey skin, but not guinea pig skin (Table 3).

In addition to sensitizing skin, IgE sensitizes human leukocytes. When isolated leukocytes from atopic patients were incubated with anti-IgE, histamine was released from the leukocytes.[16] Furthermore, previous incubation of the leukocytes with IgE myeloma protein increased the sensitivity of the leukocytes to anti-IgE, indicating that IgE actually bound to the cells. Similarly, monkey lung tissues sensitized with the myeloma protein released histamine and slow-reacting substance A (SRS-A) by exposure to anti-IgE.[17] That finding suggests that IgE antibodies are involved in allergic reactions in lung tissues.

Immunochemical properties of IgE antibodies have been studied *in vitro*. IgE antibodies against ragweed antigen agglutinated erythrocytes coated with antigen. On the basis of antigen-binding activity, the IgE and IgG antibodies obtained from the same serum had comparable hemagglutinating activity. Hemagglutination by IgE antibodies suggested that the antibodies are multivalent.

Participation of complement in anaphylactic reactions and reaginic hypersensitivity has been discussed for a long time. Complement fixation by IgE antibodies could not be detected. It has been shown that aggregated IgG can initiate complement fixation, and that the reaction medi-

TABLE 3   Immunologic Properties of IgE

Reaction	Minimal Concentration of Antibody, μgN/ml	Activity
In vivo		
P-K in human	4×10^{-5}	+
PCA in monkey	10^{-3}	+
PCA in guinea pig	>100	−
In vitro		
Agglutination	10^{-2}	+
Complement fixation	$>800^a$	−

^{a}Aggregated IgE.

ated by aggregated IgG is identical with that mediated by antigen–antibody complexes.[15] It was also found that nonspecific aggregates of IgM, as well as specific-antigen–IgM-antibody complexes, could initiate complement fixation, whereas neither aggregated IgA nor antigen–IgA-antibody complexes could initiate the reaction.[18] Recent studies with aggregated IgE myeloma proteins have shown that even a dose of 800 μgN of aggregated IgE does not fix any significant amount of complement.[14] It was also shown that aggregated IgE does not fix C1a and that it fails to form anaphylatoxin from C3.* These findings suggest that complement is not involved in reaginic hypersensitivity by IgE antibodies (Table 3).

The most important characteristic of IgE antibodies is their activity in sensitizing homologous species. The property is probably due to affinity of IgE molecules for target cells that are involved in reaginic hypersensitivity. In fact, it was found that nonantibody IgE blocked passive sensitization with reaginic antibodies. When reaginic sera were mixed with nonantibody IgE and injected into normal persons, skin sites were not sensitized for P-K reactions.[13] Stanworth and his coworkers showed that IgE myeloma protein also blocks passive sensitization.[23] The blocking of passive sensitization is a characteristic property of IgE; myeloma proteins of the other four immunoglobulin classes and subclasses did not show the blocking effect (Table 4). More recently, evidence was presented that the Fc fragment of IgE myeloma protein blocked passive sensitization, indicating that the structure essential for tissue affinity is present in the Fc portion of the IgE molecules.[22]

It is well known that reaginic antibody is inactivated by heating at 56 C for 4 hr. The skin-sensitizing activity of IgE antibodies and their affinity for target cells were lost by heating. After heating, IgE lost the ability to block passive sensitization with reaginic antibodies. Further studies on the effect of heating IgE antibodies have shown that the antibody-combining sites remained intact after heating, whereas the structures essential for passive sensitization, as well as IgE antigenic determinants, were destroyed.[12]

Reaginic antibody is inactivated by reduction in 0.1M mercaptoethanol followed by alkylation. The skin-sensitizing activity of IgE antibodies is also greatly diminished by reduction and alkylation. Antigenic deter-

---

*However, aggregated IgE induced erythema–wheal reactions in normal persons with only 1 ngN.

TABLE 4   Blocking of Passive Sensitization by Immunoglobulins

Proteins Injected with Reaginic Antibody	Dose, μgN	Wheal, mm	Erythema, mm
IgG			
IgG1	2.0	8.5	30×32
IgG2	2.0	9.5	35×42
IgG3	2.0	10.5	30×43
IgG4	2.0	10.0	30×49
IgA[a]			
Fu	2.0	9.5	30×41
Ma	2.0	9.5	34×37
He	2.0	10.0	31×45
IgD	1.6	9.5	31×34
IgM	2.0	9.5	34×36
	0.06	0	0
IgE + IgG	0.03	5.0	20×22
	0.015	6.0	21×25
IgE + IgG (heated)	2.8	9.0	30×32
Saline	0	9.5	36×42

[a]Fu and Ma (reported by Terry and Robert) are subclass IgA1 (Le); He is subclass IgA2.

minants in the IgE molecules were not destroyed. Both the antigen-binding activity of IgE antibodies and their affinity for tissues were diminished by the treatment[5] (Table 5).

TABLE 5   Effect of Heat and Reduction–Alkylation on IgE Antibodies

Structure	Effect of Heat (56 C, 4 hr)	Effect of Reduction–Alkylation
Antibody-combining sites	Intact	Diminished
Antigenic determinant	Destroyed	Intact
Affinity for target cells	Lost	Diminished

SITE OF FORMATION

Experiments were done by the fluorescent-antibody technique to measure the distribution of IgE-forming cells.[24] Frozen sections from human and monkey tissues were treated with one of the guinea pig antibodies specific for each immunoglobulin class and then stained with fluoresceinated antibody specific for guinea pig immunoglobulin. Among the various lymphoid tissues studied, tonsils and adenoid tissues obtained by surgical operation possessed the greatest numbers of plasma cells stained by anti-IgE. These cells were predominant around follicles under the epithelial capsules (Figure 6). Some germinal centers in these tissues were also stained by anti-IgE. In tonsils, IgE-staining plasma cells account for about 5–6% of all plasma cells stained by anti-L chain. Bronchial and peritoneal lymph nodes also contained IgE-forming plasma cells. Compared with these lymph nodes, IgE-forming cells were barely seen in spleen and subcutaneous lymph nodes. IgE plasma cells were found in nasal, bronchial, and tracheal mucosa, especially around the mixed glands. The gastrointestinal tract, stomach, small intestine, and rectum have been studied. In all the tissues, IgE-forming plasma cells were observed in the lamina propria, especially around the crypts of Lieberkühn. The IgE-forming plasma cells in the stomach, for example, were about 3–4% as plentiful as the IgA-forming cells, which represent more than 90% of total plasma cells. The distribution of plasma cells and germinal centers stained by anti-IgE is summarized in Table 6, which also contains the distribution of IgE-staining cells in monkey tissues. The distribution of IgE cells in the monkey tissues was very similar to that in humans.

It should be noted that tonsils of normal monkeys contained germinal centers stained by anti-IgE, although no sign of inflammation was de-

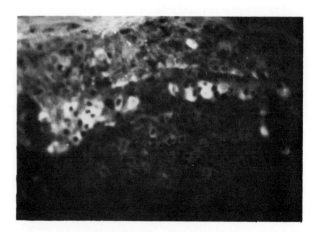

FIGURE 6   Fluorescent staining of IgE-forming plasma cells in human tonsil. Some plasma cells under epithelial capsule and around follicles were stained by anti-IgE.

TABLE 6   Distribution of IgE-Forming Cells in Lymphoid Tissues

Lymphoid Tissue	Human		Monkey	
	Plasma Cells	Germinal Center	Plasma Cells	Germinal Center
Tonsil	+ ∼ +++	+ ∼ ++	+	++
Adenoid	+ ∼ +++	+ ∼ ++		
Bronchus and peritoneum	++	+[a]	++	+[a]
Lymph node	± ∼ +	–	±	–
Spleen	± ∼ +	–	+ ∼ ++	±
Respiratory mucosa	+	–	+	–
Gastrointestinal mucosa	+ ∼ ++	–	+ ∼ ++	+[b]
Lung	–	–	–	–
Blood	–	–	nd	
Bone marrow	–	–	nd	

[a]Negative in some cases.
[b]+ in Peyer's patches.

tected in the tissues. In addition to the lymphoid tissues, peripheral leukocytes, bone marrow cells, and lung tissues from nonatopic persons have been studied. However, the lymphoid cells in the specimens were not stained by anti-IgE.

One exceptional case involved peripheral leukocytes from an atopic patient who had about 50 times as much serum IgE as normal. A few medium and small lymphocytes were stained by anti-IgE.

IgE-forming cells are present in respiratory and gastrointestinal mucosa and their regional lymph nodes. These findings strongly suggest that IgE antibodies may be formed locally in the respiratory and gastrointestinal tracts and participate in allergic diseases in these organs.

SUMMARY

Reaginic antibodies in sera of atopic persons are associated with IgE, which represents a distinct immunoglobulin class. This protein is a γ_1 glycoprotein with a sedimentation coefficient of 8.2S and a molecular weight of 200,000. The protein presumably is composed of two H and two L chains, and the IgE antigenic determinants are present in the Fc portion of the H chain.

The IgE antibody agglutinated erythrocytes coated with antigen, indicating that the antibodies are polyvalent. They do not initiate complement fixation. They are responsible for P-K reactions in humans and PCA reactions in monkeys, and they sensitize human leukocytes and monkey lung tissues. IgE combines with the tissue cells that are involved in reaginic hypersensitivity reactions through the Fc portion of the molecules.

IgE-forming cells localize in the respiratory and gastrointestinal tracts. Locally formed IgE may play an important role in allergic diseases.

REFERENCES

1. Bennich, H., K. Ishizaka, T. Ishizaka, and S. G. Johansson. A comparative antigenic study of γE-globulin and myeloma-IgND. J. Immun. 102:826–831, 1969.
2. Bennich, H., and S. G. Johansson. Studies on a new class of human immunoglobulins. II. Chemical and physical properties, pp. 199–205. In J. Killander, ed. Gamma Globulins. Structure and Control of Biosynthesis. Nobel Symposium 3. New York: John Wiley & Sons, Inc., 1967.
3. Franklin, E. C. The immune globulins: Their structure and function and some techniques for their isolation. Progr. Allerg. 8:58–148, 1964.
4. Ishizaka, K., and T. Ishizaka. Identification of gamma-E-antibodies as a carrier of reaginic activity. J. Immun. 99:1187–1198, 1967.
5. Ishizaka, K., and T. Ishizaka. Physicochemical properties of human reaginic antibodies. 8. Effect of reduction and alkylation on gamma E antibodies. J. Immun. 102:69–76, 1969.
6. Ishizaka, K., and T. Ishizaka. Physicochemical properties of reaginic antibody. 1. Association of reaginic activity with an immunoglobulin other than gammaA- or gammaG-globulin. J. Allerg. 37:169–185, 1966.
7. Ishizaka, K., T. Ishizaka, and M. M. Hornbrook. Allergen-binding activity of gamma-E, gamma-G and gamma-A antibodies in sera from atopic patients. In vitro measurements of reaginic antibody. J. Immun. 98:490–501, 1967.
8. Ishizaka, K., T. Ishizaka, and M. M. Hornbrook. Physico-chemical properties of human reaginic antibody. IV. Presence of a unique immunoglobulin as a carrier of reaginic activity. J. Immun. 97:75–85, 1966.
9. Ishizaka, K., T. Ishizaka, and M. M. Hornbrook. Physicochemical properties of reaginic antibody. V. Correlation of reaginic activity with gamma-E-globulin antibody. J. Immun. 97:840–853, 1966.
10. Ishizaka, K., T. Ishizaka, and E. H. Lee. Physiochemical properties of reaginic antibody. II. Characteristic properties of reaginic antibody different from human gamma-A-isohemagglutinin and gamma-D-globulin. J. Allerg. 37:336–349, 1966.
11. Ishizaka, K., T. Ishizaka, E. H. Lee, and H. Fudenberg. Immunochemical properties of human γA isohemagglutinin. I. Comparisons with γG- and γM-globulin antibodies. J. Immun. 95:197–208, 1965.
12. Ishizaka, K., T. Ishizaka, and A. E. Menzel. Physicochemical properties of reaginic antibody. VI. Effect of heat on gamma-E-, gamma-G- and gamma-A-antibodies in the sera of ragweed sensitive patients. J. Immun. 99:610–618, 1967.

13. Ishizaka, K., T. Ishizaka, and W. D. Terry. Antigenic structure of gamma-E-globulin and reaginic antibody. J. Immun. 99:849–858, 1967.
14. Ishizaka, T., K. Ishizaka, H. Bennich, and S. G. Johansson. Biologic activities of aggregated immunoglobulin E. J. Immun. (in press)
15. Ishizaka, T., K. Ishizaka, and T. Borsos. Biological activity of aggregated γ-globulin. IV. Mechanism of complement fixation. J. Immun. 87:433–438, 1961.
16. Ishizaka, T., K. Ishizaka, S. G. Johansson, and H. Bennich. Histamine release from human leukocytes by anti-gamma E antibodies. J. Immun. 102:884–892, 1969.
17. Ishizaka, T., K. Ishizaka, R. P. Orange, and K. F. Austen. The capacity of human immuno-globulin E to mediate the release of histamine and slow reacting substance of anaphylaxis (srs-A) from monkey lung. J. Immun. 104:335, 1970.
18. Ishizaka, T., K. Ishizaka, S. Salmon, and H. Fudenberg. Biologic activities of aggregated gamma-globulin. 8. Aggregated immunoglobulins of different classes. J. Immun. 99:82–91, 1967.
19. Johansson, S. G., and H. Bennich. Immunological studies of an atypical (myeloma) im-munoglobulin. Immunology 13:381–394, 1967.
20. Johansson, S. G., H. Bennich, and L. Wide. A new class of immunoglobulin in human serum. Immunology 14:265–272, 1968.
21. Ogawa, M., S. Kochwa, C. Smith, K. Ishizaka, and O. R. McIntyre. Clinical aspects of IgE myeloma. New Eng. J. Med. 281:1217, 1969.
22. Stanworth, D. R., J. H. Humphrey, H. Bennich, and S. G. Johansson. Inhibition of Prausnitz-Küstner reaction by proteolytic-cleavage fragments of a human myeloma protein of immunoglobulin class E. Lancet 2:17–18, 1968.
23. Stanworth, D. R., J. H. Humphrey, H. Bennich, and S. G. Johansson. Specific inhibition of the Prausnitz-Küstner reaction by an atypical human myeloma protein. Lancet 2:330–332, 1967.
24. Tada, T., and K. Ishizaka. Distribution of gamma-E forming cells in the human and monkey lymphoid tissues. J. Immun. 104:377, 1970.

DISCUSSION

DR. MILLS: Have you looked at the concentration of IgE in secretions, compared with the concentration of IgA?

DR. ISHIZAKA: We could not detect IgE in secretions, but we did not use micro-measurements, which may be necessary for its detection. With fluorescent anti-bodies, some of the mucus was specifically stained. I think some IgE is found in secretions, but I do not know its concentration.

DR. SOOTHILL: Recently, however, IgE was detected in the nasal washings and sputum of some asthmatic patients. Its concentration is lower than that of IgA and lower than that of the patient's serum IgE.

DR. ROWE: We have taken some steps at the International Reference Center for Immunoglobulins to make reagents available for IgE. We have obtained by cour-tesy of Drs. Johansson and Bennich some sheep antiserum to the Fc fragments of

ND IgE myeloma protein. This has been observed to be specific for IgE, by gel-diffusion analysis. That reagent is available for general use.

We have also observed that there are increases in IgE in African sera, which should become a useful source of IgE. In collaboration with Dr. Anderson of the Division of Biological Standards of the National Institute for Medical Research (Mill Hill, London) and others, we have lyophilized a fairly large pool of African serum. At the moment, we have 1-ml aliquots of antiserum specific to IgE and of African serum with high IgE content; these are available for limited distribution. The supply will not last long. This is not an incentive for everyone to write for them, but to obtain this material only if it is of value. I am sure that more materials will become available shortly, with more myeloma proteins becoming generally available. The serum pool is sufficient to give a precipitin line on diffusion analysis, so we feel that with the specific antiserum and a source of IgE at this increased concentration, there should not be much difficulty in identifying IgE on gel diffusion.

DR. WHITE: You said that IgE is involved in histamine release when it combines with anti-IgE, as well as when it combines with an antigen. Is that true of the Fc fragment? Will this induce histamine release when it is combined with anti-Fc, or must the IgE molecule be intact?

DR. ISHIZAKA: Fc fragments will sensitize monkey lungs for the release of both histamine and SRS-A—i.e., lung fragments sensitized with Fc derived from IgE released both mediators when they were exposed to anti-IgE.

DR. WHITE: Is the Fc fragment immunogenic?

DR. ISHIZAKA: Yes.

HENRY G. KUNKEL *and* WILLIAM J. YOUNT

Heavy-Chain Subgroups of γG and γA Globulins

Primarily through the use of myeloma proteins, a variety of different subgroups of γG and γA globulins have been delineated. These have been differentiated primarily on the basis of antigenic differences and fill the following two important criteria:

1. The antigenic specificities are localized to the Fc area of the molecule.
2. They are found in all normal individuals of different population groups.

The first criterion serves to distinguish subgroup antigens from those in the variable area of the molecules which can entirely mimic subgroup antigens particularly if only one antiserum is available. The second criterion rules out possible genetic antigens. Multiple antisera giving the same specificity are highly advantageous. In addition, it is also extremely helpful to recognize the negative proteins in a positive fashion with an antiserum giving the opposite distribution. Finally, it is extremely helpful to exchange samples with other workers in the field to avoid the mistakes of the past. It was extremely helpful in our work to exchange samples relating to the γG subgroups with Drs. Terry and Fahey and in the case of the γA proteins with Dr. Heremans. Despite at least four publications on subgroups of γM proteins, the above criteria have not been fulfilled and the problem with respect to γM subgroups remains unresolved.

Classification into subgroups as distinct from classes is a somewhat artificial way of differentiation. Both depend on differences primarily in the Fc area of the heavy chains; the differences are simply less marked among the subgroups than between classes. Thus, the subgroups cross-react in the Fc portion while the classes do not. However, recent chemical analysis has indicated that, despite this lack of cross-reaction between classes such as γG and γM, many homologies in sequence are evident. Table 1 illustrates the 10 different types of heavy chains that have been clearly demonstrated from work in different laboratories[2,5,8,14,15] which are found in all normal individuals. The major types of genetic variants of these heavy chains that are now recognized in different populations are also shown. For example, at least five types of γG3 chains are known and the Gm (g) type differs considerably from the various Gm (g) types.[9,10] It is important to appreciate the fact that genetic mutations

TABLE 1   Different Types[a] of Heavy Chains Found in All Normal Individuals and the Major Genetic Variants

1. γG1	Gm az, Gm azx Gm f Gm af
2. γG2	Gm n Gm n–
3. γG3	Gm g Gm b^0 b^1 b^3 b^4 b^5, Gm b^0 b^1 c^3 c^5 Gm b^0 s b^3 b^5 , Gm b^0 st b^3 b^5
4. γG4	
5. γA1	
6. γA2	
7. γM	
8. γD	
9. γE	

[a]Based on differences in the Fc fragment.

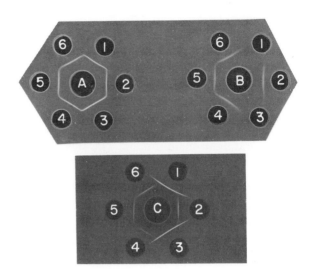

FIGURE 1   Agar-plate analyses showing the reaction of three different antisera with the subgroups of γA proteins. Central well A contains a γA1 antiserum that fails to distinguish subgroups. Central well B contains a γA2 antiserum absorbed with γA1 proteins. It reacts only with γA2 proteins. Central well C contains a γA1 unabsorbed antiserum that shows the γA2 proteins deficient. Outer wells 1 and 3 contain γA1 proteins; wells 2, 4, 5, and 6 contain different γA2 proteins.

are always limited to one type of heavy chain irrespective of subgroups or class. This indicates that all the types of heavy chains shown in Table 1 are the products of independent although closely linked genetic loci. Thus far, genetic markers are only available for three of the four subclasses of γG.

SUBGROUPS OF γA GLOBULINS

Recent interest in the subgroups of the immunoglobulins has centered primarily on the γA globulins. Two types were delineated several years ago,[2,8,15] γA1 and γA2 by means of specific antisera to the major γA1 type. The γA2 was recognized as antigenically deficient. Numerous attempts to gain antisera specific for the minor γA2 type were unsuccessful. However, recently specific γA2 antisera have become available in nonhuman primates. Figure 1 illustrates the results with such antisera. The new antisera are particularly important in order to quantitate the levels of γA2 in different biologic fluids with special reference to the external secretions where the γA proteins assume major significance. Quantitative analysis indicates that the γA2 is present at a level of approximately 15% of the total γA in serum but has a considerably higher relative level in certain external secretions.[3] In these studies, evidence was obtained that the γA2 class could be further subdivided into two genetic types.

The most interesting feature of the γA2 subgroup is that it lacks disulfide bonds linking the heavy and light chains.[3] These are present in the γA1 and all the other human immunoglobulins. In addition, the light chains are disulfide bonded as dimers in these molecules. Starch gel or polyacrylamide electrophoresis without reduction yields heavy chains and light-chain dimers. The significance of these unique features remains unclear. However, the γA in the mouse appears to be entirely of the γA2 type[1] and it is possible that this is a more primitive type in the phylogenetic scale.

DETERMINATION OF THE γG AND γA SUBGROUPS

The initial studies on delineation of the subgroups were carried out with specific antisera by agar-plate precipitin analysis. In the case of the γG subgroups, only γG3 readily yielded strong precipitating antisera in rabbits. The others occasionally gave weak antisera on immunization with heavy chains but it was clear that primate antisera were much better for all but the γG3 type. Evidence has been obtained recently[12] that better rabbit antisera can be obtained by making adult animals tolerant before immunization by injection of aggregate-free preparations of the subgroups other than the one desired. Another approach to the problem has been through the use of nonprecipitating systems. It has been observed that many antisera after absorption with heterologous subgroups fail to give precipitin reactions but still agglutinate cells coated with the specific type under study. Inhibition of such a system can be shown to be highly specific and also semiquantitative. Table 2 illustrates the results for the determination of γG1 Fc antigens. Protein Cr, a heavy-chain disease protein, which proved difficult to type by precipitin analyses in several laboratories, is clearly a γG1 protein from the inhibition results. Table 3 shows various antigens that have been determined by the inhibition system. Proteins coupled to red cells by bis-diazotized benzidine (BDB) can be used in all instances. However, anti-Rh are employed as coats whenever possible because of their clearer agglutination. The antigens "non a" and "non g" are of special interest because of their relationship to the genetic antigens.[11] "Non a" is present in all γG2 and γG3 proteins but

TABLE 2　γG1 Fc System: Inhibition of Agglutination by Isolated Proteins or Sera[a]

	mg/cc of Protein or Serum Dilution Added			
	0.5	0.12	0.03	0.008
M[b] - γG1 (El)	0	0	0	tr
M - γG1 (Dr)	0	0	0	1
γG1 (Cr)	0	0	0	±
M - γG2	2	3	3	3
M - γG3	1	3	3	3
M - γG1 - Fc	0	0	0	0
M - γG1 - Fab	2	3	3	3
	$\frac{1}{10}$	$\frac{1}{40}$	$\frac{1}{160}$	$\frac{1}{640}$
Serum Ko	0	0	0	tr
Serum Jo	0	0	0	1
Serum Fe	0	1	3	3

[a]Coat: anti-Rh 3083; antiserum: rabbit anti-γG1 heavy chains absorbed with γG2 + pepsin Fr II.
[b]M = myeloma protein.

only in the Gm (a–) γG1 proteins. It never occurs in the γG4 type. "Non g" is found in all γG2 proteins and in the Gm (g–) proteins of the γG3 class. It is totally absent in γG1 and γG4. These various markers have proved of special value in delineating unusual types of γ globulins. For example, a "Lepore type" of hybrid γ globulin has been described recently which represents a combination of γG3 and γG1 in the same molecule.[7] Also, some gene defects have been detected in parents of agammaglobulinemic children through the use of these antigenic markers as well as the classical genetic type.

SPECIAL BIOLOGIC PROPERTIES

One of the most striking characteristics of the γ globulin subgroups is their difference in enzymatic splitting. For example, under the classical Porter conditions the γG3 type is split into Fab and Fc fragments in 30 min and is broken down much further in 24 hr. However, the γG2 type is very resistant to papain digestion and remains as an intact 7S

TABLE 3 Various Antigens Detected by Hemagglutination Inhibition Systems

	γG1 Fc	γG1 Fab κ	γG1, γG3, γG4 Fc	γG3 Fc	γG3 Fab	γG2 Fc	γG2, γG3 Fc
Coat							
Antiserum	anti-Rh Rabbit γG1 H	anti-Rh Monkey γG1	anti-Rh Rabbit γG1 Monkey γG4	anti-Rh Rabbit γG3	anti-Rh pepsin Rabbit γG3	BDB Monkey γG2	BDB Monkey γG2
	γG2 Fab κ	Non a (γG1 Gma$^-$, γG2, γG3)			Non g (γG3 Gmg$^-$, γG2)		γG4 Fc
Coat	BDB	anti-Rh BDB			anti-Rh	BDB	
Antiserum	Monkey γG2	Rabbit γG1, Rabbit γG2			Monkey γG2		Monkey γG4

142

molecule after 24 hr. The other subgroups fall in between these two in this property.

The γG4 type clearly has a faster mobility than the others and perhaps corresponds to some of the γ_1 proteins of other species. On papain splitting, it has a fast Fc fragment which is clearly different from the Fc fragments of all other γ globulins. It also differs to the greatest degree from the other subgroups in both antigenic and structural features. The most striking biologic feature is its failure to fix complement in contradistinction to the other subgroups.[6, 13]

The γG2 subgroup is notable in its failure to give a passive cutaneous anaphylaxis reaction in guinea pigs.[13] It also contains selectively a number of special human antibodies. Most of the antidextrans and antilevans are almost entirely γG2. A possible relationship to carbohydrate antigens appears to exist.

The γG3 proteins have been of special interest because of their general tendency to aggregate. This is most evident in their partial localization near the point of application in agar electrophoresis. It is evident in the normal γG3 proteins as well as in the myeloma proteins. Some also behave as cryoglobulins but here some evidence suggests that they represent γG3–anti-γG3 complexes.[4] Rheumatoid factors in general, however, react poorly with γG3 proteins and many fail to react at all in striking contrast to the other subgroups which all appeared to react similarly and completely.

REFERENCES

1. Abel, C. A., and H. M. Grey. Studies on the structure of mouse gamma-A myeloma proteins. Biochemistry 7:2682–2688, 1968.
2. Feinstein, D., and E. C. Franklin. Two antigenically distinguishable subclasses of human A myeloma proteins differing in their heavy chains. Nature 212:1496–1498, 1966.
3. Grey, H. M., C. A. Abel, W. J. Yount, and H. G. Kunkel. A subclass of human γA-globulins (γA2) which lacks the disulfide bonds linking heavy and light chains. J. Exp. Med. 128: 1223–1236, 1968.
4. Grey, H. M., P. F. Kohler, W. D. Terry, and E. C. Franklin. Human monoclonal γG-globulins with anti-γ-globulin activity. J. Clin. Invest. 47:1875–1884, 1968.
5. Grey, H. M., and H. G. Kunkel. H chain subgroups of myeloma proteins and normal 7S γ-globulin. J. Exp. Med. 120:253–266, 1964.
6. Ishizaka, T., K. Ishizaka, S. Salmon, and H. Fudenberg. Biologic activities of aggregated gamma-globulin. 8. Aggregated immunoglobulins of different classes. J. Immun. 99:82–91, 1967.

7. Kunkel, H. G., J. B. Natvig, and F. G. Joslin. A "Lepore" type of hybrid γ globulin. Proc. Nat. Acad. Sci. USA 62:144–149, 1969.
8. Kunkel, H. G., and R. A. Prendergast. Subgroups of gamma-A immune globulins. Proc. Soc. Exp. Biol. Med. 122:910–913, 1966.
9. Loghem, E. van, and L. Martensson. Genetic (Gm) determinants of the γ_{2c} (Vi) subclass of human IgG immunoglobulins. Vox Sang. (in press)
10. Natvig, J. B., and H. G. Kunkel. Genetic markers of human immunoglobulins. The Gm and Inv systems. Series Haematol. 1:66–96, 1968.
11. Natvig, J. B., H. G. Kunkel, and F. G. Joslin. Delineation of two antigenic markers, "non a" and "non g" related to the genetic antigens of human γ globulin. J. Immun. 102:611–617, 1969.
12. Spiegelberg, H. L., and W. O. Weigle. The production of antisera to human γG subclasses in rabbits using immunological unresponsiveness. J. Immun. 101:377–380, 1968.
13. Terry, W. D. Skin-sensitizing activity related to γ-polypeptide chain characteristics of human IgG. J. Immun. 95:1041–1047, 1965.
14. Terry, W. D., and J. L. Fahey. Subclasses of human gamma-2-globulin based on differences in the heavy polypeptide chains. Science 146:400–401, 1964.
15. Vaerman, J.-P., and J. F. Heremans. Subclasses of human immunoglobulin A based on differences in the alpha polypeptide chains. Science 153:647–649, 1966.

DISCUSSION

DR. BALLIEUX: What is the relationship between IgA2' and IgA2? Are these antigenic differences?

DR. KUNKEL: Yes, there is a clear antigenic difference. But both showed the lack of disulfide bonds, so they are related to each other.

DR. BALLIEUX: Do you have the ratio of the two IgA subclasses?

DR. KUNKEL: Quantitative analyses indicate that IgA2 is between 5% and 15% of the total. This figure is slightly higher than that obtained from the incidence of myeloma proteins of the IgA2 type.

DR. BALLIEUX: Is IgA2' antigenically deficient with your antiserum?

DR. KUNKEL: No; it was positively recognized.

DR. FAHEY: Do agammaglobulinemics and hypogammaglobulinemics have an equal deficiency?

DR. KUNKEL: I think, as you might anticipate in view of the discrepancies between IgG, IgA, and IgM concentrations, there would also be a discrepancy in terms of the subclasses. In particular, we have found that IgG3 in many instances stays very close to normal, whereas the others go down. The reason for this relative insensitivity to depression of the IgG3 in some cases of acquired agammaglobulinemia is not clear.

DR. FAHEY: Have you tested commercial gamma globulin preparations for their content of the subclasses?

DR. KUNKEL: We have. They are pretty close to normal serum IgG's, with the exception of IgG4. IgG4 is the most acidic and in many instances is quite low in gamma globulin preparations. But the other three seem to be, at least in our hands, fairly close to the expected in the normal serum. I do not know whether that has been the experience of Dr. Terry's group.

DR. TERRY: IgG3 tends to be low sometimes, as well as IgG4.

DR. FAHEY: Dr. Kabat, you had some data on the restriction of carbohydrate antibodies in the IgG2 subclass. Was that accidental because of the subject, or is it universal?

DR. KABAT: The response of a group of persons to dextran and levan tends to be the formation of IgG2 H chains (γ_2 chains) primarily. Some respond exclusively by formation of IgG2 molecules. We have had subjects who have made some IgG1 and IgG3 antibodies to dextran. Why this selection occurs is anyone's guess. It could be that these cells respond in a given order to various levels of stimulation. We always do polysaccharide immunizations under very restricted conditions; that is, we inject 1 mg of dextran—0.5 mg/day on 2 successive days. The antibody level goes up and remains high for many years. So far as we can tell, there are no particular changes in the distribution. It seems that, once there is a given response, the same kinds of antibody molecules remain for quite a while.

DR. KUNKEL: I think this has something to do with the carbohydrate nature of the antigen. Most of the protein antigens that we have studied have been primarily IgG1. It is also of some interest that Dr. Kabat knew many years ago that his dextran antibodies did not give a passive cutaneous anaphylaxis (PCA) reaction, and he always thought that was a very strange phenomenon. Now it is easily explainable by the fact that it is fairly pure IgG2, which does not give a PCA reaction.

WILLIAM D. TERRY

Antibody Activity of Myeloma Proteins

The intensive studies of serum immunoglobulins carried out over the last few decades have been motivated primarily by a desire to understand the nature of antibody activity demonstrated by some of these proteins. Normal immunoglobulins are heterogeneous. The immunoglobulins of man consist of five major classes of proteins, three of which can be further divided into subclasses. Proteins of most of these classes and subclasses contain L chains of two different types (κ and λ), and the H chains of each subclass and L chains of each type occur in many alternative forms. Molecules carrying antibody activity that are generated in an immune response are also heterogeneous. Animals immunized with even simple immunogens develop antibody activity expressed in proteins of many of the classes, subclasses, and L-chain types.

Such heterogeneity frustrates studies that attempt to define the structure of antibody molecules and the nature of antibody–antigen interactions. This problem is circumvented by studying myeloma proteins, which are homogeneous and provide suitable material for structural studies. Until recently, this approach was not considered useful for studying antibody–antigen interactions, because myeloma proteins were considered to lack antibody activity. This assumption was accepted de-

146

spite numerous observations, during the last decade, of antibody-like activity in myeloma proteins. The apparent presence of cold agglutinins,[7,11,15] rheumatoid factors,[4,12,13] antistreptolysins,[14,21,24] anti-"aged" erythrocytes,[18] antiheparin,[17] and antilipoproteins[2] in the macroglobulin fraction isolated from the sera of some patients with Waldenström's macroglobulinemia was not pursued vigorously, perhaps because of the ill-defined nature of the putative antigens. In the last few years, however, several instances of interactions between human and murine myeloma proteins and well-defined ligands have been described. Careful study has shown that these interactions are similar to or identical with those between antigen and antibody when the antibody was induced by the same ligand in experimental animals. The criteria for accepting binding of ligands to myeloma proteins as a reflection of antibody activity include demonstration that (1) binding is restricted to the Fab fragment; (2) the number of binding sites is that expected for the particular immunoglobulin; (3) the binding shows specificity; and (4) binding energies are in the expected range.

Research in this area was given great impetus by a report that a survey of a relatively small number of human myeloma sera had led to the discovery of one IgG myeloma protein that specifically bound dinitrophenyl (DNP) haptene.[5] Extension of this work revealed that seven of 116 murine myeloma proteins had significant binding activity for DNP haptene and one of the seven had an association constant (K_A) of 10^7 liters/mole, a value equal to the mean association constant of conventionally induced rabbit antibodies to DNP.[6] The simultaneous report of a human macroglobulin that behaved in all respects like an antibody to the Fc fragment of IgG[16,22] lent further support to the idea that at least some of the homogeneous immunoglobulins produced by patients with multiple myeloma and macroglobulinemia are antibodies.

A search for additional ligands that would interact with myeloma proteins was carried out in several laboratories. In general, the approach was to test human or murine myeloma sera or proteins with a number of ligands by double diffusion in agar. Results of such a survey of human myeloma sera carried out in our laboratory are seen in Table 1. Positive reactions with DNP bound to bovine serum albumin (DNP-BSA) were found in 9% of IgG myeloma (GMP) sera, 25% of IgM Waldenström's sera (WM), and 15% of IgA myeloma (AMP) sera. Occasional reactions were seen with other test antigens. The immunoelec-

TABLE 1 Ouchterlony Analysis of Sera Containing Myeloma Proteins[a]

Source of Serum	No. Sera Tested			Haptene–BSA Conjugates						
	Total	Group 1	Group 2	DNP	TNP	Both	Pipsyl	Tosyl	Ars	Polysaccharides
GMP	133	72		6	2	12	1	0	1	3
			61	6	NT	–	0	0	0	NT
WM	24	17		2	0	7	0	1	1	0
			7	4	NT	–	0	0	0	NT
AMP	39	20		4	1	1	0	0	0	0
			19	2	NT	–	0	0	0	NT
DNP	5			0	0	0	0	0	0	0
BJ	18			0	0	1	1	0	1	0
Normal donors	100	–		12	NT	–	NT	NT	0	5

[a] Sera containing myeloma proteins, Waldenström's macroglobulin, or Bence Jones proteins were tested with the five haptene–BSA conjugates and with a mixture of polysaccharides by double diffusion in agar at pH 8.5 in 0.05M barbital buffer. Unstained plates were examined after 4 and 20 hr. DNP = 2,4-dinitrophenyl BSA; TNP = 2,4,6-trinitrophenyl BSA; pipsyl = p-iodobenzylsulfonyl BSA; tosyl = p-toluenesulfonyl BSA; ars = arsanyl BSA.

trophoretic patterns produced by several of the DNP-positive sera and some controls are shown in Figure 1. IgG myeloma protein from sera Ta and Va precipitated with DNP-BSA. A weaker reaction is seen between DNP-BSA and the IgM myeloma protein of Fr. The IgG myeloma protein in serum Be and that in serum Al do not precipitate with DNP-BSA.

Serum Va was selected for further study. The myeloma protein was

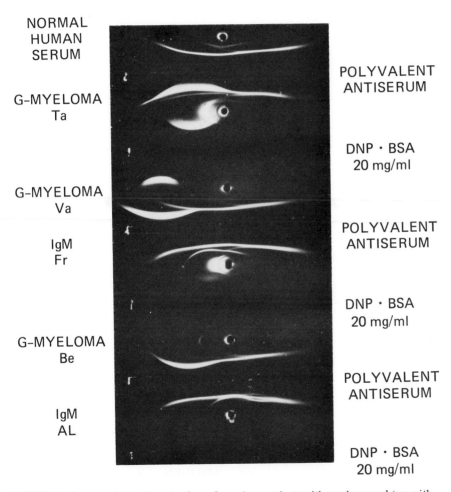

FIGURE 1 Immunoelectrophoresis of sera from three patients with myeloma and two with Waldenström's macroglobulinemia. Patterns were developed with antiserum to IgG, IgA, IgM, κ, and λ (polyvalent antiserum) or with DNP-BSA (20 mg/ml). Anode is to the right.

isolated, and it precipitated with DNP-BSA. The isolated Va protein was labeled with ^{125}I, and precipitin analyses were performed with DNP-BSA. The degree of precipitation was estimated by measurement of radioactivity in the precipitate. A precipitin curve was obtained with DNP-BSA and several other haptene protein conjugates; the controls of BSA alone were negative (Figure 2). Attempts were made to inhibit

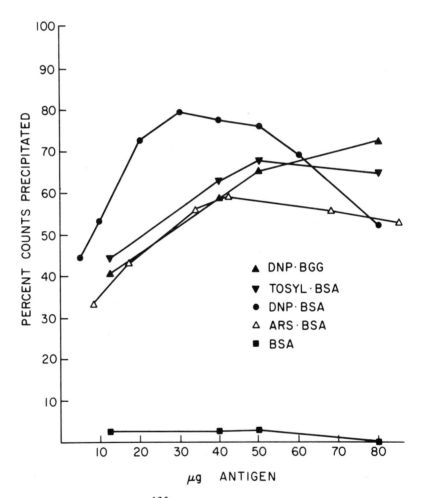

FIGURE 2   Precipitin analysis of ^{125}I-labeled GMP Va. A constant amount of Va protein (0.13 mg) was mixed with increasing quantities of antigen in 0.01 M PO_4 buffer, with a pH of 7, in a total volume of 0.2 ml. Reactants were incubated at 37 C for 30 min and 4 C for 60 min and centrifuged at 4 C for 45 min. Supernatant fluid was analyzed for radioactivity.

TABLE 2   Precipitation of ^{125}I-Labeled Va MP by DNP-BSA Inhibited by Va Fab Fragment[a]

Va MP, mg/200 λ	Inhibitor, mg/200 λ	% Inhibition
0.13	–	–
0.13	Fc 0.93	0
0.13	Fab 0.31	23.8
0.13	Fab 0.52	48.6
0.13	Fab 0.63	65.7
0.13	Fab 0.75	100

[a]DNP-BSA (20 μg) was incubated with the inhibitor for 30 min at 37 C. Va protein was added and additional incubations, centrifugations, and analyses were carried out, as indicated in Figure 2.

the precipitation of labeled Va by DNP-BSA with the Fc and Fab fragments of unlabeled Va protein. Fab inhibited precipitation, whereas Fc did not (Table 2), indicating that the reaction between Va and DNP-BSA was via the Fab portion of the molecule. Va protein therefore meets two of the criteria for antibody: it shows specificity (no precipitation with BSA) and the reactivity is via the Fab fragment. Attempts to establish the number of combining sites and the binding energies by equilibrium dialysis of Va with DNP epsilon-aminocaproic acid (EACA) showed, however, that the K_A for this interaction was less than 10^2 liters/mole. In other words, binding was very weak, so that one cannot consider this a true antibody–antigen interaction. Further studies showed that the precipitation reactions between the IgG Va protein and DNP protein conjugates depend on ionic strength. As the NaCl concentration approached 0.14M, a precipitin curve could no longer be demonstrated.

Many other examples of myeloma proteins that precipitate well at low ionic strength with DNP protein conjugates but that do not have appreciable binding of DNP haptenes under physiologic conditions have been encountered. The opposite problem has also been encountered: a human Waldenström's macroglobulin has been shown to have a K_A of 4×10^4 liters/mole for DNP EACA but does not precipitate in agar double diffusion with DNP protein conjugates.[1] This illustrates the need for careful interpretation of precipitation reactions and for the use of direct binding assays, as opposed to those that depend on secondary effects, such as precipitation, in screening for antibody activity among myeloma proteins.

The range of materials that have been examined for reactivity with myeloma proteins is somewhat limited, and this reflects the nature of the screening process. DNP and some other haptenes are easily detected. They have therefore been extensively investigated, and binding assays indicate that about 5% of mouse myeloma proteins show significant binding of DNP.[6] Reactions have also been found, by agar gel diffusion and other techniques, with these additional reactants: polysaccharides and lipopolysaccharides, IgG, DNA, purines, pyrimidines, pyridines, and cardiolipin.[3,8,10,19,20] All these will require verification by binding or other studies to ensure that they are truly antibody–antigen reactions.

Some observations of interactions between human myeloma proteins and "antigens" reflect the fact that patients with myeloma are treated by physicians who notice unusual clinical laboratory results or unexpected disease processes. Clinicians have the opportunity to establish causal relationships between the presence of myeloma proteins and some unusual sign or symptom. For example, patients with macroglobulinemia do not always have a hemolytic process. Some do, and this has been shown to be due to cold agglutinin activity in the abnormal macroglobulin.[7,11,15] This homogeneous protein has all the characteristics of antibody with specificity for erythrocyte antigen I. In this case, antibody activity was looked for on the basis of clinical observations. Another example concerns the simultaneous presence in a patient of multiple myeloma and a disorder of lipid metabolism leading to tissue deposition of lipid. It has been shown that the myeloma protein of a patient combined with heparin or heparin-like substances.[9] Heparin is apparently required for the activation of lipoprotein lipase, and the failure of this activation leads to abnormal metabolism of lipid with tissue accumulation. Whether this binding of heparin by the myeloma protein represents an antigen–antibody interaction remains to be proved, but it illustrates the general point that alert clinicians have an opportunity to detect biologically significant interactions between myeloma proteins and ligands.

At present, the significance of the binding activity of human and murine myeloma proteins is obscure. Some points, however, are clear. Considering the limited spectrum of antigens tested, a remarkably high percentage of proteins have shown activity. Interactions with IgG, erythrocytes, streptolysin, lipoproteins, pneumococcal C polysaccharide, nitrophenyl derivatives, purines, and pyrimidines have been found repeatedly in one or both species.

There are as yet no explanations either for the unexpected frequency with which a single reactivity has been encountered (5–10% reactivity with DNP haptenes) or for the large number of proteins that have demonstrable activity with this limited panel of antigens. It is generally assumed that malignant plasma cells represent a random selection of the population of lymphoid cells that have differentiated for immunoglobulin production. If myeloma cells have been committed to produce antibody of a given specificity before they become neoplastic, the frequency of antibody specificities of myeloma proteins should reflect the occurrence in the host of lymphoid cells committed to that specificity. From logical considerations, it seems highly unlikely that a significant number of human or murine lymphoid cells are committed to the production of antibody to DNP haptenes. Alternative explanations must be sought.

One possibility is that the specificity of myeloma proteins depends on some aspect of the pathogenesis of plasma-cell tumors. Tumor induction may be associated with the destruction of cells present at the site of induction, the generation of a local immune response to these cells and their products, and the subsequent neoplastic transformation of a lymphoid cell committed to the synthesis of antibody to cell antigens or products.[20] This suggests that myeloma proteins should frequently have specificity for "host" antigens and materials that cross-react with host antigens, and this hypothesis is consistent with the observation of many proteins that interact with IgG and nucleic acid derivatives. The reactions with DNP could be ascribed to cross-reactivity between DNP and nucleic acid derivatives and might therefore reflect the antigenic relationships between the true inducing antigen and the fortuitously chosen test antigen. If that is correct, it follows that a single antibody molecule may have significant binding activity for a number of "antigens." This would be of theoretical importance, in that it would markedly decrease the number of variable amino acid sequences that must be generated to account for antibody activity against all possible antigens. Studies of the range of specific activities shown by a single myeloma antibody should provide information on this point.

Another possibility for the nonrandom distribution of myeloma protein specificities implies that the site of plasma-cell tumor induction is important. It is postulated that lymphoid cells that have previously differentiated for the production of antibody to specific antigens migrate into the adjacent area, where neoplastic induction is taking place, and that one of the cells becomes neoplastic there. It would then synthesize and secrete a myeloma protein with specificity directed against the original antigen. The antibody activity of a myeloma protein would be dictated by the kind of antigens present in areas near the point of tumor induction. If, for example, the myeloma tumor is being induced in the peritoneal cavity of a mouse, then intestinal wall lymphoid cells, previously sensitized to intestinal bacteria, might migrate into the peritoneal cavity, become neoplastic, and secrete myeloma protein with specificity for an intestinal bacterium.

Insufficient information is available to permit critical evaluation of the speculations presented here or to determine whether all myeloma proteins have antibody-like activity. It is clear, however, that several myeloma proteins that have been extensively investigated are found to bind ligands in a manner indistinguishable from conventionally induced antibodies. These homogeneous proteins with defined binding activity open new possibilities for the investigation of structure–function relationships in immunoglobulin molecules. When coupled with recent advances in the crystallization and x-ray diffraction studies of myeloma proteins,[23] the availability of myeloma proteins with binding activity for well-defined antigens should make possible the construction of a three-dimensional model of an antibody-combining site.

REFERENCES

1. Ashman, R. F., and H. Metzger. A Waldenström macroglobulin which binds nitrophenyl ligands. J. Biol. Chem. 244:3405–3414, 1969.
2. Beaumont, J. L., B. Jocotot, C. Vilain, and V. Beaumont. Présence d'un auto-anticorps anti-beta-lipoprotéine dans un sérum de myélome. C.R. Acad. Sci. 260:5960–5962, 1965.
3. Cohn, M. Natural history of the myeloma. Cold Spring Harbor Symp. Quant. Biol. 32:211–221, 1967.
4. Curtain, C. C., A. Baumgarten, and J. Pye. Coprecipitation of some cryomacroglobulins with immunoglobulins and their fragments. Arch. Biochem. 112:37–44, 1965.
5. Eisen, H. N., J. R. Little, C. K. Osterland, and E. S. Simms. A myeloma protein with antibody activity. Cold Spring Harbor Symp. Quant. Biol. 32:75–81, 1967.

6. Eisen, H. N., E. S. Simms, and M. Potter. Mouse myeloma proteins with antihapten antibody activity. The protein produced by plasma cell tumor MOPC-315. Biochemistry 7:4126-4134, 1968.

7. Fudenberg, H. H., and H. G. Kunkel. Physical properties of the red cell agglutinins in acquired hemolytic anemia. J. Exp. Med. 106:689-702, 1957.

8. Gisler, R., and J. Pillot. Activité anticardiolipide LIEE à un complexe macroglobuline de Waldenström–IgG cryoprecipitant. Immunochemistry 5:543-555, 1968.

9. Glueck, C. J., R. I. Levy, H. Greten, A. P. Kaplan, H. I. Glueck, H. Gralnick, and D. S. Fredrickson. Exogenous fat intolerance, low post heparin lipolytic activity, and heparin binding globulins. Clin. Res. 16:550, 1968. (abstract)

10. Grey, H. M., P. F. Kohler, W. D. Terry, and E. C. Franklin. Human monoclonal γG-globulins with anti-γ-globulin activity. J. Clin. Invest. 47:1875-1884, 1968.

11. Harboe, M. Proceedings of the Tenth International Congress, International Society of Haematology, p. 65. Stockholm: Munksgaard, 1965.

12. Heimer, R., and C. J. Nosenzo. Pseudoglobulin rheumatoid factors. J. Immun. 94:502-509, 1965.

13. Kritzman, J., H. G. Kunkel, J. McCarthy, and R. C. Mellors. Studies of a Waldenstrom-type macroglobulin with rheumatoid factor properties. J. Lab. Clin. Med. 57:905-917, 1961.

14. Kronvall, G. Ligand-binding sites for streptolysin O and staphylococcal protein A on different parts of the same myeloma globulin. Acta Path. Microbiol. Scand. 69:619-621, 1967.

15. Mackay, I. R. Macroglobulins and macroglobulinaemia. Aust. Ann. Med. 8:158-170, 1959.

16. Metzger, H. Characterization of a human macroglobulin. V. A Waldenström macroglobulin with antibody activity. Proc. Nat. Acad. Sci. USA 57:1490-1497, 1967.

17. Miller, D. Heparin precipitability of the macroglobulin in a patient with Waldenström's macroglobulinemia. Blood 16:1313-1317, 1960.

18. Ozer, F. L., and H. Chaplin, Jr. Agglutination of stored erythrocytes by a human serum. Characterization of the serum factor and erythrocyte changes. J. Clin. Invest. 42:1735-1752, 1963.

19. Potter, M., and M. A. Leon. Three IgA myeloma immunoglobulins from the BALB/c mouse: precipitation with pneumococcal C polysaccharide. Science 162:369-371, 1968.

20. Schubert, D., A. Jobe, and M. Cohn. Mouse myelomas producing precipitating antibody to nucleic acid bases and/or nitrophenyl derivatives. Nature 220:882-885, 1968.

21. Seligmann, M., F. Danon, A. Basch, and J. Bernard. IgG myeloma cryoglobulin with antistreptotysin activity. Nature 220:711-712, 1968.

22. Stone, M. J., and H. Metzger. The valence of a Waldenström macroglobulin antibody and further thoughts on the significance of paraprotein antibodies. Cold Spring Harbor Symp. Quant. Biol. 32:83-88, 1967.

23. Terry, W. D., B. W. Matthews, and D. R. Davies. Crystallographic studies of a human immunoglobulin. Nature 220:239-241, 1968.

24. Zettervall, O., J. Sjöquist, J. Waldenström, and S. Winblad. Serological activity in myeloma type globulins. Clin. Exp. Immun. 1:213-222, 1966.

III
IMMUNOGLOBULIN
FRAGMENTATION

F. ŠKVAŘIL

Fragmentation of Gamma Globulin Preparations

In the last few years, a systematic study has been performed in several institutions concerning the stability of gamma globulin solution.[7,13-22] It was found that during storage the IgG molecule splits, as if digested by papain, into two fragments analogous to the Fab and Fc fragments. This is generally accepted, and it is presumed that the proteolytic enzyme plasmin is responsible for the fragmentation.

Some typical pictures of fragmented gamma globulin are shown in Figures 1 through 3. Immunoelectrophoresis of six lots of placental gamma globulin, of which four are fragmented and the other two intact, is shown in Figure 1; the same samples have been analyzed by starch gel electrophoresis in formate–urea buffer (Figure 2). In the centrifuge, fragmented gamma globulin appears as two peaks (the lower part of Figure 3). In the same preparations stabilized with epsilon-aminocaproic acid (EACA), a fast-moving peak is detectable, corresponding to the 10S dimer of gamma globulin. When filtered through Sephadex G-100 or G-200 columns, the fragments can be separated from the remaining IgG (Figure 4), and this method is often used for quantitating fragmentation.

A schematic outline of a mechanism that could account for the fragmentation has been proposed by James and co-workers.[7] It postulates

159

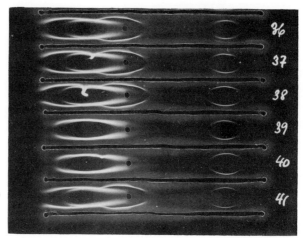

FIGURE 1 Immunoelectrophoresis of gamma globulin preparations after storage for 5 months. Samples from lots 36, 37, 38, and 41 were stabilized with glycine, and samples from lots 39 and 40, with EACA.

formation of a dimer and fragmentation of the complex first to a 5S subunit and finally to Fab- and Fc-like 3.5S fragments.

FACTORS INFLUENCING THE RATE OF FRAGMENTATION

With venous plasma, placental serum, and placental extracts, the most decisive factor influencing fragmentation is the quality of the starting material. Placental gamma globulin, isolated from placental extracts and from placental serum, is most easily fragmented, but fragmentation was

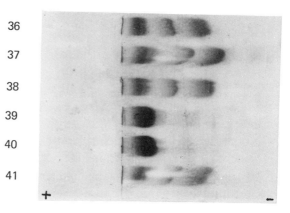

FIGURE 2 Starch gel electrophoresis of gamma globulin preparations (from same lots as in Figure 1) in formate–urea buffer.

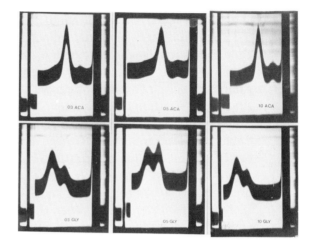

FIGURE 3 Sedimentation analyses of three gamma globulin preparations. The preparations were stored for 5 months in solutions of epsilon-aminocaproic acid (ACA) and glycine (GLY) and then centrifuged at 52,000 rpm for 56 min.

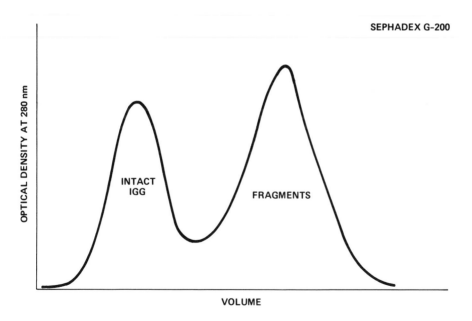

FIGURE 4 Separation of components of fragmented gamma globulin by Sephadex G-200 filtration: optical density at 280 nm expressed as a function of the eluted volume.

demonstrated also in preparations obtained from venous plasma,[5,7,15,16,22] and even in IgG in three normal or pathologic sera before fractionation.[3]

Fragmentation in placental preparations occurs regularly and rapidly. Only exceptionally can we find a placental gamma globulin that is not fragmented. However, only very rarely can fragmentation be detected in gamma globulin of venous origin within its expiration period. The quantitative distribution of components in three batches of our placental gamma globulin, stabilized with glycine and with EACA, is shown in Table 1. After 5 months of storage, a high concentration of fragments can be detected in the preparations stabilized with glycine; the stabilizing effect of EACA is notable. The content of fragments in the same preparations stored for 3 years increased to approximately 70% (Table 1); there is still a difference between the preparations stabilized with glycine and with EACA. After 5 years (Table 1), the difference between preparations with the two agents is small, the concentration of fragments reaching probably a maximal level of around 75%. We assume that some gamma globulin remains intact indefinitely. That would suggest some similarity between papain-resistant and plasmin-resistant gamma globulin molecules. It is not clear whether this resistance to plasmin is a function of the subclass of IgG, as is the case with resistance to papain.

The rate of fragmentation is influenced by the fractionation proce-

TABLE 1   Distribution of Components in Placental Gamma Globulin Preparations after Storage for 5 Months, 3 Years, and 5 Years

| | | Concentration of Components, %[b] | | | | | |
| | | Stored for 5 Months | | Stored for 3 Years | | Stored for 5 Years | |
Preparation[a]	Stabilizing Agent	4S	7S	4S	7S	4S	7S
A	EACA	9	84	45	49	71	29
D	Glycine	62	38	72	28	76	24
B	EACA	6	88	51	47	63	37
E	Glycine	58	42	71	29	78	22
C	EACA	6	87	51	47	62	38
F	Glycine	61	39	70	30	76	24

[a]Members of a given pair of preparations (A–D, B–E, and C–F) are always from the same original freeze-dried gamma globulin and differ only in stabilizing agent.
[b]Deficits from 100% are represented by a 10S dimer of gamma globulin.

dure. By various methods, proteases are removed in varying degrees, generally unknown.[4,9,12,13,23]

The influence of temperature on storage and the rate of fragmentation was studied by Art et al.[2] and by Sgouris and Matz.[16] More degradation occurs at 24 C than at 37 C. Heating at 45 or 50 C, as well as keeping the pH of the preparation below 7.6, minimizes the rate of cleavage.

THE FATE OF ANTIBODIES DURING IMMUNOGLOBULIN G FRAGMENTATION

Some data seem to indicate a decrease of antibody titers with fragmentation,[10,11] especially of antipolio and antimeasles antibodies; other data fail to confirm this decrease.[5,14] In collaboration with the virus laboratory of our institute, we compared three lots of placental gamma globulin in the early stage of storage, from zero to 5 months, at 1-month intervals, and we observed a statistically significant decrease in antipolio antibodies.[20] In another three lots, examined 1 month and 5 months after preparation, a difference in antimeasles antibody titer has been demonstrated in preparations stabilized with glycine and with EACA (Table 2).

The data can be summarized as follows:

1. In fragmented gamma globulin, antibody activity doubtless remains; it is present in intact IgG, as well as in Fab fragments. It is not clear whether fragmentation is connected with antibody decrease.

2. Antibodies that remain in the fragmented gamma globulin and are associated with intact IgG can be considered "fully valuable." Those associated with the Fab fragment are, as described by Painter et al.,[14] "less valuable," owing to their rapid turnover.

INHIBITION OF IMMUNOGLOBULIN G FRAGMENTATION

It was suggested by James et al.[7] that fragmentation could result in alterations in antigenicity and accelerated removal of gamma globulin from the circulation. Although there is no evidence that such preparations, even when administered repeatedly, can be harmful, the problem of stabilization is still of great importance.

Some suitable methods of stabilization—e.g., freeze-drying of the

TABLE 2   Results of Neutralization Tests of Gamma Globulin Preparations Stabilized with
EACA and Glycine and Stored for 1 Month and 5 Months

Preparation	Stabilizing Agent	Neutralization Titers of Antimeasles Antibodies	
		Stored for 1 Month	Stored for 5 Months
A	EACA	1,420	1,250
D	Glycine	982	560
B	EACA	1,320	1,550
E	Glycine	1,024	630
C	EACA	1,024	1,450
F	Glycine	780	450
Reference[a]	–	1,320	1,200

[a]Reference preparation: nonfragmented venous gamma globulin.

final product and production of plasminogen-free gamma globulin—
are technically difficult and expensive. For those reasons, we tried to
use EACA to inhibit fragmentation.

Potential malformation of the fetus in pregnant women given EACA[9]
provided the main reason for the reluctance to introduce the stabilizer
into the product. At present, there are two reports refuting the terato-
genicity of EACA. One concludes that only a decrease in pregnancy rate
was demonstrated after increasing doses of EACA; the other[6] is similar
in content.

After it had been demonstrated by Adam *et al.*[1] that there was a difference in effectiveness in the prevention of measles between preparations stabilized with EACA and glycine, EACA inhibitor was introduced
into large-scale production of placental gamma globulin. Gamma globulin of venous origin is stabilized with glycine.

EFFECTIVENESS OF PLACENTAL GAMMA GLOBULIN IN
THE PREVENTION OF MEASLES

I would like to report the results of one investigation on the effectiveness of placental gamma globulin in the prevention of measles. The

study was performed by Dr. Adam and co-workers from the Clinical-Epidemiological Department of the Research Institute of Immunology in Prague.

Three batches of 16% human gamma globulin were prepared from placental materials. Each was divided in half. To one half, 2.25% glycine was added, and to the other half, 3% EACA. The field trial began after 5 months of storage of the products. The working team performing the experiment was not acquainted with the codes of the preparations. Only when the experiment was finished were the codes disclosed for statistical evaluation. Fragmentation was assessed by sedimentation analysis at the beginning of the experiment (after 5 months of storage), at the end of the field trial (after 3 years), and again 2 years later.

Gamma globulin was administered at 46 institutions in which measles had erupted. There were a total of 948 administrations of gamma globulin (given in injections of 0.3 ml/kg of body weight). In 23 institutions (accounting for 494 children), no further case of the disease was recorded. The institutions were divided as follows:

1. Those in which contact of the children with the ill child was dubious, because of either timing or space (five, with 121 children)

2. Those in which gamma globulin was administered, but the clinical course of the disease or the epidemiologic case history of the infective source did not favor diagnosis of measles (four, with 100 children), or those in which serologic examination was negative (three, with 44 children)

3. Those in which the circumstances described above were not known to obtain, but where the children did not fall ill (11, with 229 children)

In 23 other institutions, with 454 children, a contact disease outbreak took place after gamma globulin administration. In only one institution was the percentage of children ill after the administration of gamma globulin with glycine lower than that after the administration of EACA-stabilized gamma globulin. The difference is not statistically significant.

The combined data from all institutions are presented in Table 3. Of 221 children treated with EACA preparations of gamma globulin, 19% contracted measles; of 223 children who were given gamma globulin with glycine, 42.9% contracted the disease. The frequencies given in parentheses are expected frequencies, assuming that the occurrence of the disease is independent of the kind of stabilizer used. The differences

TABLE 3   Evaluation of Effect of Gamma Globulin on Prevention of Measles in 23 Institutions in Relation to Stabilizing Agent

Stabilizing Agent	No. Children Exposed	Measles after Administration of Gamma Globulin[a]			
		With Measles		Without Measles	
		No.	%	No.	%
EACA (3%)	221	42 (69.1)	19.0	179 (151.9)	81.0
Glycine (2.25%)	233	100 (72.9)	42.9	133 (160.1)	57.1
Totals	454	142	31.3	312	68.7

[a]Numbers in parentheses are numbers of cases expected if choice of stabilizing agent has no effect.

between the values with and without that assumption are statistically significant at the 0.1% level (the value X^2 is greater than 20).

I would like to express my appreciation to Dr. Johanovsky, Head of the Research Institute of Immunology (Prague), for his consultative and critical assistance; to Dr. Adam and co-workers for their cooperation in performing the effectiveness studies; and to Dr. Kyncl for assistance in the sedimentation studies.

REFERENCES

1. Adam, E., E. Kubátová, M. Kratochvílová, V. Burian, and F. Škvařil. Preparáty placentárního gamaglobulinu stablizované kyselinou epsilon-aminokapronovou. Studie reaktogennosti a účinnosti. Cas. Lek. Cesk. 104:1093–1100, 1965.
2. Art, G. P., E. H. Mealey, and J. S. Finlayson. Studies on the stability of human gamma globulin. Vox Sang. 13:59, 1967.
3. Augustin, R., and B. J. Hayward. Cleavage of human γ-globulin. Nature 187:129–130, 1960.
4. Cohn, E. J., L. E. Strong, W. L. Hughes, Jr., D. J. Mulford, J. N. Ashworth, M. Melin, and H. L. Taylor. Preparation and properties of serum and plasma proteins. IV. A system for the separation into fractions of the protein and lipoprotein components of biological tissues and fluids. J. Amer. Chem. Soc. 68:459–475, 1946.
5. Connell, G. E., and R. H. Painter. Fragmentation of immunoglobulin during storage. Canad. J. Biochem. 44:371–379, 1966.
6. Eneroth, G., and C. A. Grant. Epsilon aminocaproic acid and reduction in fertility of male rats. Acta Pharm. Suec. 3:115–122, 1966.
7. James, K., C. S. Henney, and D. R. Stanworth. Structural changes occurring in 7S γ-globulins. Nature 202:563–566, 1964.
8. Johnson, A. J., L. Skoza, and E. Claus. Observations on epsilon aminocaproic acid. Thromb. Diath. Haemorrh. 7:203–204, 1962. (abstract)

9. Kuška, J., and J. Krěmer. Czechoslov. Patent Spec. No. 89170/56.
10. Mosley, J. W., D. M. Reisler, D. Brachott, D. Roth, and J. Weiser. Comparison of two lots of immune serum globulin for prophylaxis of infectious hepatitis. Amer. J. Epidem. 87: 539–550, 1968.
11. Murray, R. Gamma globulin for clinical use based on antibody titers of the preparation, pp. 92–101. In M. Mannik, Ed. Symposium on Gamma Globulin. Washington, D.C.: National Academy of Sciences–National Research Council, 1962.
12. Oncley, J. L., M. Melin, D. A. Richert, J. W. Cameron, and P. M. Gross, Jr. The separation of the antibodies, isoagglutinins, prothrombin, plasminogen and β-lipoprotein into sub-fractions of human plasma. J. Amer. Chem. Soc. 71:541–550, 1949.
13. Painter, R. H. Observations on the preparation and testing of stable and unstable immune serum globulin preparations. XI International Congress of Microbiological Standardization, Milan, 1968.
14. Painter, R. H., M. J. Walcroft, and J. C. Weber. The efficacy of fragmented immune serum globulin in passive immunization. Canad. J. Biochem. 44:381–387, 1966.
15. Sgouris, J. T., D. W. Brackenbury, K. B. McCall, and H. D. Anderson. The effect of fibrino-lysin on human gamma globulin. Fed. Proc. 21:35, 1962. (abstract)
16. Sgouris, J. T., and M. J. Matz. Observations on the fragmentation of venous and placental immune serum globulins. Vox Sang. 13:59–71, 1967.
17. Škvařil, F. Changes in human gamma globulin preparations during storage. Folio Microbiol. 5:264–271, 1960.
18. Škvařil, F. Changes in outdated human γ-globulin preparations. Nature 185:475–476, 1960.
19. Škvařil, F., and V. Brummelová. Isolation of components of fragmented normal human γG immunoglobulin. Collection Czech. Chem. Commun. 33:2316–2321, 1968.
20. Škvařil, F., D. Grünberger, M. Dřevo, D. Slonim, and J. Strauss. Osud protilátek v průběhu samovolné ho štrěpení placentárního epsilon-aminokapronovou (EACA). Cesk. Epidem. 13:343–350, 1964.
21. Škvařil, F., D. Grünberger, and F. Kyncl. Inhibition of the spontaneous splitting of human γ-globulin preparations by epsilon-aminocaproic acid. Collection Czech. Chem. Commun. 28:644–651, 1963.
22. Strauss, A. J., P. G. Kemp, Jr., W. E. Vannier, and H. C. Goodman. Purification of human serum γ-globulin for immunologic studies: γ-globulin fragmentation after sulfate precipi-tation and prolonged dialysis. J. Immun. 93:24–34, 1964.
23. Taylor, H. L., F. C. Bloom, K. B. McCall, L. A. Hyndman, and H. D. Anderson. The preparation of γ-globulin from placental blood by ethanol fractionation. J. Amer. Chem. Soc. 78:1356–1358, 1956.

JAMES T. SGOURIS

Stability Studies on Gamma Globulin

Millions of doses of gamma globulin prepared from plasma by the ethanol method of Cohn *et al.*[4] and Oncley *et al.*[9] have been used in the last 25 years. During that time, fractionation by the cold ethanol method has undergone modifications and has also been applied to placental extracts. These variations in procedures may have an effect on the stability of the molecule and, in part, account for the differences observed between products from different manufacturers.

Development of antibodies to gamma globulin after injection of gamma globulin[17] or to aggregated gamma globulin in patients with hypogammaglobulinemia[6,7] has been reported. We have studied chromatographically a number of venous gamma globulin preparations. Analysis on Sephadex G-200, at pH 8.0, of two heat-treated and outdated preparations revealed the presence of polymers of gamma globulin (Table 1). One of the lots contained over 40% dimer (10S). Whether heating or storage, or both, contributed to this aggregation has not been determined.

In addition to aggregation, gamma globulins may undergo fragmentation into relatively low-molecular-weight components during storage.

TABLE 1 Chromatographic Analysis[a] of Outdated Heat-Treated Preparations of Venous Gamma Globulin

Run	Peak 1, %[b]	Peak 2, %[c]
A	29	71.0
B	41.5	58.5

[a]Sephadex G-200 at pH 8.0 in a Tris buffer.
[b]10S component.
[c]7S component.

Several years ago, it was observed by Škvařil[15] that a number of outdated human gamma globulin preparations prepared by the cold ethanol method fragmented during storage at 4 C. The breakdown of gamma globulin obtained from venous blood was slow, whereas placental preparations fragmented more readily. Similar instability was observed[3] with aged human sera and gamma globulins prepared by fractionation on DEAE cellulose. The latter product fragmented after storage at 4 C for only a few weeks. We have observed[13] breakdown of venous gamma globulin prepared by the Oncley procedure and stored at 4 C for over 5 years. Fragmentation of a number of gamma globulins from several producers was assessed in our laboratory several years ago.[12] These lots, stored at 4 C, had expired or were close to the expiration date. Six of the seven lots were found to have undergone fragmentation comparable with that which we reported on our outdated lots. Painter and co-workers[5,10,11] also reported that some gamma globulin preparations of venous origin had fragmented within the prescribed dating period.

Clinical evaluation of two lots of gamma globulin for prophylaxis against infectious hepatitis was recently reported by Mosley et al.[8] They noted that one of the lots that had undergone considerable fragmentation had an efficiency for protection of exposed household contacts of only 47%, compared with 87% for the second lot, which contained intact gamma globulin.

Clinical trials on the prevention of measles by Adam and Škvařil[1] gave convincing evidence that gamma globulin in which proteolysis had been inhibited by epsilon-aminocaproic acid (EACA) was more effective in the prevention of measles than that in which it had not.

The producer is, then, faced with the need for preparing a gamma

TABLE 2 Effect of pH on Fragmentation of Placental Gamma Globulin at Three Temperatures[a]

pH	Peak		Storage at 37 C			Storage at 25 C			Storage at 4 C		
			0 Days	30 Days	60 Days	0 Days	30 Days	60 Days	0 Days	30 Days	60 Days
7.2	1 (10S)	%	16.3	17.9	23.5[b]	16.3	17.2	9.9	16.3	15.0	16.2
	2 (7S)	%	83.7	79.5	70.0	83.7	75.8	69.9	83.7	83.7	74.3
	3 (3.5S)	%	—	2.6	6.5	—	7.0	20.2	—	1.3	9.5
6.4	1 (10S)	%	16.3	17.1	20.7	16.3	16.6	23.2	16.3	15.9	18.7
	2 (7S)	%	83.7	80.4	79.3	83.7	73.5	73.3	83.7	82.4	77.3
	3 (3.5S)	%	—	2.5	—	—	9.9	3.5	—	1.7	4.0

[a]Fragmentation determined by chromatographic analysis on Sephadex G-200 at pH 8.0; 0.1M Tris, 0.5M NaCl buffer.
[b]Includes 3.5% of a faster-eluting component.

170

globulin that is free of aggregates and fragments and that will remain so during its shelf life. Three problems arise: (1) What factors contribute to the instability of the product? (2) How can unstable lots be distinguished from stable lots? (3) What can be done to avoid instability?

Fragmentation of gamma globulin into Fab-like and Fc-like components is caused by proteolytic enzymes. Plasminogen is present in fraction II + III[9] and is ordinarily removed in subsequent fractionation. Trace quantities of proteolytic activity have been detected in gamma globulins,[13] and this activity was enhanced by the addition of streptokinase. We have shown that fragmentation similar to that seen in outdated lots of gamma globulin can be achieved in a few hours with fresh lots by the addition of highly purified human plasmin.

The stability of placental gamma globulin was studied[14] at pH 6.4 and 7.2 and at storage temperatures of 4, 25, and 37 C. Samples were taken at 0, 30, and 60 days and subjected to starch gel electrophoresis at pH 8.9. Starch gel electrophoresis at pH 8.9 revealed that a greater degree of fragmentation occurred at pH 7.2 than at pH 6.4 over the 60-day period at all temperatures. Optimal temperatures for fragmentation was 25 C, and minimal fragmentation occurred at 4 C. This agrees with the observations of Art et al.[2] Starch gel electrophoresis revealed that placental gamma globulin at 4 C undergoes less fragmentation if stored at pH 6.4. Fragmentation was also assessed by chromatography on Sephadex G-200 at pH 8.0. The effects of pH, storage time, and temperature are shown in Table 2. These data agree with those obtained by starch gel electrophoresis.

The use of EACA as an inhibitor of plasmin activity has been recommended by Škvařil and Grunberger.[16] The effect of EACA on 16.5% venous gamma globulin to which 5 caseinolytic units (C.U.) of plasmin were added is shown in Table 3. Fragmentation determined qualitatively by starch gel electrophoresis revealed that the effect of plasmin was reduced but not completely inhibited by EACA.

Another inhibitor, Trasylol, was more effective in inhibiting the action of extrinsic plasmin added to gamma globulin (Table 4). Eight kallikrein inhibitor units (K.I.U.) of Trasylol completely inhibited the action of one unit of plasmin on samples of 16.5% venous gamma globulin.[14]

In summary, starch gel electrophoresis was found[14] to be an excellent

TABLE 3   Effect of EACA on Cleavage of Gamma Globulin[a]

	Lot			
	1	2	3	4
Gamma globulin (16.5%), ml	5.0	5.0	5.0	5.0
Plasmin, C.U.	–	5	5	5
EACA, %	–	1.0	2.0	4.0
Incubation time				
96 hr	–	+++	+++	++
240 hr	–	++++	++++	+++

[a]Cleavage (fragmentation) determined by chromatography or starch gel electrophoresis on 5.0-ml samples of venous gamma globulin. (–, no cleavage; +, cleavage.)

TABLE 4   Effect of Trasylol on Cleavage of Gamma Globulin[a]

	Lot				
	1	2	3	4	5
Gamma globulin (16.5%), ml	5.0	5.0	5.0	5.0	5.0
Plasmin, C.U.	–	5	5	5	5
Trasylol, K.I.U./ml	–	–	10	20	40
Incubation time					
96 hr	–	+++	++	+	–
240 hr	–	++++	++	+	–

[a]Cleavage (fragmentation) determined by starch gel electrophoresis on 5.0-ml samples of venous gamma globulin. (–, no cleavage; +, cleavage.)

screening tool for detecting fragmentation. Fragmentation, as well as aggregation, can be determined by Sephadex G-200 chromatography. Because we are interested in what happens to gamma globulin during its shelf life, these tests should be conducted at various intervals during the dating period to determine the extent of fragmentation or aggregation. It is desirable to maintain the pH of the final preparation at the lower allowable limit of 6.4, where gamma globulin is less likely to undergo fragmentation. The addition of proteolytic inhibitors, such as EACA and Trasylol, to the product should be evaluated further. Finally, additional data are needed to determine the maximal degrees of aggregation and fragmentation allowable for this product.

The work reported here was supported in part by Public Health Service grant HE 07585 from the National Heart Institute.

REFERENCES

1. Adam, E., and F. Skvaril. The use of placental gamma globulins stabilized with the epsilon-aminocaproic acid for the prevention of measles. Arch. Ges. Virusforsch. 16:220–221, 1965.
2. Art, G. P., E. H. Mealey, and J. S. Finlayson. Studies on the stability of human gamma globulin. Vox Sang. 13:59, 1967.
3. Augustin, R., and B. J. Hayward. Cleavage of human γ-globulin. Nature 187:129–130, 1960.
4. Cohn, E. J., L. E. Strong, W. L. Hughes, Jr., D. J. Mulford, J. N. Ashworth, M. Melin, and H. L. Taylor. Preparation and properties of serum and plasma proteins. IV. A system for the separation into fractions of the protein and lipoprotein components of biological tissues and fluids. J. Amer. Chem. Assoc. 68:459–475, 1946.
5. Connell, G. E., and R. H. Painter. Fragmentation of immunoglobulin during storage. Canad. J. Biochem. 44:371–379, 1966.
6. Ellis, E. F., and C. S. Henney. Adverse reactions following administration of human gamma globulin. J. Allerg. 43:45–54, 1969.
7. Henney, C. S., and E. F. Ellis. Antibody production to aggregated human γ-G-globulin in acquired hypogammaglobulinemia. New Eng. J. Med. 278:1144–1146, 1968.
8. Mosley, J. W., D. M. Reisler, D. Brachott, D. Roth, and J. Weiser. Comparison of two lots of immune serum globulin for prophylaxis of infectious hepatitis. Amer. J. Epidem. 87:539–550, 1968.
9. Oncley, J. L., M. Melin, D. A. Richert, J. W. Cameron, and P. M. Gross, Jr. The separation of the antibodies, isoagglutinins, prothrombin, plasminogen and β_1-lipoprotein into subfractions of human plasma. J. Amer. Chem. Soc. 71:541–550, 1949.
10. Painter, R. H., and G. E. Connell. Instability of immune serum globulin preparations. Vox Sang. 10:355–356, 1965.
11. Painter, R. H., M. J. Walcroft, and J. C. Weber. The efficacy of fragmented immune serum globulin in passive immunization. Canad. J. Biochem. 44:381–387, 1966.
12. Sgouris, J. T. Stability of immunoglobulin G preparations. Fed. Proc. 25:726, 1966. (abstract)
13. Sgouris, J. T., D. W. Brackenbury, K. B. McCall, and H. D. Anderson. The effect of fibrinolysin on human gamma globulin. Fed. Proc. 21:35, 1962. (abstract)
14. Sgouris, J. T., and M. J. Matz. Observations on the fragmentation of venous and placental immune serum globulins. Vox Sang. 13:59–71, 1967.
15. Škvaril, F. Changes in outdated human γ-globulin preparations. Nature 185:475–476, 1960.
16. Škvaril, F., and D. Grunberger. Inhibition of spontaneous splitting of γ-globulin preparations with epsilon-aminocaproic acid. Nature 196:481–482, 1962.
17. Stiehm, E. R., and H. H. Fudenberg. Antibody to gamma-globulin in infants and children exposed to isologous gamma-globulin. Pediatrics 35:229–235, 1965.

ROBERT H. PAINTER

Fragmentation of Serum Gamma Globulin and Its Prevention

It is well established that gamma globulin solutions undergo breakdown during storage, resulting in the formation of Fab- and Fc-like fragments, probably as a result of the proteolytic action of traces of plasmin remaining in fraction II.[2,4-6] The effects of this process are twofold: a fall in the titer of bivalent antibody in the preparation and a reduction in the half-life of the antibody represented by the Fab fragment. In a series of experiments, we have used gamma globulin preparations in which approximately 50% of the protein was present as low-molecular-weight (3.5S) component. When comparable doses were injected into monkeys, the level of circulating polio antibody induced by the fragmented material was only 15% of that induced by the unfragmented material. Between 40% and 60% of the antibody was recovered in the urine within 8 hr after intravenous injection of the fragmented material. Similarly, fragmented material failed to protect guinea pigs against subsequent challenge with doses of tetanus toxin that were not lethal in pigs protected with a similar number of units of tetanus antitoxin contained in unfragmented gamma globulin.

Until now, it has not been possible to assess the significance of these findings in medical practice because of the lack of quantitative data on

174

the extent to which fragmentation occurs in production lots of gamma globulin. Art and Finlayson have reported the presence of fragmentation to varying extents in gamma globulin from several manufacturers in the United States (unpublished data). Table 1 shows the results of our own investigations into fragmentation in gamma globulin prepared at the Connaught Laboratories in Canada from venous plasma and stored for various periods at 2 C. Fragmentation has been quantitated by gel filtration on Sephadex G-200. It can be seen that the extent of fragmentation varies. Samples of each lot, frozen at the time of manufacture, showed no fragmentation, indicating that fragmentation occurred during storage.

It is difficult to know at what level fragmentation becomes clinically significant. It will depend largely on the dose of antibody administered and the amount of antibody necessary to effect protection in a given instance. Adam and Škvaříl[1] have reported finding a significant difference in the protection afforded children against measles by normal gamma globulin, presumably degraded, and by gamma globulin in

TABLE 1   Occurrence of Fragmentation in Production Lots of Gamma Globulin Held for Various Periods at 2 C and for 1 Month at 20 C

Lot	Percent Fragmented[a] at 2 C		Rate of Fragmentation at 2 C, % per month	Rate of Fragmentation at 20 C, % per month
205	6.1	(4)	1.5	6.6
201	8.2	(6)	1.4	11.3
197	9.6	(10)	1.0	8.6
194	13.4	(13)	1.0	5.5
192	11	(15)	0.7	1.9
191	7.6	(19)	0.4	6.9
189	14.6	(24)	0.6	7.4
185	32.5	(27)	1.2	7.2
181	11.5	(28)	0.4	not tested
173	17	(30)	0.6	3.8
179	37	(31)	1.2	15.7
171	22	(37)	0.6	12.1
166	8.2	(42)	0.2	10.2
159	4.0	(49)	0.1	5.3

[a]Estimated by gel filtration on Sephadex G-200; numbers in parentheses are numbers of months of storage.

which proteolysis was inhibited by epsilon-aminocaproic acid (EACA). The most critical situations are probably those in which specific or rare antibody preparations are used, such as tetanus and vaccinia immune globulins, and in the treatment of hemolytic disease of the newborn with anti-D immune globulin. In some of these cases, perhaps as little as 10% fragmentation becomes critical. The fragmentation shown in Table 1 occurred during storage at 2 C. Under different conditions, the amount of fragmentation could be higher and more variable.

Several proposals have been made for the preparation of gamma globulin solutions that are not prone to fragmentation. Chemical inhibitors of plasmin, such as EACA, have been used effectively in Czechoslovakia.[7] Some manufacturers in the United States have apparently avoided the problem by heating the gamma globulin solution at 45 C for 72 hr, which is effective in inactivating plasmin. We have elected to avoid fragmentation by introducing a modification in fractionation method 9,[3] to ensure the complete removal of plasmin into fraction III. This can be achieved by precipitating fraction III at pH 5.4 instead of pH 5.2. The effect is shown in Table 2. Gamma globulin solutions, prepared after the removal of fraction III at one of a series of pH values from 4.8 to 5.6, were examined by gel filtration for fragmentation after storage at 2 C for 3 months or at 20 C for 1 month. It can be seen that there is a relationship between the pH at which fraction III is removed and the stability of the gamma globulin solution

TABLE 2   Effect of pH at Which Fraction III is Separated on Stability of Fraction II Solution

pH at Which Fraction III is Removed	Gamma Globulin Fragmentation, %[a]		
	Control, No Storage	3 Months at 2 C	1 Month at 20 C
4.5	–	29	–
4.8	0	22	18.7
5.15	0	8.8	9.6
5.4	–	1.0	–
5.6	0	1.0	1.8
5.8	–	0	–

[a]Estimated by gel filtration.

TABLE 3   Effect of pH at Which Fraction III is Separated on Yield of Protein and Quantity of Antibody in Fraction II

pH at Which Fraction III is Removed	Total Protein[a]	Antibody Titer[b]		
		Tetanus, hemagglutinating units/ml	Log Measles Titer	Log Polio Titer
4.5	110	–	3.01	3.31
4.8	113	–	3.31	3.76
5.1	100	–	3.01	3.76
5.4	85	–	3.01	4.06
5.8	74	–	3.01	3.46
4.8	125	13	2.44	3.76
5.2	100	12	2.62	3.76
5.5	85	15	2.44	3.69

[a]Expressed as percent of that recovered at pH 5.2.
[b]10% protein solution w/v.

prepared. If fraction III is removed at pH 5.4, there is little or no fragmentation during storage, whereas if it is removed at pH 4.8, there is considerable fragmentation.

The effects of these changes in fractionation on the quality and quantity of antibody recovered are shown in Table 3. It is evident that antibody titers are not changed by this process. Quantitative estimation by radial immunodiffusion of the classes of antibody found in these preparations showed that the levels of IgA and IgM found when fraction III was removed at low pH were approximately 20 and 40 mg/g of protein, respectively. These values were reduced by a factor of 10 when fraction III was removed at pH 5.6. The effect on the overall yield of antibody in fraction II can be seen from the second column of Table 3, where the protein is expressed as percent of that recovered at pH 5.2, the usual pH for precipitation of fraction III. At pH values below this, the yield of protein is increased; at values above it, the yield is reduced. At pH 5.4, the recovery is 85% of that at pH 5.2.

Thus, it appears possible to prepare stable gamma globulin by a simple modification of the fractionation procedure that involves a 15% loss of production. Conversely, by precipitating fraction III at pH 4.8, it is possible to prepare gamma globulin solutions that are prone to fragmentation.

REFERENCES

1. Adam, E., and F. Škvařil. The use of placental gamma globulins stabilized with the epsilon-aminocaproic acid for the prevention of measles. Arch. Ges. Virusforsch. 16:220–221, 1965.
2. Connell, G. E., and R. H. Painter. Fragmentation of immunoglobulin during storage. Canad. J. Biochem. 44:371–379, 1966.
3. Oncley, J. L., M. Melin, D. A. Richert, J. W. Cameron, and P. M. Gross, Jr. The separation of the antibodies, isoagglutinins, prothrombin, plasminogen, and β_1-lipoprotein into subfractions of human plasma. J. Amer. Chem. Soc. 71:541–550, 1949.
4. Painter, R. H. Instability of immune serum globulin solutions. II. In vivo studies on solutions which have fragmented during storage and on those fragmented by digestion with plasmin. Vox Sang. 13:57–58, 1967.
5. Painter, R. H., M. J. Walcroft, and J. C. Weber. The efficacy of fragmented immune serum globulin in passive immunization. Canad. J. Biochem. 44:381–387, 1966.
6. Škvařil, F. Changes in outdated human γ-globulin preparations. Nature 185:475–476, 1960.
7. Škvařil, F., and D. Grünberger. Inhibition of spontaneous splitting of γ-globulin preparations with epsilon-aminocaproic acid. Nature 196:481–482, 1962.

DISCUSSION

DR. DEUTSCH: Dr. Sgouris observed a decrease in some of the 3.5S material following digestion for periods of over 60 days. I wonder whether some of this material is being converted to lower-molecular-weight material, which is not included in your analysis. I think one might also comment on Dr. Škvařil's observation that it appears that plasmin is degrading the 8S–10S IgG preferentially to the 7S form.

DR. PAINTER: I think you are right. We have begun to look for F′c, as well, and to include it in our analyses. I noticed in Dr. Škvařil's immunoelectrophoresis a beautiful F′c arc at the anodic end of each pattern. The breakdown obviously does not cease with the formation of Fc and Fab; it continues. The small amount of fragment found in the older samples might indicate complete breakdown of Fab and Fc.

DR. SCHWICK: We have also done some experiments with plasmin fragmentation of gamma globulins. Our attempts to inhibit fragmentation were not too successful. We used Trasylol in large amounts and EACA. There is some inhibition, but after several years, spontaneous fragmentation still occurs. We looked for new procedures to remove plasminogen in the early stages of fractionation. Last year, we tried absorption with Pharmasol or Aerosil. Aerosil at pH 7.8 removes plasminogen. In the last few months, we succeeded in preparing an insoluble substrate for plasminogen that removes practically all the plasminogen from plasma. It is a copolymer of lysine dimer. It reacts like EACA, but it is insoluble. With this material, we were able for the first time to prepare a plasminogen-free fibrinogen. That was the starting point of our work.

JOAN D. CRAIN, FRED S. ROSEN, *and*
CHARLES A. JANEWAY

Clinical Experience with Intravenous Fragmented Gamma Globulins

The intravenous administration of gamma globulin is frequently followed by adverse reactions, especially in patients with antibody deficiency syndromes[1] and in children with acute infections (W. Berenberg and C. A. Janeway, unpublished data). These reactions, which vary in severity, are manifested by flushing, pallor, hypotension, muscle pains, nausea and vomiting, brief collapse, chills, and fever.[1] Aggregates of gamma globulin present in the preparation are thought to be responsible for these anaphylactoid reactions, and it has been shown that preparations from which the aggregates have been removed can be safely administered. Treatment with proteolytic enzymes[6] or some hydrolytic procedure[2] to disaggregate the gamma globulin while retaining its biologic properties intact is more practical for large-scale production.

In 1968, Janeway *et al.*[3] reported on the metabolism of two preparations of gamma globulin rendered suitable for intravenous use by digestion with either pepsin or plasmin. Plasmin digestion of pooled human gamma globulin leaves 60–80% of the gamma globulin nearly unfragmented (6.5S) and 20–40% converted to Fc-like and Fab-like fragments.[7] Pepsin digestion of gamma globulin results in a major 5S fraction, F(ab')2, and the remainder of the digest is changed to small fragments.[5]

179

The metabolic fate of the digests and their components was studied in normal volunteers who were given ^{131}I-labeled fragments with ^{125}I-labeled gamma globulin. The half-life of gamma globulin varied from 17.5 to 22.1 days, whereas the 6.5S gamma globulin component of the plasmin-treated digest had a half-life of 15–17 days. The other fragments were rapidly excreted in the urine. The F(ab')2 fragments, which accounted for 90% of the pepsin digest, had a half-life of 10½ hr. The half-life of the plasmin-digested gamma globulin was 17–19 days in five patients with agammaglobulinemia[3] (Figure 1).

The plasmin-digested pooled human gamma globulin in a 16% solution was supplied by Dr. Sgouris. Agammaglobulinemic patients were given 100–150 mg/kg of body weight every 3 weeks. Seven patients are children with congenital sex-linked disease who were 7–17 years old when the study began. Three patients are adults with acquired agammaglobulinemia. Before the study, all patients had been on intramuscular

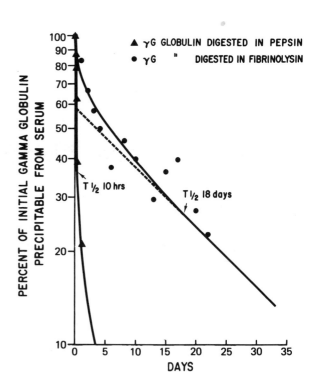

FIGURE 1 Half-life of plasmin and pepsin digests of gamma globulin in a patient with congenital agammaglobulinemia.

gamma globulin in doses of 100 mg/kg every 4 weeks, except one 7-year-old boy with congenital sex-linked disease, who had never been treated.

Infusions were given as a 5% solution of gamma globulin diluted with saline and were given at a rate of 100 cc/hr. Vital signs were checked every 15 min during the initial infusion and at the beginning and end of subsequent ones.

During the 28 months of this study, a total of 166 infusions have been given to seven children with congenital agammaglobulinemia without any serious side effects. No fever, nausea, abdominal or flank pains, tachycardia, angioedema, or hypotension has occurred. At the end of the infusion period, the serum concentration of gamma globulin varied between 175 and 390 mg/100 ml, with an average of 275 mg/100 ml. Serum complement levels, determined by the CH50 method, did not vary significantly before and after infusions. A more sensitive stoichiometric C1 assay also showed no change. No abnormalities have been found in the urine analyses or liver-function studies.

During the 28-month period of study that represents 115 infusion-months for six of the children with agammaglobulinemia, nine bacterial infections occurred. In a comparable 115 months before they received the digest, while they were receiving intramuscular gamma globulin, there were 11 bacterial infections. Thus, there was no significant difference in prophylactic effect with regard to infection. The child who had not been on any gamma globulin before this study had repeated episodes of otitis media and two episodes of pneumonia. In the 19 months of therapy, he has had otitis media twice.

In contrast with the 166 infusions given to the children without any reactions, the digest has been given to three adults with acquired agammaglobulinemia. All three had reactions to the material; two had had reactions to intramuscular gamma globulin before they were given the intravenous preparation; the other patient had the initial infusion without any problems, but after the second infusion, 3 weeks later, adverse reactions were noted. One of the patients had an adverse reaction after the first infusion, and the other patient after the third. These reactions were similar in all patients and occurred at the end of the infusion. They started with chills, vomiting, and hypotension. There followed flank pain, leg pain, and tachycardia. Temperature increased immediately in one patient and within an hour in the other two. Symptoms subsided in 45–60 min, with chills and pain decreasing first. Temperature remained high for 2–3 hr. Hypotension decreased in 1–3 hr. All patients were given intravenous Benadryl; no other treatment was required. Blood cultures and cultures of all materials used during the infusion were sterile. Serum-complement levels did not change during the reactions, nor did C1 levels.

To ascertain whether these reactions were induced by *in vivo* complex formation, one patient was given ^{131}I-labeled 6.5S gamma globulin added to 40 ml of unlabeled digest. When he developed a reaction similar to the one described, blood samples were taken every 15 min during the infusion, during the reaction, and 1 and 2 hr afterwards. Serum samples were fractionated by gel filtration on a Sephadex G-200 column. No evidence of *in vivo* complex formation was noted.

The goal of therapy in agammaglobulinemia is the prevention of infections. Although some favor continuous chemoprophylaxis as a means of preventing bacterial illnesses, experience at the Children's Hospital Medical Center in Boston has shown that prophylaxis with gamma globulin is more efficient.[4] In patients without tissue damage, 0.1 g of gamma globulin per kilogram of body weight per month is adequate after a loading dose of two to three times this amount. The major problem with this treatment is the large volume of the injections. The pain involved is psychologically traumatic, especially in younger children. Giving the medication intravenously has been found to be a readily accepted, if not welcome, mode of treatment.

In conclusion, during a 28-month study, which represents 115 infusion months for six children with congenital agammaglobulinemia, there have been nine bacterial infections. This does not represent any significant difference in prophylactic effect when compared with the 11 bacterial infections that occurred in a comparable period before the study. Three adults with acquired agammaglobulinemia have had adverse reactions to the intravenous administration of plasmin-digested gamma globulin. No evidence of *in vivo* complex formation could be demonstrated. The mediators of these reactions are not understood.

The work reported here was supported by Public Health Service grants AM-05877 and FR-00128, research career development award 5 K3 AM 19,650 (Dr. Rosen), and postdoctoral fellowship grant F2 HD 36 525 (Dr. Crain).

REFERENCES

1. Barandun, S. Die Gammaglobulin-Therapie. Chemische, immunologische und klinische Grundlagen. Bibl. Haemat. 17 (Suppl.):1–134, 1964.
2. Barandun, S., P. Kistler, F. Jeunet, and H. Isliker. Intravenous administration of human γ-globulin. Vox Sang. 7:157–174, 1962.
3. Janeway, C. A., E. Merler, F. S. Rosen, S. Salmon, and J. D. Crain. Intravenous gamma globulin: Metabolism of gamma globulin fragments in normal and agammaglobulinemic persons. New Eng. J. Med. 278:919–923, 1968.
4. Janeway, C. A., F. S. Rosen, E. Merler, and C. A. Alper. The Gamma Globulins. Boston: Little, Brown and Company, 1967. 148 pp.
5. Nisonoff, A., F. C. Wissler, and L. N. Lipman. Properties of the major component of a peptic digest of rabbit antibody. Science 132:1770–1771, 1960.
6. Schultze, H. E., and G. Schwick. Über neue Möglichkeiten intravenöser Gammaglobulin-Applikation. Deutsch. Med. Wschr. 87:1643–1650, 1962.
7. Sgouris, J. T. The preparation of plasmin treated immune serum globulin for intravenous use. Vox Sang. 13:71–84, 1967.

DISCUSSION

DR. MANNIK: I wish to remark on the possibility of a different way of removing aggregates from gamma globulin preparations, because it appears that the clinical reactions observed are caused by soluble aggregates. It has been shown that, after reducing and alkylating the interchain disulfide bonds, the ability of the protein to fix complement is lost. Furthermore, reduced and alkylated molecules have in rabbits a half-life identical with that of native IgG, in contrast with the half-life of pepsin-digested IgG.

DR. ROSEN: The clinical reactions observed are not complement-mediated. Despite these anaphylactoid reactions in patients, we cannot demonstrate any change in C1, C4, or C2. I do not see how we can work on the presumption that these are complement-mediated reactions.

H. G. SCHWICK

Pepsin-Disaggregated Gamma Globulins

Eight years ago, we found a relationship between the side effects of intravenous administration of human gamma globulin and the complement-fixation capacity of normal gamma globulin preparations. Since then, we have attempted to modify the gamma globulin molecule without changing its antibody activity, to make it suitable for intravenous administration. Schultze and I studied many potential methods and finally found that pepsin, if allowed to digest gamma globulin long enough, will remove the ability to fix complement.[1] Pepsin is thus a suitable enzyme for transforming gamma globulin, with no loss of antibody activity, into a substance that can be administered intravenously.

A gamma globulin obtained by this procedure was first tested clinically and then made available for clinical use under the name of Gamma-Veinine 6 years ago. Table 1 shows the composition of five batches of Gamma-Veinine.

Removal of the ability of a gamma globulin preparation to initiate complement fixation during enzymatic splitting of the gamma globulin molecule can be easily examined with a simple plate test. A more sensitive method is the testing of the influence of gamma globulin on individual complement factors, such as C1 and C4.[1]

184

TABLE 1   Composition of Five Batches of Gamma-Veinine (on the Basis of Ultracentrifugal Analysis)

Lot	7S, %	5S, %	3.5S, %
68 XII 3	11	80	9
69 II 5	11	81.5	7.5
69 II 6	11	80.5	8.5
69 II 9	13.5	77.5	9
69 III 6	14	80	6

Extensive antibody determinations, in which Gamma-Veinine preparations were compared with nondisaggregated gamma globulins, have demonstrated that the antibody activities of modified and original gamma globulins are practically identical (Table 2).

Gamma-Veinine has been used increasingly for several years and has been found to be extremely well tolerated. If Gamma-Veinine is stored

TABLE 2   Antibody Activities in Gamma Globulin and Gamma-Veinine

Antigen	Antibody Titers Measured by Agglutination or Neutralization	
	Gamma Globulin	Gamma-Veinine
Diphtheria	+++	+++
Tetanus	+++	+++
Pertussis	++	++
Typhoid O	++	+
Typhoid H	++	+
Paratyphoid	++	++
Staphylococci	+++	+++
Pneumococci	+++	+++
Escherichia coli	++	+
Streptolysin O	+++	+++
Varicella	++	++
Herpes simplex	++	++
Rubella	+++	+++
Measles	+++	+++
Infectious mononucleosis	++	++
Poliomyelitis, types I, II, and III	+++	+++
ECHO viruses	+++	+++
Mumps	+++	+++
Influenza	+++	+++
Smallpox	++	++

TABLE 3   Indications and Dosages for Gamma-Veinine

Disease	Dose, ml/kg of body weight
Hypogammaglobulinemia or agammaglobulinemia (acute phase)	1.0–2.0
Herpes zoster	1.0
Bacterial infections (e.g., sepsis caused by pneumococci, streptococci, staphylococci, *Escherichia coli*, Proteus, or Pseudomonas)	1.0–2.0
Recurrent infections (if antibody deficiency syndrome is suspected)	1.0–1.5
Measles encephalitis	2.0–3.0
Purulent meningitis	3–6 ml total dose, intrathecally
Temporary hypogammaglobulinemia, especially in premature infants	1.0–2.0 every 3 weeks

or heated at 60 C for 2 hr, no reaggregation occurs. The main fields of use for intravenously administrable Gamma-Veinine are:

1. Temporary hypogammaglobulinemia in premature births
2. Viral encephalitis (intrathecal application)
3. All cases in which gamma globulin should be given at short intervals over a long period (cytostatic therapy)
4. All cases in which large amounts of gamma globulin are necessary (acute septic general infections)

Because of the shortened half-life of gamma globulins disaggregated by pepsin, in comparison with normal gamma globulins, Gamma-Veinine is used more in therapy than in prophylaxis. Indications and dosages are shown in Table 3.

REFERENCE

1. Schultze, H. E., and G. Schwick. Über neue Möglichkeiten intravenöser Gammaglobulin-Applikation. Deutsch. Med. Wschr. 87:1643–1650, 1962.

DISCUSSION

DR. SMOLENS: What is the half-life of Gamma-Veinine?

DR. SCHWICK: The half-life is 4–6 days. As I mentioned, we do not like to give this preparation for prophylaxis, because of its short half-life. It has been given to agammaglobulinemic children. It was found that Gamma-Veinine has to be given every 2 weeks, instead of every 4 weeks, as with normal gamma globulin. That means that there is no linear correlation between the half-life of labeled Gamma-Veinine and its limit of protection.

DR. WARD: I wish to report our experience with gamma globulin, modified by the Swiss method, which has been added directly to blood before transfusion. We wanted to know whether the addition of gamma globulin had any effect on the incidence of posttransfusion hepatitis with jaundice. That is, could IgG in one-fifth the amount that had been shown to be effective in two previous studies, but modified for intravenous use, promote neutralization of hepatitis viruses before they passed the portal of entry, and thus prevent or modify the disease? We have studied this, since April 1965, with Dr. Ricardo Koch, in Santiago, Chile. Gamma globulin was modified by hydrolysis at pH 4 by Drs. Hessig, Isliker, Barandun, and Kistler at the Swiss Red Cross Blood Transfusion Service.

In the course of the study, this modified gamma globulin has been added to blood given to 1,500 patients, without a single adverse reaction. The subjects were women 20–75 years old admitted to various medical and surgical services of the Hospitale del Salvador in Santiago, Chile. To each unit of blood required by a patient whose hospital number ended with an even digit 10 ml of a 6% solution of modified gamma globulin was added. Those patients constituted group A. The gamma globulin was added to the blood 60–70 hr before transfusion. Group B consisted of patients whose record numbers ended with an odd digit and who needed a transfusion; they received blood alone and were the controls. Group C consisted of patients who were admitted to the same services at the same time but who received neither blood nor gamma globulin; they served as environmental or background hepatitis controls.

All the patients were examined. Blood was drawn right after transfusion and 30, 50, 70, 90, 120, and 150 days after transfusion. It was used to assess liver function and then frozen.

Over 4,000 patients were included in the study: 1,367 patients in group A, over 1,500 in group B, and about 1,400 in group C. Five patients in group A, 14 in group B, and only one in group C acquired hepatitis and were jaundiced.

Thirteen patients in group A, 10 in group B, and five in group C acquired hepatitis but were not jaundiced. The p value for these results (in this case, the difference between 5 and 14) is 0.05.

I should like to emphasize that there were four serious cases of hepatitis in group A—one with coma that ended fatally and three with precoma symptoms but eventual recovery—but no severe cases in group B.

IV
CELLULAR AND
CLINICAL ASPECTS OF
IMMUNOGLOBULINS

ROBERT A. GOOD

Immunoglobulin Deficiency Syndromes in Man

It is appropriate to discuss immunologic deficiency diseases by considering the cellular aspects that characterize them; the processes that we are concerned with are basically cellular processes.

In the development of understanding of the immunologic deficiency diseases of man, there has been a remarkable interplay between the experimental laboratory and the clinic, with the clinic providing the questions and the direction for the investigations and the laboratory providing at least approximations to answers.

CELLULAR DIFFERENTIATION

Some basic facts about the initiation of the immunologic process and its development are known. Evidence has accumulated to indicate that there is a basic progenitor cell that during embryonic development resides in the fetal liver and perhaps in the yolk sac and in adult life in the marrow of the bone. This lymphoid stem cell can be in a variety of microchemical environments and be induced by them to differentiate into different cell lines. The products of these cell lines are the hema-

191

topoietic elements that we recognize in the peripheral blood and in the connective and hematopoietic tissues of the body. Erythrocytes, granulocytes, platelets, eosinophils, and so on, are such products.

The prototype of cell-mediated immune responses is the tuberculin reaction, an example of delayed hypersensitivity. But this same process is also responsible for the recognition and rejection of "non-self," inasmuch as tissue homografts are rejected largely by the actions of the cells that mediate cellular immunity. These same cells also initiate but probably do not execute graft-versus-host reactions in man and experimental animals. They play a major role in the recognition and elimination of some viruses, fungi, and bacterial pathogens, like mycobacteria and other pathogens of low-grade virulence, and probably also constitute a line of defense against the development of malignant cell lines.

Lymphoid cells can be expanded indirectly by thymic influence, perhaps in a way analogous to the way erythropoietin can expand the erythrocyte population after the initial step in differentiation.

Thymic-dependent lymphocytes occupy in the peripheral lymphoid tissue areas that are distinct from those in which another set of lymphoid cells may be found. The other lymphoid cells seem also to develop from a basic stem cell, but they differentiate into a separable population of lymphocytes and plasma cells. I think the argument as to whether plasma cells or lymphocytes form antibody is no longer relevant; both lymphocytes and plasma cells form antibodies. Lymphocytes develop along a particular line of differentiation. In birds, this differentiation occurs in the bursa of Fabricius, a lymphoepithelial organ lying along the posterior end of the gastrointestinal tract. We do not know whether an equivalent organ exists in man. There is evidence that in some mammals this activity resides in lymphoid accumulations associated with gut epithelium, appendix, Peyer's patches, and sacculus rotundus. Other cells that can be recognized as belonging to this population are the cells of the germinal centers.

The thymus is the organ in which thymic-dependent cells develop. These cells are responsible for cell-mediated immunologic responses. In man, the thymus develops largely from the epithelial anlagen of the third and fourth pharyngeal pouches. In many animals, it develops much more broadly in the pharyngeal region from anlagen that represent the second through sixth pharyngeal pouches. The thymus is a composite organ, containing central lymphoid tissue, peripheral lymphoid elements, and cells in various stages of differentiation. The thymus stroma is unlike the stroma of most of the other lymphoid organs. It is epithelial in origin, and it has a stromal epithelial characteristic that can be differentiated from that of the lymph nodes, spleen, etc. Some components of the thymus are still poorly understood. Hassall's corpuscles seem to derive largely from ectodermal epithelium, whereas the basic stromal component is derived largely from the endodermal epithelium at the ectodermal–endodermal junction. But the thymus also contains blood vessels, and along the blood vessels are plasma cells and mature lymphocytes that have the capacity to exercise immunologic functions.

The thymus is the first organ to become truly lymphoid; its lymphoid tissue develops before that of the spleen and the lymph nodes.

Germinal centers develop in the far cortical regions of the thymus. Lymphocytes in these areas are more sessile than those in the deep cortical areas (the paracortical region). The far cortical regions are related functionally to the medullary cords, and it is in the medullary cords of the node that plasma cells are found. These plasma cells are derived from cells that are thymic-independent. Similarly, the deep cortical regions contain areas that are thymic-independent. Clearly, there are cells of thymic-dependent origin in regions called thymic-independent, and, conversely, thymic-independent cells in thymic-dependent regions. These are broad areas that are somewhat differentiated from one another, but not separable.

The bursa of Fabricius is not the avian equivalent of the thymus, inasmuch as birds have a well-developed thymus. Rather, it is a lymphoepithelial organ that is essential to development of the plasma-cell population; it seems to have nothing to do with the development of cell-mediated immunities.

There is evidence that a circulating cell is necessary for the development of the lymphocytes of the bursa of Fabricius. These lymphocytes become antigen-reactive within the bursa and emigrate to the peripheral lymphoid tissue. While in the bursa, their number expands within the germinal centers.

EXPERIMENTALLY INDUCED IMMUNOLOGIC DEFICIENCIES

Cooper, in our laboratory, irradiated chickens at hatching and took out either the bursa or the thymus. Animals that had been thymectomized when newly hatched lacked cells capable of executing cell-mediated im-

mune responses but retained intact the ability to synthesize immunoglobulins. Near-lethally irradiated bursectomized animals, however,
lacked cells in the germinal centers and lacked plasma cells. He produced
agammaglobulinemic chickens that could not form circulating antibodies. Recently, with Van Alten, we have taken out the bursa of
Fabricius at various stages of embryonic life and before hatching. The
earliest we can remove the bursa is at 15 days of embryonation in an
animal that has a 21-day embryonation period. Removal of the bursa at
day 15 produced agammaglobulinemic animals. Removal at day 19 prevented development of germinal centers but not of all plasma cells. The
animal formed 19S, but not 7S, immunoglobulins. The mechanism under-
lying this bursal influence has not yet been elucidated.

It has been shown with many animals that removal of the thymus immediately after birth prevents development of immunologic competence.
This has been demonstrated in mice, rats, hamsters, and rabbits. Thymectomized and irradiated animals do not, however, form antibodies to
all antigens. It is clear from the work of Mitchell, Miller, Nossal, Claman,
Talmage, and others that antibodies are not produced by thymic-
dependent or thymic-derived cells. The nature of the influence of
thymic-dependent cells on a thymic-dependent antibody response is
being investigated, but is best visualized in terms of the mechanism of
delivery of antigenic stimulation to the antigen-sensitive cells of the
thymic-independent system. After neonatal thymectomy and irradiation, the mouse has markedly deficient lymphoid cellularity of the deep
cortical areas of the node. It has well-developed far cortical regions and
medullary cords. It has plasma cells and, on antigenic stimulation, it
develops germinal centers.

Rabbits approximately 1 month old were deprived of one or several
lymphoid organs. They were irradiated at lethal dosages but were
kept alive with stem cells from fetal livers of rabbits. The only animals
that failed to develop a capacity for immune responsiveness were those
in which lymphoepithelial tissue along the posterior end of the gastrointestinal tract was removed. Animals lethally irradiated and given stem
cells developed far cortical regions, deep cortical regions, and plasma
cells. Animals lethally irradiated and thymectomized failed to rede-
velop cellular immunities and deep cortical areas. Animals that had been
lethally irradiated and had the lower intestinal lymphoid tissue removed
failed to develop far cortical regions, where germinal centers derive, and

plasma cells responded to primary antigenic stimulation, but they had fairly well-developed deep cortical areas.

IMMUNOLOGIC DEFICIENCY DISEASES OF MAN

With this as a background, let us consider the immunologic deficiency diseases of man. Many observations on these diseases antedated some of the experimental results outlined, but I chose to present them in the reverse order because it is only now that the immunologic deficiency diseases of man are becoming clear. We are beginning to understand them and to devise improvements in therapy. The lid of Pandora's box was lifted in 1952, when Bruton described patients whose circulation lacked gamma globulins but in whom most of the proteins in the classical electrophoretic pattern were present in normal amounts. Hitzig and Gitlin in Dr. Janeway's laboratory and others demonstrated that these patients lack not only IgG, but also IgM, IgA, IgE, and IgD. They fail to develop the immunoglobulin-producing cell system normally, and they cannot make antibodies in response to a variety of antigenic stimulations.

The form of this disease that I think is the most revealing is associated with an X-linked recessive genetic inherited trait. These patients are susceptible to infection—but largely infection with the high-grade pyogenic pathogens. If they are untreated, their lives are a succession of infections with pneumococci, hemophilus, streptococci, occasionally Pseudomonas, and, to a lesser extent, staphylococci. They are also susceptible to other infections. Given gamma globulin, they are free of infection with these pathogens.

These patients are able to resist some kinds of infection, such as viral infections. They can contract measles, but they recover from measles and resist recurrences. They will show immunity to measles in the absence of demonstrable antibody in their circulation. Similarly, they develop immunity to a variety of other viral infections. They are also more resistant to low-grade pyogenic pathogens than to the high-grade ones. They develop delayed hypersensitivity as well as normal persons. These patients have in their circulation lymphocytes that, if transferred to immunologically normal unimmunized recipients, will immunize the recipients with the cell-mediated immunity. They have the ability to develop immunity, but not the ability to form antibodies. They reject a skin homograft and show a second set rejection, but are slower at this than normal persons. We have seen the thymus in eight of these patients, and it is normal. These patients lack the lymphocyte population that is capable of developing plasma cells, but they have lymphocytes in their deep cortical regions. The tonsils of patients with Bruton agammaglobulinemia do not have germinal centers or plasma cells, but they have a lymphocyte population.

These patients develop malignancies and many other diseases with inordinate frequency. Among these diseases are mesenchymal diseases. They have rheumatoid arthritis and tenosynovitis and they have a tendency to develop vasculitis and possibly dermatomyositis. Their malignancies are generally in the thymus or in the thymic-dependent lymphocyte population. They are not generally susceptible to other forms of malignancy.

An opposite type of deficiency was described by DiGeorge, who interpreted a condition first observed by Harrington around the turn of the century in patients who had an endocrinologic abnormality—namely, hypocalcemic tetany of the newborn. But it is not the hypocalcemic tetany that prevents these patients from growing up and surviving. It is that they have failed to develop not only their parathyroid glands, but the other organ derived from the third and fourth pharyngeal pouches, namely, the thymus. These patients have normal levels of immunoglobulins and have plasma cells, and their far cortical regions contain lymphocytes that are capable of developing germinal centers. But their deep cortical regions are essentially lacking small lymphocytes. Their circulating lymphocyte populations are peculiar, in that, although they are roughly normal in number, the small lymphocytes are not normal in number. These patients cannot execute cell-mediated immunities. They do not reject a homograft and will not develop delayed hypersensitivity.

If these patients are given the thymus from an embryo, their lymphoid tissues and immunologic responses are reconstituted. Two such cases have been reported. Cleveland, with Humphrey, Kay, and others, was able to reconstitute one of these patients by thymic transplantation. After transplantation, the deep cortical areas enlarged and the total lymphocyte population began to accumulate; by 1 month, the patient was exhibiting vigorous cell-mediated immunity. He had many cells in the deep cortical areas and within 6 months had normal cell-mediated immunity and thymic-dependent lymphocyte population. August,

Rosen, and their co-workers in Boston have observed a similar case.

There are two perplexing things about these cases. One is the speed with which the first evidence of immune responsiveness to the lymphoid cells seems to be reconstituted after thymic transplantation. Another is the characteristics of the DiGeorge patient in the immediate neonatal period, when he is under maternal influence but does not have a thymus of his own.

Another form of immunologic deficiency disease of man that has told us a great deal is lymphopenic agammaglobulinemia. Waldenstrom and I have called this "Swiss agammaglobulinemia," because the original definition and most of the important discoveries relating to it were made in Switzerland by Tobler and Cottier and by Hitzig and Willi. These patients are extraordinarily susceptible to infection. They are susceptible to overwhelming viral infections, to fungal infections, and to persistent Candida infections. They may succumb to inoculation with live vaccinia virus, when they develop the disseminated vaccinia infection. They can become overwhelmingly infected with measles virus but do not show a skin rash; they do not express measles in the usual way. Their lymphoid tissue lacks lymphocytes in the far cortical areas, in the medullary cords, and in the deep cortical areas. Plasma cells and germinal centers are also lacking. These patients fail to develop and generally do not survive beyond 1 year of age.

This disease is transmitted as autosomal recessive, and it has been seen both in the United States and in Switzerland. There is a variant form of this disease that is X-linked recessive, and this was originally reported by Gitlin and Rosen. X-linked affected persons lack lymphoid cells and plasma cells, but they have a thymus that is almost entirely epithelial.

Many have tried to correct the defect in these patients with peripheral lymphoid cells, spleen, and blood transfusions. These patients are very susceptible and are often killed by a blood transfusion, because they cannot resist the graft-versus-host reaction. We attempted to correct the defect in one patient with stem cells that were derived from fetal liver and that we obtained from Humphrey and Kay. We succeeded in reconstituting him. He had kept a skin graft for 2 months before stem-cell infusion, but he rejected it after the administration of the stem cells. However, the patient died from a graft-versus-host reaction.

We had the opportunity to treat a patient with the X-linked variant
of this disease, a little boy from the family described by Gitlin and
Rosen. We had been experimenting on mice with a system of transplantation immunity in which recipients and donors are matched at the
H-2 histocompatibility locus only. With this system, adults can be made
tolerant to the cells of the donor. We could not induce a graft-versus-
host reaction if the recipient did not differ from the donor at the H-2
histocompatibility locus, even if the cell donor had been immunized.

We thought it would be interesting to transplant into a patient cells
from a donor within the family. It has become apparent that both men
and experimental animals inherit their histocompatibility characteristics
according to the pattern of a single major genetic locus at which multiple alleles may operate. In that case, the chances of getting a match at
that locus in the general population are very small. In the family in
question, the patient had four sisters, one of whom matched him in all
the antigens of the HL-A locus, except for one disputed antigen, and
their cells matched in mixed leukocyte cultures. We therefore gave the
patient stem cells from the female donor. He was promptly reconstituted
immunologically and developed a graft-versus-host reaction. He developed a skin rash, had hepatosplenomegaly, and developed hemolytic
anemia, presumably because the donor differed from the recipient at
the ABO locus (O cells to A). The graft-versus-host reaction subsided,
the fever and the hepatosplenomegaly went away, and the hemolytic
anemia went away. The child remained completely reconstituted immunologically. Reactivity to phytohemagglutinin became positive; it
had been negative. The patient became capable of reacting to dinitro-
fluorobenzene; he had not been. Small lymphocytes appeared in the
circulation. He began forming anti-B isohemagglutinins. Immunoglobulin levels rose to normal within 2–3 months, and secretory IgA, which
had not been present before, was produced. He even developed a thymic
shadow in the mediastinum. But he developed antibodies to his A cells,
because the donor's lymphocytes were in his marrow; 25% of the cells
in the marrow were donor cells, which could be identified by female
karyotype. He had hemolytic anemia first, and then a complete aplastic
pancytopenia; all the cells of the hematopoietic system were lacking. We
transplanted more marrow from the same donor, and promptly reestab-
lished hematopoietic cells. The patient now is chimeric: all the cells in

his marrow are female cells, and all the cells in his peripheral blood are A cells with female karyotype.

Diseases of immunologic deficiency can be considered as a block in the development of stem cells, and this has been observed in the Duval syndrome, in which erythrocytes and granulocytes, as well as lymphoid cells, fail to develop. Or they can be considered as a failure of development of lymphoid stem cells, a result of either the X-linked recessive or the autosomal recessive form of inheritance of thymic alymphoplasia. Finally, they can be considered as a failure of development of the thymus, and that is the DiGeorge syndrome. Moreover, interferences along the line of development may give some of the confusing, incomplete pictures of immunologic diseases.

There are, furthermore, patients who are immunologically defective and have a tumor in the mediastinum. These are stromal epithelial thymomas, which do not contain many lymphoid cells. Removal of the thymoma does not correct the immunologic deficiency. These patients seem to lose the cells of the thymic-dependent system progressively. What causes this, what the thymic tumor is, what its response is, and what its response means are questions that remain unanswered.

Finally, there are patients with late-occurring immunologic deficiencies. These patients may have hyperplastic lymphoid tissues and marked developments of germinal centers. Their deficiencies are expressed as deficiencies of cell-mediated, as well as humoral, immunities. They cannot reject homografts normally, and they have all sorts of bizarre immunoglobulin patterns. Their gamma globulins look like myeloma proteins, with restricted heterogeneity.

These are examples of the immunologic deficiency diseases of man. They are only the primary immunologic deficiencies; there are also secondary deficiencies—those which occur in Hodgkin's disease, in which there is a primary deficit of functions of cell-mediated immunity; those which occur in myeloma, in which there is a primary deficit of humoral immunity and immunoglobulin synthesis; and the diseases in the leukemias.

I have tried to present an approach to the study of the immunologic deficiency diseases of man that is useful because it classifies the deficits that one observes and presents possible systems for correcting these deficits.

DISCUSSION

DR. ROSEN: Have you had a chance to study some patients with the Swiss type of agammaglobulinemia who have immunoglobulins in their serum and who can form antibodies?

DR. GOOD: Yes. In the late-occurring hypogammaglobulinemias, there are tremendous variations from time to time within a patient, and from patient to patient within a family, in level of immunoglobulins and in degrees of deficit of cell-mediated immunity and humoral immunities. That is also true in patients who have maldevelopment of the thymic system. Among patients with lymphopenic hypogammaglobulinemia, you may see some who have nearly normal levels of lymphocytes, at least at some times, and some who have gamma globulins and form antibodies somewhat feebly. In a few instances, they may even have hypergammaglobulinemia, for example, of IgM. I think, though, that they generally have deficits of both the antibody-producing apparatus and cellular immunity.

DR. POULIK: Do you have any opinion as to why patients with hemolytic anemia lack IgA? We have about 27 cases of hemolytic anemia in children, of whom many have absence of IgA.

DR. GOOD: That may very well be a signal that there is something wrong with the development of the lymphoid and immunologic systems. It may be a very delicate signal. There is no question that in patients with rheumatoid arthritis there is frequently an absence of IgA. The same is true of patients with a variety of mesenchymal diseases and hemolytic anemia. I do not know whether this has to do with the fact that what we have thought to be mesenchymal diseases are in reality infections, or whether it is a signal of what Dr. Fudenberg and I have emphasized—that when there is a deficit of immunologic function, there is very likely to be a perturbation of the immunologic adaptation with the development of autoimmune phenomenon. But I consider the lack of IgA often as a signal of the immunologic malfunction that needs further analysis.

DR. BRUNELL: Have you been able to correlate any of these immunologic defects with maintenance of viruses in a latent state, as manifested by recurrence of herpes simplex or herpes zoster in a particular group of patients?

DR. GOOD: Our observations about latent viruses are not critical, because we do not have enough information. We have, however, observed that patients with deficits of cell-mediated immunities seem to be fair game for progressive viral infection without expressing them in the normal way. Patients with skin lesions who have become exposed to the virus may not recover from herpes simplex infection. One of the most interesting groups of patients in this regard consists of those who constantly have skin lesions, such as patients with the Wiskott-Aldrich syndrome. This is a very interesting disease, in which the deficit is primarily in the handling of some polysaccharide antigens. But there are also other deficits.

I think in this instance crucial information derives from experimental animals. If, in mice, you selectively depress cell-mediated immunity with antilymphocyte serum, you markedly shorten the interval and increase the incidence of latent viruses of the oncogenic type. This could be true with the polyoma virus in neonatally thymectomized mice or mice treated with antilymphocyte serum. It is true of a number of other oncogenic agents. We think the maintenance of latent viral infections, preventing them from expressing themselves (at least as malignancies), is related to cell-mediated immunologic function.

J. F. SOOTHILL

Treatment of Immunoglobulin Deficiency Syndromes

There are seven possible lines of treatment for specific immunity deficiency.[23] Some entail replacement supplementation or passive transfer of defective systems and are best considered in terms of the different patterns of deficiency of immunity mechanisms—the different immunity deficiency syndromes summarized in Figure 1. Some are related to prevention or treatment of etiologic processes and are best considered in terms of etiologic mechanism (Table 1), although their particular application in each of the various immunity deficiency diseases, extensively reviewed recently,[3] is, with rare exceptions, open to conjecture. The classifications, as presented here, do not consider the possibilities of local deficiency of specific immunity mechanisms, such as deficiency of secretory IgA, or the treatment of deficiencies of nonspecific immunity mechanisms. The deficiencies are frequently complex, and therapeutic success can sometimes provide evidence, of the classic passive-transfer type, of the particular defect resulting in symptoms; but it is possible that immunologic mechanisms overlap, so that, although one may normally predominate in conferring immunity to a particular infection, another may well be able to take over from it in the event of

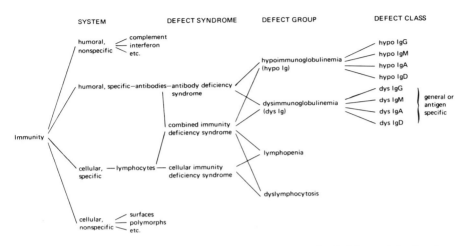

FIGURE 1   A functional or syndrome classification of the immunity deficiency states, based on the current concept of the duality of specific immunity. (Adapted from Soothill.[23])

its deficiency. Such overlapping may explain why deficiencies of isolated immunity mechanisms are often symptomless. An important exception is the phenomenon of chronic granulomatous disease, in which the failure of bacterial killing of phagocytosed organisms is associated with sequestering of the organisms, surviving in polymorphs, from specific immunity mechanisms and from antibiotics,[22] so that a failure of one mechanism indirectly invalidates others, although they are functioning normally. This illustrates the importance of "compartment" concepts in approaches to the treatment of immunity deficiency. Clearly, immunoglobulin treatment would be of no value here.

CHEMOTHERAPY OF INDIVIDUAL INFECTIONS

Antibiotics were recognized by Gitlin and Janeway[10] as effective in individual infections in hypogammaglobulinemia. With some exceptions, this generalization may be accepted for the whole range of immunity deficiency, but such measures do not avoid chronic tissue damage, which in itself results in liability to repeated infections, disability, and death.

TABLE 1   Etiologic Classification of Immunity Deficiency States[a]

Genetic
     Sex-linked → ADS
     ? Autosomal recessive (? other) → ADS, CIDS, and combined IDS
     Reticular dysgenesis
     Aldrich's disease
     With ataxia-telangiectasia
     DiGeorge's disease (with hypoparathyroidism)
     Late-onset ADS with familial immunologic abnormalities

Physiologic
     Neonatal IgM and IgA ADS
     IgG trough

Transient ADS

Loss
     Urine, gut, etc. → ADS
     Experimental thoracic duct cannulation → CIDS

Environmental
     Drugs, poisons, x-rays → ADS or combined IDS
     Congenital rubella → ADS (? combined IDS)

? Autoimmune (? genetic)

Associated with neoplasia → ADS, CIDS, and combined IDS

---

[a]Adapted from Soothill[23]; ADS = antibody deficiency syndrome; CIDS = cellular immunity deficiency syndrome; IDS = immunity deficiency state.

PROPHYLACTIC CHEMOTHERAPY

The role of prophylactic antibiotics has not been explored in great detail. It must be suspected that the special susceptibility of patients with deficient immunity to molds may arise not only from the immunity deficiency, but also as a result of the continued use of antibiotics.

REPLACEMENT OF GAMMA GLOBULIN

Gitlin and Janeway[10] recorded an impression of obvious benefit from injecting gamma globulin intramuscularly into patients with hypogamma-globulinemia. The benefit seems to be confined largely to patients with antibody deficiency syndrome but relatively little deficiency of cellular immunity. Severe forms of combined immunity deficiency are fatal, in spite of continued gamma globulin treatment. The Medical Research Council (MRC) Working Party on Hypogammaglobulinaemia has made a long-term study of the effect of gamma globulin in patients with less than 200 mg/100 ml of IgG (or less than 100 mg/100 ml in patients less than 6 months old). Patients with obvious secondary hypogamma-globulinemia were excluded. In the study, a dose equivalent to Gitlin and Janeway's (although more frequently administered) of 0.025 g/kg of body weight per week was compared with a dose of 0.05 g in treatment periods of 4 months or a year on each dose. In spite of the heterogeneity of patients and the decision to seek a purely dose-related effect to obviate an untreated control group, there was significant evidence of difference between the two groups, including a difference of concentration of C-reactive protein in the serum, a nonspecific quantitative index of incidence of infection.[17] In spite of this effect, there was a considerable mortality, mainly in girls, which probably resulted from the fact that many had a considerable degree of cellular immunity deficiency, in addition to antibody deficiency.

Far greater than the demonstrated difference of effect of the two dose periods was the impression of improvement after the onset of gamma globulin treatment in many patients, as had been reported in previous studies. It is impossible to be sure that such improvement is neither the effect of the spontaneous improvement likely in patients who survive a particularly bad period (which has led to diagnosis) of a chronic fluctuating illness, nor the effect of more rigorous medical care, but I believe that this probably is an effect of gamma globulin treatment.

Meningitis was common before diagnosis, but only two patients had meningitis after gamma globulin treatment was started. Hobbs et al.[16] have suggested that meningitis is particularly common in patients with isolated IgM deficiency, and postulate that the efficient IgM-complement-dependent bactericidal antibody in the blood compartment prevents the bacteremic episode. In this series, meningitis was confined to patients lacking IgM antibodies (whether the IgM was quantitatively or qualitatively defective). It is therefore surprising that the injected gamma globulin, which contained virtually no IgM, appeared to be successful in preventing recurrent meningitis in our patients. Perhaps this is an example of the overlapping of different immunity mechanisms.

Gitlin *et al.*[11] have suggested that the low concentration of IgM present in newborn children may be the reason for their special susceptibility to coliform infections. If my deduction from the meningitis incidence is sound, there might be a case for large doses of gamma globulin here, too, but it seems that abnormal susceptibility to infection due to lack of secretory IgA is not likely to be amenable to any form of long-term prophylactic replacement. Gamma globulin injections lead to effective serum concentrations of IgG because of the long half-life of IgG. IgG is not likely to be of use in secondary hypogammaglobulinemia due to loss or in the immunoglobulin deficiency of myotonia atrophica, in which there is accelerated catabolism.[27] Transient hypogammaglobulinemia, so clearly described by Gitlin and Janeway,[10] can be associated with severe infection, which may lead to chronic damage or even death. Protection of children with this condition is perhaps the most important field of treatment in immunity deficiency, in view of their long-term prospect of good health; injection of gamma globulin probably has a place. That at least some of these patients are close relatives of patients with hypogammaglobulinemia of other than the sex-linked form may permit early recognition of risk.[24] Hobbs and Davis[15] have reported evidence that gamma globulin injections into very premature babies, born before the placental transfer of IgG reaches effective levels, may be of value.

Reactions were rare in the experience of the MRC Working Party series (85 in 40,000 injections), but they were severe enough to warrant review of continued gamma globulin treatment in those affected. A brief description of the reactions has been published, as has the finding that reactions were significantly more rare in boys with affected male relatives and in patients with lymphatic leukemia who were treated with identical material in an identical fashion.[26]

The pain of injection of gamma globulin is a problem, and the possibility of using intravenous IgG also needs consideration.

REPLACEMENT WITH IMMUNOLOGICALLY COMPETENT CELLS

The failure of graft rejection in patients with severe combined immunity deficiency led to the consideration of the possibility that grafting of immunologically competent tissue might be a satisfactory mode of treatment.[11,13,19] Early attempts with lymph nodes and other tissue met with only limited success; but when it was suspected that patients with severe combined immunity deficiency were suffering from thymus deficiency, attempts were made to graft thymuses to such patients. Graft-versus-host disease has been a significant problem,[20] although this can to some extent be precluded by use of fetal tissue, which may produce some evidence of return of both cellular and humoral immunity function to the recipient. Death of the recipient, however, usually follows these procedures.[14] Recently reported successes[1,6] with fetal thymus grafts in DiGeorge's syndrome (human thymus deficiency[7]) have added impetus to this approach and the clear difference in the results in severe combined immunity deficiency provides support for the view[12,23] that the latter may be a stem-cell defect, rather than thymus deficiency. The thymus abnormality is presumably disuse dystrophy, secondary to lack of cells for the thymus to work on—thymus grist. This is confirmed by the recently reported success of transplantation of closely tissue-matched related bone marrow into a patient with severe combined immunity deficiency[9]; presumably, there was restoration of immunologic competence and the development of a radiologic thymus shadow, which occurred as a result of the graft. Graft-versus-host disease remains a major problem in such treatment, and precise tissue matching, cross-matching using the mixed-lymphocyte reaction, attempts at enhancement with specific antibodies to any particularly dangerous antigen system that may operate, and elimination of mature lymphocytes from the graft should all help to minimize this risk. The report by Bach et al.[2] of similar success in a patient with Wiskott-Aldrich syndrome (although in this patient the graft did not result in restoration of the platelet count) suggests that this measure may have a role in a number of the disease processes associated with cellular immunity deficiency, whether combined or isolated.[8,21] In all such cases, the risk of graft-versus-host disease after blood transfusion must always be recalled, and the handling of blood used for this purpose must be appraised, including aging, cell separation, and radiation.

IMMUNIZATION

Immunization would be irrational in a person with no capacity to mount specific immunity responses. But, because the available evidence suggests that all immunity deficiencies are indeed quantitative phenomena, all safe immunizations should be undertaken. Progressive necrotic vaccinia, in cellular or combined immunity deficiency,[8] generalized nonprogressive vaccinia in IgM deficiency,[5] and disseminated BCG infection[4] point to the risk of live vaccines for such patients. Our present tests of different mechanisms and our knowledge of their relevance for protection against each individual infection are not yet adequate to justify the use of any live vaccines in any patients with immunity deficiency, unless direct exposure to infection creates a very strong special case for doing so.

TREATMENT OF CAUSATIVE MECHANISMS

In secondary immunity deficiency, treatment of etiologic mechanisms may be possible—e.g., with steroids in the nephrotic syndrome, or cytotoxic drugs in leukemia, myelomatosis, and possibly autoimmune immunity deficiency.[18]

PREVENTION

Until recently, a eugenic approach seemed to be the only possible way of preventing immunity deficiency, but the association of congenital rubella with IgG deficiency[25] and abnormal susceptibility to other infection leads to the possibility of eliminating this condition by immunizing all susceptible women against rubella.

REFERENCES

1. August, C. S., F. S. Rosen, R. M. Filler, C. A. Janeway, B. Markowski, and H. E. Kay. Implantation of a foetal thymus, restoring immunological competence in a patient with thymic aplasia (DiGeorge's syndrome). Lancet 2:1210–1211, 1968.
2. Bach, F. H., R. J. Albertine, P. Joo, J. L. Anderson, and M. M. Bortin. Bone-marrow transplantation in a patient with the Wiskott-Aldrich syndrome. Lancet 2:1364–1369, 1968.
3. Bergsma, D., and R. A. Good, Eds. Immunologic Deficiency Diseases in Man. Birth Defects Original Article Series, Vol. IV, No. 1. New York: The National Foundation, 1968. 473 pp.

4. Bouton, J., D. Mainwaring, and R. W. Smithells. B.C.G. dissemination in congenital hypo-gammaglobulinaemia. Brit. Med. J. 1:1512–1515, 1963.
5. Chandra, R. K., B. Kaveramma, and J. F. Soothill. Generalized non-progressive vaccinia associated with IgM deficiency. Lancet 1:687–689, 1969.
6. Cleveland, W. W., B. J. Fogel, W. T. Brown, and H. E. Kay. Foetal thymic transplant in a case of DiGeorge's syndrome. Lancet 2:1211–1214, 1968.
7. DiGeorge, A. M. Congenital absence of the thymus and its immunologic consequences: Concurrence with congenital hypoparathyroidism. Birth Defects, Orig. Artic. Series 4:116–121, 1968.
8. Fulginiti, V. A., C. H. Kempe, W. E. Hathaway, D. S. Pearlman, O. F. Sieber, Jr., J. J. Eller, J. J. Joyner, Sr., and A. Robinson. Progressive vaccinia in immunologically deficient individuals. Birth Defects, Orig. Artic. Series 4:129–145, 1968.
9. Gatti, R. A., H. J. Meuwissen, H. D. Allen, R. Hong, and R. A. Good. Immunological re-constitution of sex-linked lymphopenic immunological deficiency. Lancet 2:1366–1369, 1968.
10. Gitlin, D., and C. A. Janeway. Agammaglobulinemia. Congenital, acquired and transient forms. Progr. Hemat. 1:318–329, 1956.
11. Gitlin, D., F. S. Rosen, and C. A. Janeway. The thymus and other lymphoid tissues in congenital agammaglobulinemia. II. Delayed hypersensitivity and homograft survival in a child with thymic alymphoplasia. Pediatrics 33:711–720, 1964.
12. Good, R. A., R. D. Peterson, D. Y. Perey, J. Finstad, and M. D. Cooper. The immunologi-cal deficiency diseases of man: consideration of some questions asked by these patients with an attempt at classification. Birth Defects, Orig. Artic. Series 4:17–34, 1968.
13. Good, R. A., R. L. Varco, J. B. Aust, and S. J. Zak. Transplantation studies in patients with agammaglobulinemia. Ann. N.Y. Acad. Sci. 64:882–924, 1957.
14. Hitzig, W. H., H. E. Kay, and H. Cottier. Familial lymphopenia with agammaglobu-linemia: an attempt at treatment by implantation of fetal thymus. Lancet 2:151–154, 1965.
15. Hobbs, J. R., and J. A. Davis. Serum γ G-globulin levels and gestational age in premature babies. Lancet 1:757–759, 1967.
16. Hobbs, J. R., R. D. Milner, and P. J. Watt. Gamma-M deficiency predisposing to menin-gococcal septicaemia. Brit. Med. J. 4:583–586, 1967.
17. Hypogammaglobulinaemia in the United Kingdom. Summary report of a Medical Research Council Working-Party. Lancet 1:163–168, 1969.
18. Kretschmer, R., C. A. Janeway, and F. S. Rosen. Immunologic amnesia. Study of an 11-year-old girl with recurrent severe infections associated with dysgammaglobulinemia, lymphopenia and lymphocytotoxic antibody, resulting in loss of immunologic memory. Pediat. Res. 2:7–16, 1968.
19. Martin, C. M., J. B. Waite, and N. B. McCullough. Antibody protein synthesis by lymph nodes homotransplanted to a hypogammaglobulinemic adult. J. Clin. Invest. 36:405–421, 1957.
20. Miller, M. E. Graft-vs.-host reactions in man with special reference to thymic dysplasia. Brith Defects, Orig. Artic. Series 4:257–263, 1968.
21. Nezelof, C. Thymic dysplasia with normal immunoglobulins and immunologic deficiency: pure alymphocytosis. Birth Defects, Orig. Artic. Series 4:104–112, 1968.
22. Quie, P. G., J. G. White, B. Holmes, and R. A. Good. In vitro bactericidal capacity of human polymorphonuclear leukocytes: diminished activity in chronic granulomatous disease of childhood. J. Clin. Invest. 46:668–679, 1967.
23. Soothill, J. F. Immunity deficiency syndromes. J. Roy. Coll. Physicians 2:67–74, 1967.

24. Soothill, J. F. Immunoglobulins in first-degree relatives of patients with hypogamma-globulinaemia. Transient hypogammaglobulinaemia: a possible manifestation of heterozygosity. Lancet 1:1001–1003, 1968.
25. Soothill, J. F., K. Hayes, and J. A. Dudgeon. The immunoglobulins in congenital rubella. Lancet 1:1385–1388, 1966.
26. Soothill, J. F., L. E. Hill, and D. S. Rowe. A quantitative study of the immunoglobulins in the antibody deficiency syndrome. Birth Defects, Orig. Artic. Series 4:71–79, 1968.
27. Wochner, R. D., G. Drews, W. Strober, and T. A. Waldmann. Accelerated breakdown of immunoglobulin G (IgG) in myotonic dystrophy: A hereditary error of immunoglobulin catabolism. J. Clin. Invest. 45:321–329, 1966.

DISCUSSION

DR. PAINTER: Is the gamma globulin pure IgG or is it commercial gamma globulin, which would contain perhaps 5% of IgM? Would the protection against meningococci be due to this residual IgM in the preparation?

DR. SOOTHILL: The material was the human gamma globulin prepared by the Lister Institute initially by the ether fractionation technique of Keckwick and MacKay, and later by the alcohol method of Cohn. There is, of course, a small amount of IgM in it, but IgM was not detectable, by sensitive immunochemical methods, in the blood of the patients who received it, who did not have any detectable IgM beforehand.

DR. ALEXANDER: Is there any evidence from the animal model or from man of interference with or blocking of interferon-inducing agents with regard to the viral producers? Has production of interferon been considered in the infections of man in these immunodeficient states?

DR. SOOTHILL: I have no data on this.

DR. GOOD: In patients with the different kinds of immunologic deficiencies that I outlined whom we and others have studied, interferon production seems to be adequate. It seems to be inducible with the inducing agents, and it seems to be produced as a consequence of viral infection.

H. HUGH FUDENBERG

Sensitization to Immunoglobulins and Hazards of Gamma Globulin Therapy

In this presentation of the hazards of gamma globulin therapy, the anaphylactic reactions that sometimes occur after intravenous administration of Cohn's fraction II will not be considered. These reactions are characterized by anxiety, blotching of the face, constricted feeling in the chest, muscular pain, fever, nausea and vomiting, and, rarely, collapse. They can occur in a person who receives gamma globulin for the first time intravenously. Similar reactions occur in persons who have become sensitized to gamma globulin.

Sensitization to gamma globulin occurs in persons who have received injections of gamma globulin and make antibodies to it. The first type of sensitization described by Henny and Ellis is caused by formation of antibodies against antigenic determinants of aggregated gamma globulin. These antibodies fail to react with native gamma globulin, but instead react with the 11S component. In three of six patients with hypogammaglobulinemia in one study, antibodies developed to the 11S IgG component. One of these patients had a severe reaction after intramuscular administration of Cohn's fraction II. Presumably, these reactions do not occur in children with congenital agammaglobulinemia, who lack antibodies. In our experience, these antibodies to aggregated gamma

211

globulin are not manifested in persons with gamma globulin levels of less than 100 mg/100 ml, but are expressed in those with levels greater than 200 mg/100 ml.

The second type of sensitization also results in the formation of antibodies that exhibit adverse biologic reactions. These are antibodies to genetic determinants of gamma globulin, the so-called Gm factors. Immunization with gamma globulin (of foreign genetic type) may result in the elaboration of anti-Gm factors; if large amounts of plasma of appropriate Gm type are later administered, homologous antibody may react with it to produce symptoms suggesting severe transfusion reaction. These reactions were also observed when plasma containing IgA was given to sensitized persons. These observations defined genetic determinants on the a chains of IgA.

As is well known, sera containing antibodies to human IgG have been used in defining genetic determinants on γ chains. These factors genetically determined the subclasses of IgG. It seemed, by analogy, that reagents that reacted with genetic antigens and IgA could be useful in defining the genetic controls of IgA.

Sera were obtained from 100 normal adult volunteers and from 150 patients suffering from a variety of disorders, including 22 with repeated sinopulmonary infections, 12 with idiopathic acquired agammaglobulinemia, 12 with IgG myeloma, 12 with Waldenstrom's macroglobulinemia, and 30 with ataxia-telangiectasia. Immunoglobulin levels were determined by radial diffusion.

For the serologic test system, we used inert indicator erythrocytes to which various antigens had been coupled. These antigens included proteins derived from sera containing 12 IgA myelomas, 12 IgG myelomas, normal IgG from persons of various Gm and Inv types, and 12 Waldenström's macroglobulinemias.

Twelve purified IgA myelomas (containing both the major and minor subgroups, that is, IgA1 and IgA2, and both κ and λ L chains), pooled macroglobulins, κ and λ Bence Jones proteins, normal L chains, a_2 macroglobulins, and transferrin were coated on human group O cells with chromic chloride. Sera were screened for antibodies to IgA at a 1 : 4 dilution by direct agglutination of the panel of coats. Agglutinators of any one protein were tested for specificity by inhibition of agglutination with the panel of proteins cited above.

The AB sera used as controls included pooled normal sera and indi-

vidual normal sera in which the IgA was isolated, commercial Cohn's
fraction II, IgM, Bence Jones proteins, pooled L chains from IgG, and
serum from a person with selective deficiency of IgA. These sera failed
to inhibit IgA–anti-IgA reactions.

Titrations are done with microtiter plates. The trays are incubated
for an hour, spun in a refrigerated centrifuge, and allowed to incline at
60 deg for 15 min. The difference between agglutination and nonagglu-
tination is easily distinguished: a smooth button indicates agglutination;
when there is no agglutination or agglutination is inhibited, the cells
streak to the bottom of the tray. One can test 24 sera at one time in
one plate.

In general, the anti-IgA sera could be divided into two groups, one
that agglutinated all IgA coats (a class-specific anti-IgA), and one that
agglutinated only some IgA coats.

These agglutinators were tested for specificity. It was shown that,
in each instance, the agglutination system was inhibited by homologous
coats; with the class-specific coats, agglutination was inhibited by all
normal sera. The agglutinating factors were antibodies, by the following
criteria: (1) they had gamma globulin mobility in a starch block, and
(2) on Sephadex columns, they eluted with either the first (IgM) peak
or the second (IgG) peak.

During this study, it became apparent that persons with IgA antibodies, especially those with class-specific anti-IgA, had a high incidence
of anaphylactic reactions to gamma globulin. One typical patient, a
40-year-old woman with refractory normoblast anemia, who is receiving
three to four units of cells each month, had an anaphylactic reaction
with diffuse skin rash, abdominal and lumbar pain, anxiety, nausea,
headache, and tachycardia. When her serum was tested, she was shown
to have antibodies against the IgA of one member of the panel. After
she volunteered for experimental transfusion, she was given 15 ml of
blood containing the IgA to which she had antibodies. The anaphylactic
symptoms were directly reproduced. In contrast, when she was given
50 ml of blood from a donor who had no IgA (with selective deficiency
of IgA), she had no reaction. She has since been receiving cells free of
plasma, washed in the cytoagglomerator of Huggins, and has had no
more reactions.

Another patient had no previous history of blood transfusion or
gamma globulin injection; she had had one abortion and two normal

pregnancies. She received three units of blood during and after hysterectomy. During transfusion of the last unit, she complained of extreme discomfort, severe headache, pain in the chest and back, and a feeling of impending doom. She had an obvious bronchial wheezing, abdominal cramps, and a diffuse erythematous rash. This rash is characteristic in patients with IgA–anti-IgA reactions. Her pretransfusion serum had no antibodies to erythrocytes, platelets, or leukocytes, but did have potent monospecific IgA antibodies. The two units that produced no reaction were compatible in the IgA system, but the unit that produced the symptoms was incompatible in the IgA system, as shown by inhibition of agglutination.

Of 250 normal adults, approximately 1–2% had antibodies to IgA. These antibodies had a limited specificity and reacted with some IgA coats, but not others. Of 32 persons with ataxia-telangiectasia—many of whom had no IgA, most of whom had deficient IgA, and only one or two of whom had normal or increased levels of IgA—class-specific antibodies were found in 13. Of 18 patients with transplanted kidneys, only one was found to have antibodies to IgA. Of 55 patients who received an average of 12 units of blood each during open-heart surgery, nine had anti-IgA antibodies, and they were of limited specificity. Two persons with dysgammaglobulinemia (IgA absent but IgG or IgM normal or high) were studied. They had received Cohn's fraction II. They both had anti-IgA antibodies and experienced severe reactions after administration of gamma globulin.

Of 27 patients exhibiting anaphylactoid transfusion reactions, 24 had anti-IgA antibodies. One of the 27 sera tested showed some inhibition patterns consistent with polymorphism. More than 95% of sera of Caucasians, 40% of sera of Negroes, and 38% of sera of Japanese inhibited the agglutination system called Am-1 (analogous to Gm-1). Family studies disclosed that this was compatible with simple Mendelian genetic inheritance. For example, an Am(1+) subject is heterozygous if one parent is Am(1−). If he marries an Am(1−) person, half their children will be Am(1+), and half Am(1−). The frequency of Am-1 in a family seems to be what would be expected if the trait were a simple genetic trait.

Transfusion reactions can occur when an Am(1−) person receives Am(1+) blood. Some persons with transfusion reactions have never re-

ceived plasma but had received Red Cross gamma globulin. Immunoelectrophoresis of the Red Cross gamma globulin used showed that the
material contained a considerable amount of IgA.

Because anti-IgG reactions are much rarer, it would seem advisable
either to eliminate IgA from the preparations, or to label the products
that contain IgA.

A person may also become sensitized to IgG if his ability to make
antibodies is not impaired. Of 12 agammaglobulinemic patients who
received either gamma globulin injections or, recently, whole plasma
(at intervals of 3 weeks for gamma globulin or 2 months for whole
plasma), none formed antibodies to IgG. However, of 13 hypogammaglobulinemic patients who were given gamma globulin repeatedly, 10
formed agglutinating antibodies to IgG. These were anti-Gm antibodies.
Four of nine children who received Cohn's fraction II because of
"allergy" also formed antibodies to gamma globulin. Of 35 newborns
who were exchange-transfused at birth, 13 formed antibodies to Gm
determinants, whereas, of their 28 normal sibling controls, only two
had such antibodies.

To assess whether anti-Gm antibodies have any deleterious consequences when corresponding Gm factors are present in infused blood,
three volunteers were each given 125 ml of Gm-incompatible plasma—
the same amount of plasma that an infant gets in an exchange transfusion. One immediately made anti-Gm(a) antibodies at a titer of 160.
The other two made no antibodies, but, when they were given 0.1 ml
of the same plasma subcutaneously, they made anti-Gm(b) and anti-
Gm(f) antibodies, showing that a minimum of two exposures is sufficient to produce anti-Gm antibodies.

We studied a hemophiliac who had received many units of plasma
over a period of several years. Recently, he developed anaphylactic reactions to some plasma, but not to others. We gave him four units of
Gm(a–) plasma, because he had anti-Gm(a) antibodies, after plasmapheresis of four units of his own blood. He had no fall in the titer of
anti-Gm(a) antibodies and had no symptoms. He was given four units
of Gm-incompatible plasma 24 hr later. His antibody titer dropped
from 128 to zero within a half-hour. He had alarming symptoms, generalized rash, abdominal pain, tachycardia, and a feeling of impending
doom. The reaction was stopped with epinephrine, cortisone, and anti-

histamines. His antibody titer remained zero for 3 weeks, and then rose to 2. At this point, he was given 1,000 ml of Gm-incompatible plasma. His antibody titer dropped from 2 to zero. He had very slight symptoms, manifest by circumoral tingling and hives. There is no doubt that the anti-Gm reaction's severity is related to the amount of plasma administered. Presumably, this reaction would be negligible except in hemophiliacs, who receive large amounts of plasma at one time.

Anti-IgA or anti-Gm antibodies in the absence of transfusions or anti-gamma globulin administration can be acquired in two ways. An infant may be immunized *in utero* by maternal gamma globulin, or a mother may be immunized by the gamma globulin produced by the fetus. The latter possibility has been demonstrated. It is equivalent to the situation that causes hemolytic disease in the newborn, when an Rh-negative mother gives birth to an Rh-positive child and consequently makes anti-Rh antibodies. In this case, a Gm(a–) mother gives birth to a Gm(a+) child and consequently makes anti-Gm(a) antibodies.

That was shown to have happened in my family. Blood was obtained from me and my wife before, during, and after each of four pregnancies. I am heterozygous Gm(a+b+), and my wife is homozygous Gm(b+), Gm(a–) (b is used here to define the whole Gmb phenotype, i.e., b_0, b_1, b_3, etc.). During the first three pregnancies, there were no agglutinators present in my wife's serum. The infants were Gm(a–). During the fourth pregnancy, however, anti-Gm(a) antibodies developed, and the cordblood serum was Gm(a+). Antibodies appeared in my wife during the seventh month of fetal intrauterine life and persisted until termination of pregnancy. They disappeared shortly after pregnancy, when the antigenic stimulus was removed. What other conclusions can we draw, other than that this Gm(a–) mother who gave birth to a Gm(a+) child is now perhaps predisposed to anaphylactic reactions if she were to receive Gm(a+) plasma? It seems possible that persons with anti-Gm determinants produce infants who develop transitional hypogammaglobulinemia of infancy. It is possible that, when IgG anti-Gm antibodies are made, rather than IgM, they cross the placenta and bind to the infant's antibody-producing cells, to blindfold these cells, so that elaboration of gamma globulin-specific antigens is delayed. The infant would not make gamma globulin initially or at 6 months, but perhaps at 1, 2, or 3 years of life, thus producing transitional hypogammaglobulinemia of infancy.

DISCUSSION

DR. BELLANTI: I wonder about the prospects of typing gamma globulins for the various specificities, so that patients could receive only type-specific gamma globulin.

DR. FUDENBERG: I think that would be worthwhile. However, the prospects are dim. We have tried, unsuccessfully, to convince one gamma globulin producer in the San Francisco Bay area (namely, Cutter) to do this. Whether other pharmaceutical firms are more interested, I do not know. There are some complications. Some laboratories are getting blood from India or from Southern convicts, who are predominantly Negro. The genetic Gm factors in such persons differ markedly from those of the Caucasian population who are receiving the product. Thus, even if these biologic reactions are rare, it still seems reasonable that the half-life of administered gamma globulin in the presence of antibody to the Gm factors would be very low. In this context, the data reported by Waldmann *et al.* earlier in these proceedings on rapid disappearance of IgA and individual IgA antibodies are of some significance.

DR. TERRY: One of the hazards in gamma globulin therapy seems to depend on the presence in these preparations of high-molecular-weight complexes resulting from chemical manipulation of the IgG molecules and expressed in improved solubility and decreased aggregation. I wonder whether there has been any experience in polyalanylating IgG preparations to reduce aggregation and increase the survival of these products *in vivo*. Are there any other means of modifying the molecule to improve its behavior?

There is a hazard in the administration of these preparations, but is the hazard great, relative to the value? I would direct you to the question of patients with hypogammaglobulinemia or agammaglobulinemia. Is this really useful therapy? I would like to address this question to Dr. Fudenberg, Dr. Rosen, and any others in the audience who have had experience with the administration of these materials in these patients. If it is useful, what is the evidence that it is useful? Assuming that it is useful, what are the criteria for determining which patients should get it and which ones should not? Dr. Good has commented that he spends a great deal of his time and energy trying to induce physicians to take their pediatric patients off gamma globulin therapy.

DR. FUDENBERG: There is no doubt that a great deal of gamma globulin is being wasted by physicians who give it to patients that they think have susceptibility to infections. We have screened many such patients for the Western Division of the Red Cross, and have found that, even in persons with gamma globulin levels 25% above normal, some ENT men were giving gamma globulin every 3 weeks.

Our own experience indicates that many infants diagnosed as having low gamma globulin levels, about 600 mg/100 ml, have been getting gamma globulin. There is a vast amount of gamma globulin being wasted.

In terms of immunologic deficiency disease, I would say that no more than 5% of the gamma globulin being given is really indicated. In patients with true agammaglobulinemia—and we have defined this as less than 200 mg/100 ml of IgG and less than one-fifth of the normal IgA or IgM—there is no doubt that gamma globulin administration prevents infection. Some of our patients had pneumonia once or twice a year before such treatment and have had no pulmonary infections during 5 years on it, although they do get occasional conjunctivitis and sinusitis.

A danger is presented by these aggregates, and we have circumvented it recently by giving whole plasma instead of gamma globulin. We give two units of plasma every 2–3 months, instead of gamma globulin every 3 weeks. First, there are no aggregates. Second, there is no pain at the site of injection, which often occurs with intramuscular injection. Third, larger quantities of immunoglobulins can be infused. We use hepatitis-free donors of the same Gm type as the patient. We try to get the same donor all the time, by plasmapheresis. We call this the "buddy treatment." Since we first described this method some years ago, other laboratories have used it (Dr. Good's, for example), and they find it to be of considerable benefit.

I might add that we used this in ataxia-telangiectasia in one instance, despite the fact that secretory IgA, rather than serum IgA, is presumably useful. An infant who had respiratory infections every 3 or 4 weeks for the 18 months before beginning plasma infusion therapy has had no respiratory infections for the last year. I am convinced that plasma infusion has a logical role to play. Perhaps it will save a lot of work in fractionation.

DR. ROSEN: I can only confirm what Dr. Fudenberg has said. There is no question that the administration of gamma globulin to children with X-linked agammaglobulinemia prevents the pyogenic infections to which these children are susceptible, which are caused mostly by *Haemophilus influenzae*, staphylococci, pneumococci, and streptococci. The greatest threat to the lives of these children is the progressive bronchiectasis that they get from recurrent pulmonary infections when they receive no replacement therapy. We have, as Dr. Fudenberg mentioned, seen an abolition or decreased incidence of these recurrent episodes of infection in agammaglobulinemic children. Dr. Good's case of a boy with conjunctivitis illustrated a very common symptom associated with agammaglobulinemia. It is amazing how this symptom is suppressed by giving IgG, which seems to keep this secretory surface uninfected. We have not had any experience with the buddy system that Dr. Fudenberg talked about, largely because of logistic problems and the number of patients we treat.

DR. KABAT: I would like to say, in response to Dr. Terry's comment about using polyalanylated materials, that our National Research Council committee has been interested in using polypeptides as plasma standards, but we felt that hazards would be introduced by their antigenicity. If you look at some of the studies by Maurer, you will see that one obtained extraordinary reactions to these antigens from very small doses in volunteers. I think that one has to proceed cautiously in the introduction of substances that could function as new antigenic determinants on the gamma globulin.

DR. ROWE: I think upwards of 150 hypogammaglobulinemics have been studied at one time in the United Kingdom. The hypogammaglobulinemia was defined in general as an IgG level of less than 200 mg/100 ml. An overall view of that series was that no statistically significant difference emerged regarding the effectiveness of two doses of gamma globulin, except for the differences in the levels of C-reactive proteins.

There is no doubt that there seemed to be a striking effect of gamma globulin therapy in some persons in the British series, but it still remains to be determined which patients are going to benefit from treatment and which are not.

In relation to the sensitization to IgG, Dr. Henney, who described antibodies in IgG aggregates that appeared in large amounts in one patient who suffered a severe reaction to IgG, has recently looked at a large number of sera. He included 16 control sera from blood banks and 46 sera from patients on repeated therapeutic gamma globulin infusions because of hypogammaglobulinemia. He measured the ability of these sera to precipitate aggregated Fc fragments from IgG. Controls showed values of around 100 μg of Fc precipitable per milliliter of serum, whereas, almost without exception, serum from persons on gamma globulin therapy showed more reactivity of this type, the amount of precipitated aggregated Fc going up as high as fivefold. Whether the ratio of antibody to aggregated Fc fragment is in fact related to the anaphylactic reaction remains to be seen, but for the moment it looks as though it is a rather consistent finding in patients on gamma globulin treatment.

DR. ROSEN: The Medical Research Council working party in the United Kingdom lumped together all the agammaglobulinemics, or the hypogammaglobulinemics, without any etiologic diagnosis.

Giving gamma globulin to children with any of the thymic deficiency syndromes that Dr. Good talked about is absolutely futile, even though these patients are hypogammaglobulinemic. Their cellular immunity is so impaired that there is no obvious benefit from giving them gamma globulin. They continue on their inexorably fatal course. We come ultimately to the fact that these diagnoses are not made on the basis of estimated serum levels of gamma globulin. They are histopathologic diagnoses. We start treating a child with gamma globulin primarily on the basis of what we see in his lymph node, and not his serum.

DR. MOSLEY: Dr. Terry suggests that we must weigh the demonstrated value of gamma globulin against its potential hazards in children with hypogammaglobulinemia. I would like to comment concerning the same problem when this material is used for the prevention of infectious hepatitis.

The American public has shifted from an attitude of relative unconcern about community-wide epidemics to one of apprehension over a few cases. They are aware that a prophylactic "shot" is available, and frequently demand such protection, even when presumed exposure is very unlikely, from an epidemiologic point of view, to result in transmission. Physicians have regarded gamma globulin as completely safe and understandably yield to demands in many instances when they may not believe there is a great need for its administration. As a result, all the children in a classroom or even an entire school may receive injections, despite the occurrence of only two or three cases of hepatitis. Similarly, co-workers in an office or medical and paramedical personnel in a hospital may receive protection against a very low risk.

Dr. Fudenberg has told us that the frequency of detectable antibodies is very low after a single dose of gamma globulin. I would point out, however, that, as a result of the situation I have described, as well as use of gamma globulin for prophylaxis for travel abroad, repeated doses are becoming much more common.

We are now beginning to realize that gamma globulin may not be so innocuous as we thought, especially when given in large and repeated doses. A brief recapitulation of the potential hazards or disadvantages of gamma globulin use seems warranted: (1) the material may become less effective when needed in future situations, through formation of antibodies that shorten the half-life of some of its constituents; (2) the incidence of future transfusion reactions may be increased in a population that receives gamma globulin repeatedly; (3) the incidence of maternal–fetal ABO or other incompatibilities may be increased in the future in girls or young women who receive gamma globulin derived from placental blood; and (4) pre-exposure prophylaxis may prevent harmless inapparent infection, leading to an accumulation of susceptibles in our population and postponing experience to an age at which the disease is more severe.

None of these considerations is sufficient to warrant the withholding of gamma globulin therapy if the risk of icteric infectious hepatitis is great. For household contacts of an icteric case, for example, the secondary attack rate among the unprotected is quite high and fully justifies routine administration of gamma globulin. But casual contact limited to the classroom or office carries too low a secondary attack rate for gamma globulin to be indicated. Similarly, travel abroad in itself is not sufficient justification, unless Americans in the area in question experience an incidence significantly above that in the United States.

V
USES OF
IMMUNOGLOBULINS
IN PREVENTION
AND THERAPY

S. KRUGMAN, J. P. GILES, *and* R. WARD

Use of Immunoglobulin in Infectious Hepatitis

Infectious hepatitis occurs in epidemic and endemic forms and constitutes one of the most important unsolved problems in the field of infectious diseases. Although it is generally believed to be caused by a virus, no virus has been isolated and identified as the etiologic agent. Hence, no specific vaccine can be prepared to prevent the disease. Even if hepatitis virus were grown in tissue culture and established today as the cause of infectious hepatitis, it would take several years before a vaccine would be available. In the case of poliomyelitis, the interval between adaptation to tissue culture and vaccine was 6 years; in measles, 9 years; in German measles, probably 7 years. Therefore, until active immunizing methods become available, one has to fall back on passive immunity.

It has been known for some time that gamma globulin is effective in preventing or modifying infectious hepatitis. Stokes and Neefe[7] were the first to report this, in 1945, followed in a few months by the confirmatory observations of Havens and Paul.[2] It is clear from the results shown in Table 1 that both pairs of investigators observed highly significant differences in favor of the groups receiving gamma globulin.

Figure 1 shows the results of another trial carried out during an epidemic of hepatitis by Stokes and his co-workers in an institution for

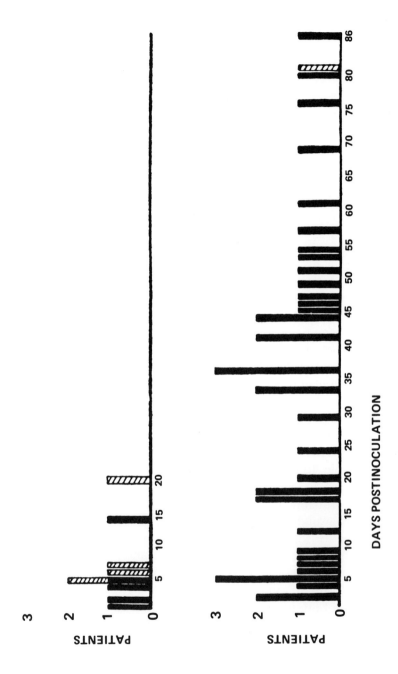

FIGURE 1 Effect of gamma globulin (0.06 ml/lb) in the prevention of infectious hepatitis with jaundice in an institution for mentally retarded males. This chart represents approximately the first 3 months of the hepatitis epidemic in the inoculated and the control groups. The solid blocks represent hepatitis with jaundice; the striped blocks, hepatitis without jaundice. The top portion represents the inoculated group (248 patients); the bottom portion, the control group (264 patients). (Reprinted with permission from Stokes et al.[6])

TABLE 1   Early Studies (1945) of Gamma Globulin in Prevention of Infectious Hepatitis

Authors	Group	No. Persons	Cases of Hepatitis with Jaundice	
			No.	%
Stokes and Neefe[7]	Gamma globulin, 0.15 ml/lb	53	3	5.7
	Control	278	125	45.0
Havens and Paul[2]	Gamma globulin, 0.08 ml/lb	97	2	2.1
	Control	155	36	23.2

mentally retarded males.[6] After eliminating from the study the patients in buildings in which no hepatitis had occurred, all men over 46 years old, Negro patients, and all those who were known to have had hepatitis, gamma globulin (0.06 ml/lb) was given to alternate patients alphabetically. In 248 patients who received gamma globulin, five cases of hepatitis with jaundice (2%) occurred, four in the first 5 days and one on the 14th day after injection. No additional cases emerged in the inoculated group, although cases with jaundice continued to appear in the controls for several months—40 cases (15%) in all. The difference is highly significant.

The studies so far described have shown the effectiveness of large doses of gamma globulin—that is, 0.15, 0.08, and 0.06 ml/lb of body weight. Table 2 shows the effectiveness of a smaller dose of gamma globulin, 0.01 ml/lb. In 1954, Hsia *et al.*[3] and, separately, Drake and

TABLE 2   Hepatitis at Rosewood: Effect of Gamma Globulin (0.01 ml/lb) in Children 4–14 Years Old Observed for 9 Months[a]

	No. Children	Cases of Hepatitis with Jaundice	
		No.	%
Gamma globulin (0.01 ml/lb)	52	2	3.8
Controls	77	42	54.5

[a]Derived from Stokes *et al.*[6]

Ming[1] confirmed the effectiveness of the small dose of gamma globulin (e.g., 0.01 ml/lb).

Additional evidence of the effectiveness of gamma globulin has been obtained from the studies at Willowbrook State School in New York, an institution for mentally retarded children, where infectious hepatitis has been endemic since 1953. The Willowbrook studies, initiated in 1956, have provided good evidence that gamma globulin does not protect against infection by hepatitis virus, but rather suppresses detectable illness and jaundice. A similar effect of suppressing overt manifestations occurs in posttransfusion hepatitis and in measles.

On admission to Willowbrook, alternate patients received gamma globulin (0.06 ml/lb). An equivalent number of patients served as uninoculated controls. The groups were comparable in regard to age range and degree of exposure. During the first 5 months, there was a striking difference in the incidence of jaundice: 31 cases in the control group and only one case in the gamma globulin group (Figure 2). In the succeeding 19 months of observation, there was no difference in incidence of hepatitis with jaundice between the two groups (18 cases in each group). The design of this study was such that only patients with frank

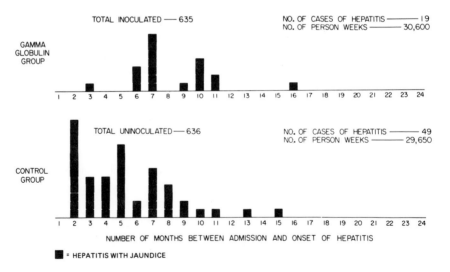

FIGURE 2   Infectious hepatitis at Willowbrook. Effect of gamma globulin (0.06 ml/lb to alternate patients on admission) on incidence of hepatitis with jaundice. (Reprinted with permission from Krugman *et al.* [5])

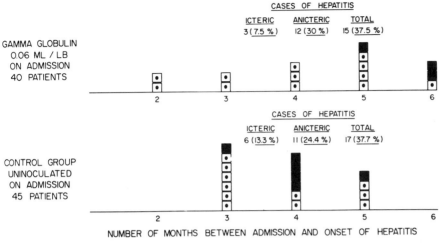

FIGURE 3   Infectious hepatitis at Willowbrook. Effect of gamma globulin on incidence of icteric and anicteric hepatitis. (Reprinted with permission from Krugman and Ward.[4])

jaundice were recognized; no attempt was made to detect anicteric cases. It was concluded that gamma globulin (0.06 ml/lb) provided protection against hepatitis with jaundice for a period of 5 months after admission to the institution.[5]

The possibility that mild or inapparent infection (anicteric hepatitis) occurred in some of those patients receiving and supposedly protected by gamma globulin was investigated in another study at Willowbrook. Of 85 newly admitted children chosen on an alternate basis, 40 received gamma globulin (0.06 ml/lb), and the remaining 45 served as uninoculated controls.[4] All patients were studied very closely for 6 months; liver-function tests were carried out at least once a week on all patients. Criteria for diagnosis of anicteric hepatitis were a crescendo-like rise in serum transaminase value and a rise in thymol turbidity. The results are seen in Figure 3. The overall incidence of hepatitis was the same in both groups—about 38%. There were six cases of jaundice in the control group and three in those who received gamma globulin. This difference obviously could have occurred by chance alone. Moreover, it is important to realize that the diagnosis of jaundice was made by one of the authors in nine patients, but the degree of jaundice was so slight that it was recognized by the regular Willowbrook staff of nurses and physicians in only one patient. The important observation made in this trial is the evidence of hepatitis infection without jaundice demonstrated in 12 of 40 patients in the gamma globulin group within 5 months of admission to the institution. This occurred despite the large dose of gamma globulin (0.06 ml/lb). It is clear that, under the conditions of these trials, gamma globulin failed to prevent hepatitis infection. It seems to have modified the disease by suppressing jaundice, thus making clinical recognition more difficult.

Another study compared the effects of two different doses of gamma globulin on the incidence of hepatitis with jaundice. Newly admitted patients were assigned in rotation to one of three groups: a group to receive gamma globulin at 0.06 ml/lb of body weight; a group to receive gamma globulin at 0.02 ml/lb; and a control group, to remain uninoculated. The results are shown in Figure 4. A comparison of the two treated groups with the controls indicates significant protection against jaundice for the first 5 months after admission to the institution. The smaller dose

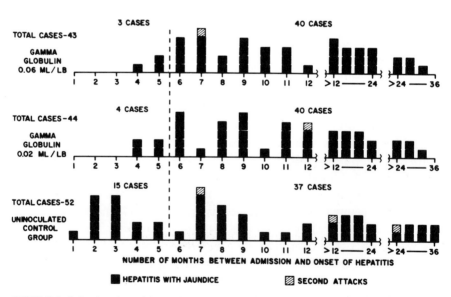

FIGURE 4   Infectious hepatitis at Willowbrook. Effect of various doses of gamma globulin on incidence of hepatitis with jaundice, July 1, 1960, through September 1, 1964.

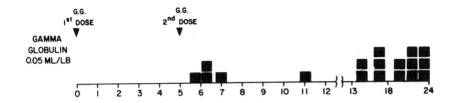

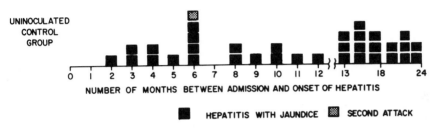

FIGURE 5   Infectious hepatitis with jaundice at Willowbrook. Prophylactic effect of two doses of gamma globulin, November 1, 1963, through November 1, 1965.

(0.02 ml/lb) seemed to be as effective as the larger dose (0.06 ml/lb). Neither of these single injections provided protection after 5 months.

For this reason, another trial was designed to determine the effect of two doses of gamma globulin given 5 months apart. This study was carried out during the 2-year period 1963–1965. Alternately admitted patients received gamma globulin, one dose of 0.05 ml/lb of body weight given on admission, and the same dose repeated 5 months later. A total of 441 patients received two doses of gamma globulin; 460 alternately admitted patients served as uninoculated controls. The results of this trial of two doses of 0.05 ml/lb of gamma globulin are shown in Figure 5. During the first year, five cases of hepatitis with jaundice were seen in the gamma globulin group, compared with 17 cases in the control group ($p=0.013$). In the treated group, at least one and possibly two patients were in the incubation period of hepatitis when the second dose was given. After 12 months, no significant difference was observed between the two groups in the incidence of hepatitis with jaundice. Under the conditions of this test, two 0.05-ml/lb doses of gamma globulin given 5 months apart provided good protection against hepatitis with jaundice for 1 year. A similar result seems likely in any endemic area in which persons would be subjected to a similar type of prolonged exposure.

Since 1960, gamma globulin has been given for the protection of nurses, hospital attendants, and kitchen and laundry workers at Willowbrook. From 1960 to 1962, gamma globulin was offered to all new employees on an optional basis; it was accepted by 177 and refused by 190. Since 1962, it has been injected routinely into all new employees. As shown in Table 3, a single 4-ml dose of gamma globulin, approximately 0.03 ml/lb of body weight, given intramuscularly, provided significant protection; that is, injection of gamma globulin was followed by an 80–85% reduction in the incidence of icteric hepatitis.

The results of the several studies described confirm the effectiveness of gamma globulin in the prevention of hepatitis with jaundice. The evidence suggests that anicteric hepatitis is *not* prevented, but that the disease is modified to the degree that jaundice tends to be suppressed.

Gamma globulin is recommended for children or adults who have had an exposure that is likely to result in infection. The available evidence suggests that the disease is transmitted chiefly by the fecal–oral route; thus, direct intimate contact is required for an adequate exposure. If a person with hepatitis were a food handler, the infection could be spread by indirect means through the ingestion of contaminated food. Infectious hepatitis may also be transmitted by the parenteral route.

Persons living in the same household as a person who has hepatitis and those subjected to intimate direct or indirect contact with such a person should receive gamma globulin. However, the routine administration of gamma globulin is not indicated for children and adults casually exposed in schools, offices, and factories. In institutions for the mentally retarded and in other closed facilities, such as prisons, gamma globulin may be indicated for new admissions or new employees if

TABLE 3   Effect of Gamma Globulin on Incidence of Hepatitis with Jaundice in Employees During First Year at Willowbrook

Years	Group	No. at Risk	Cases of Hepatitis with Jaundice	
			No.	%
1960–1962	No gamma globulin	190	11	5.8
	Gamma globulin, 4 ml	177	2	1.1
1962–1965	Gamma globulin, 4 ml	1,560	8	0.5

TABLE 4   Recommended Dose of Gamma Globulin for Prophylaxis against Infectious Hepatitis

Type of Exposure	Dose, ml/lb
Single or short-term	0.01–0.02
Prolonged or continuous	0.03–0.06

hepatitis is endemic in the institution. Hospital employees caring for infected patients will not require gamma globulin if diligent handwashing procedures are carried out and if there is no obvious break in the application of such procedures.

The dose of gamma globulin depends on the type of exposure—for example, a single or brief contact (less than 2 months) or a more prolonged and continuous type (more than 3 months). The recommended dose in milliliters per pound of body weight is shown in Table 4.

REFERENCES

1. Drake, M. E., and C. Ming. Gamma globulin in epidemic hepatitis. Comparative value of 2 dosage levels, apparently near the minimal effective level. JAMA 155:1302–1305, 1954.
2. Havens, W. P., Jr., and J. R. Paul. Prevention of infectious hepatitis with gamma globulin. JAMA 129:270–272, 1945.
3. Hsia, D. Y., M. Lonsway, Jr., and S. S. Gellis. Gamma globulin in prevention of infectious hepatitis; studies on use of small doses in family outbreaks. New Eng. J. Med. 250:417–419, 1954.
4. Krugman, S., and R. Ward. Infectious hepatitis: Current status of prevention with gamma globulin. Yale J. Biol. Med. 34:329–339, 1961-62.
5. Krugman, S., R. Ward, J. P. Giles, and A. Jacobs. Infectious hepatitis. Studies on the effect of gamma globulin and on the incidence of inapparent infection. JAMA 174:823–830, 1960.
6. Stokes, J., Jr., J. A. Farquhar, M. E. Drake, R. B. Capps, C. S. Ward, Jr., and A. W. Kitts. Infectious hepatitis. Length of protection by immune serum globulin (gamma globulin) during epidemics. JAMA 147:714–719, 1951.
7. Stokes, J., Jr., and J. R. Neefe. The prevention and attenuation of infectious hepatitis by gamma globulin; preliminary note. JAMA 127:144-145, 1945.

DISCUSSION

DR. MOSLEY: It seems quite logical that larger doses of gamma globulin would protect longer against icteric infectious hepatitis. But the available evidence lends

Gamma Globulin Prophylaxis against Infectious Hepatitis in Scandinavian Troops of the United Nations Emergency Force, Gaza Strip, 1956–1961[a]

Dose, ml/lb	Frequency within 6-Month Tour	Nationality	No. Men	Cases of Hepatitis		Efficiency of Protection, %[b]
				No.	%	
No gamma globulin		Danish, Norwegian, Swedish	11,373	132	1.16	—
0.063	Every 3 months	Norwegian	1,373	1	0.07	94
0.018	Once	Swedish	1,168	1	0.09	92
0.018 0.013	On arrival 3 months later	Swedish	3,529	3	0.09	92
0.018	Every 3 months	Norwegian	1,820	0	0	100
0.018	Every 6 weeks	Swedish	1,625	1	0.06	91
0.021	Every 4 weeks	Norwegian	363	3	0.83	28
0.066	Once	Danish	550	1	0.18	84

[a] Adapted from T. Kluge, Acta Med. Scand. 174:469–477, 1963.
[b] Recalculated on the basis of attack rate in all Scandinavian contingents.

no support to this concept. To emphasize how poorly the duration of protection correlates with the size and frequency of dose, I have rearranged Kluge's data (Acta Med. Scand. 174:469–477, 1963) in the accompanying table. Among Scandinavian troops in the Gaza Strip, small and infrequent doses seemed as effective as large or more frequent doses. Kluge's observations are supported by the finding at Willowbrook that gamma globulin in a dose of 0.02 ml/lb of body weight protected as well and as long as 0.06 ml/lb. Therefore, should the recommendation of the larger dose for long-term protection be modified?

DR. WARD: I think the smaller of the two doses should be the one that is recommended—i.e., 0.02 ml/lb of body weight (3 ml for adults), rather than 0.06. This is also the dose recommended for persons exposed over long periods, provided it is repeated every 5 months.

JAMES W. MOSLEY *and* DANIEL BRACHOTT

Variations in Effectiveness of Gamma Globulin Preparations for Prophylaxis against Infectious Hepatitis

That gamma globulin can be of value in prophylaxis against infectious hepatitis is adequately established. There is evidence that not all lots are equivalent in potency. We would like to call attention to this question.

During the early 1940's, when the cold-ethanol technique was being developed, there was concern about the uniformity of batches of gamma globulin. Enders[3] found variability of lots in titers of antibodies to various antigens. The differences, however, were not large. This conclusion was reinforced by the initial field trials of prophylaxis against measles and infectious hepatitis.

Table 1 presents the results of four major studies[2,4,11,12] of gamma globulin prophylaxis against infectious hepatitis from 1944 through 1952. Levels of effectiveness ranged from 83% to 95%, even with doses as small as 0.005–0.01 ml/lb of body weight. These evaluations included both pre-exposure and postexposure inoculations and indicated that passive protection lasted for several months.

The studies by Krugman and associates at Willowbrook State School constituted the first significant failure to obtain good protection against infectious hepatitis.[6] The results of their first and second trials are given

TABLE 1 Selected Studies on Effectiveness of Gamma Globulin in Prophylaxis against Infectious Hepatitis, United States, 1944–1952

Year of Study	Investigators	Type of Prophylaxis[a] and Study Situation	Dose, ml/lb	Results Inoculated No. Persons	Cases of Icteric Hepatitis[b] No.	%	Control No. Persons	Cases of Icteric Hepatitis[b] No.	%	Effectiveness, %
1944	Stokes and Neefe[12]	Predominantly post-exposure: water-borne epidemic at a summer camp	0.15	53	3	5.7	278	125	45.0	87
1945	Havens and Paul[4]	Predominantly post-exposure: person-to-person spread in an orphanage	0.08	97	2	2.1	155	36	23.2	91
1950	Stokes et al.[11,c]	Predominantly pre-exposure: person-to-person spread in an institution	0.01	106	3	2.8	83	45	54.2	95
1952	Drake and Ming[2]	Predominantly pre-exposure: person-to-person spread in an institution	0.005–0.01	157	5	3.2	267	49	18.4	83

[a]Prophylaxis is defined as "pre-exposure" or "postexposure," depending on whether most susceptible persons were presumed to have been infected at the time of inoculation.
[b]Includes all cases with onset of symptoms a day or more after inoculation.
[c]Refers only to study at State Training School ("Third Institution").

235

TABLE 2 Summary of First Two Trials of Gamma Globulin in Prophylaxis against Infectious Hepatitis, Willowbrook State School, New York[a]

Year of Study	Trial of Pre-exposure Prophylaxis	Study Group	Dose, ml/lb	Results Inoculated			Control			Effectiveness, %
				No. Persons	Cases of Icteric Hepatitis		No. Persons	Cases of Icteric Hepatitis		
					No.	%		No.	%	
1956	First	Inmates	0.01	1,224	9	0.7	2,988	61	2.0	64
1957–1958	Second[b]	Inmates	0.06	1,182	3	0.3	1,771	39	2.2	89

[a]Derived from Krugman et al.[6]
[b]Summary of data for first year only.

in Table 2. With the conventional dose of 0.01 ml/lb in pre-exposure
prophylaxis, they obtained only 64% efficiency. In their second trial, a
much larger dose yielded an efficiency of 89%. Better protection during
the second trial was attributed to the fact that a larger dose was used.
The preparations used in the two trials, however, may have had different
characteristics. Unfortunately, no opportunity to evaluate the hypothesis that the gamma globulin used in the first trial had low levels of antibody was immediately available.

Systematic exploration of possible differences among lots of gamma
globulin became possible with the establishment by Brachott and associates of a project to study hepatitis in Israel. Children between 2 and 9
years old were inoculated after household exposure to an icteric sibling.
In each trial, two gamma globulin preparations were evaluated against
albumin as a placebo. The inoculated children were visited periodically
for 8 weeks to determine the secondary attack rate of symptomatic,
clinically apparent disease.

Table 3 lists characteristics of the two preparations of gamma globulin
used in the first trial in Israel.[8] The reference material (globulin B) was
a special preparation made from blood collected in 1961 by the American National Red Cross. Titers of antibodies to measles virus and polio-
viruses were high, and no fragmentation was detected at the end of the
trial. Only two of 238 children who received 0.01 ml of this material
per pound of body weight became ill, compared with 16 of 250 controls,
a statistically significant difference. The estimated effectiveness of 87%
makes it comparable with gamma globulins used in most other trials.

The other preparation (globulin A) used in the first trial was produced
by the manufacturer of the gamma globulin used in the first trial at
Willowbrook. The gamma globulin was prepared by precipitation with
ammonium sulfate. Antibody levels were relatively low (Table 3), and
fragmentation was extensive. It was "outdated" at the time of use, although that was not known to be significant. Eight cases of hepatitis occurred among 236 children who received the material; this represented
an effectiveness of 47%. The result suggests that this preparation differed from the reference material ($p=0.07$), although exhaustion of the
supply of globulin A precluded determination of whether this trend
would have become significant at the 5% level of confidence.

In the second trial in Israel, use of reference preparation B from the
United States was continued. Because no data were available concerning

TABLE 3   Characteristics of Gamma Globulin Preparations Used in First Comparison in Israel, 1965-1966[a]

Characteristic	Reference Preparation	Gamma Globulin Prepared by Precipitation (Ammonium Sulfate)
Source of globulin	Plasma	Plasma
Geographic area in which blood was collected	Entire U.S.	? Entire U.S.
Year of plasma collection	1961	? 1953-1954
Year of release for distribution	1961	1957
Neutralizing antibodies to measles virus[b]	1:260	1:71
Neutralizing antibodies to poliovirus type 1[b]	1:4,200	1:370
Fragmentation[c]	Trace	Extensive
Effectiveness (compared with placebo group)	87%	47%
Statistical significance of level of protection (compared with placebo group)	$p < 0.01$	$p = 0.06$

[a]Derived from Mosley *et al.*[8]
[b]Assays for neutralizing antibodies carried out at National Communicable Disease Center during time of first comparison.
[c]Results of electrophoretic studies carried out at conclusion of first comparison.

gamma globulin produced in Israel, we studied an Israeli preparation (globulin C) having the characteristics listed in Table 4. Preliminary laboratory results showed antibody titers generally comparable with or higher than those of the American reference preparation, and only a trace of fragmentation was present at the end of the study. The Israeli material achieved a statistically significant reduction in the attack rate among inoculated children. The 56% efficiency of the Israeli preparation, despite the statistical significance of the result, is well below the levels listed in Table 1. Unfortunately, the characteristics of the preparation to date suggest no reason for the relatively poor potency.

The American reference preparation also showed strikingly lower effectiveness in the second comparison (65%) than in the first (87%). This suggested that some change occurred in the preparation with time.

Table 5 presents a preliminary assessment of this hypothesis, examining
efficiency estimates for three successive years. It appears that the material retained a high level of effectiveness through the first year of the
second trial (September 1966 through August 1967) and then declined
in potency during the third year (September 1967 through August 1968).
Further evaluations are now in progress to determine the changes that
may have been responsible.

To the experience in Israel should be added that of Cervenka in
Czechoslovakia.[1] In a field trial of pre-exposure prophylaxis in school-
children, a poor result was obtained in one of four districts. Analysis revealed that a placental gamma globulin was used in the district in which
no protection was achieved, but plasma-derived gamma globulin was
used in the areas in which the material was effective. Two attempts have
since been made to compare directly the efficacy of placental gamma
globulin, placental gamma globulin stabilized with epsilon-aminocaproic

TABLE 4   Characteristics of Gamma Globulin Preparations Used in Second Comparison in
Israel, 1966–1968

Characteristic	Reference Preparation	Israeli Preparation
Source of globulin	Plasma	Plasma
Geographic area in which blood was collected	Entire U.S.	Israel
Year of plasma collection	1961	1966
Year of release for distribution	1961	1966
Neutralizing antibodies to measles virus[a]	1:640	1:640
Neutralizing antibodies to poliovirus type 1[a]	>1:1,400	1:1,200
Fragmentation[b]	Minimal	Trace
Effectiveness (compared with placebo group)	65%	56%
Statistical significance of level of protection (compared with placebo group)	$p < 0.01$	$p < 0.01$

[a]Assays for neutralizing antibodies carried out at Hebrew University–Hadassah Medical School
during the second comparison. Techniques were not similar to those during first comparison;
therefore, titers should not be compared with those obtained during first comparison (Table 3).
[b]Results of electrophoretic studies by J. T. Sgouris, Lansing, Michigan, and R. H. Painter,
Toronto, Ontario, Canada, at conclusion of second comparison.

TABLE 5   Effectiveness During Successive Years of Reference Gamma Globulin Used in Comparisons in Israel, 1965–1968

Period of Use	Population Inoculated with Reference Preparation			Control Population			Effectiveness, %
	No. Persons	Cases of Icteric Hepatitis No.	%	No. Persons	Cases of Icteric Hepatitis No.	%	
September 1965–August 1966[a]	238	2	0.8	250	16	6.4	87
September 1966–August 1967[b]	118	1	0.8	137	13	9.5	91
September 1967–August 1968[c]	369	11	3.0	358	22	6.1	51

[a]First comparison.[8]
[b]First year of second comparison.
[c]Second year of second comparison.

acid, and plasma-derived gamma globulin. Trends in the results suggested that unstabilized placental gamma globulin was indeed less effective. In both Czech comparisons, however, the attack rates in all groups were too low to permit statistically valid conclusions.

These field observations, scattered and inconclusive though they may be, have the support of several considerations that suggest that differences in gamma globulin preparations could, in fact, be expected. Factors of potential importance can easily be suggested:

Antibody levels   Review of the increasingly available data indicates wide variations among some preparations with respect to several antibodies. This is perhaps best illustrated by the data of Meyer and co-workers[7] concerning antibodies to measles virus in 64 lots of commercially prepared gamma globulin. Their findings are summarized in Table 6. Differences of eightfold or greater were found, approximately one third of the lots tested having either very low or very high titers. Requirements with respect to minimal levels of measles antibodies have since been established in the United States. Antibodies to the infectious hepatitis agent may show the same spectrum of values seen in measles antibodies. Recent data from the National Communicable Disease Center indicate that this is true for antibodies to viral antigens (Table 7).

Fragmentation   The discovery by Škvařil[10] that IgG undergoes cleavage opened a new direction in investigations of lot variations. Painter and co-workers[9] reported that fragmentation resulted in failure to protect guinea pigs against tetanus toxin. As pointed out in the first trial in Israel and in Cervenka's experience in Czechoslovakia, fragmentation may alter the effectiveness of gamma globulin in pre-exposure prophylaxis against infectious hepatitis. In the third trial in Israel, now in progress, the two preparations being used differ only in this respect, the fragmented material having been prepared by Sgouris by addition of fibrinolysin to a portion of an unfragmented batch.

Aggregation   Various lots of gamma globulin differ not only in extent of fragmentation, but also in the extent to which IgG molecules are aggregated. Whether this change is significant with respect to clinical potency remains to be determined.

Minor components   Gamma globulin preparations have been found to differ widely in their concentrations of plasma proteins other than IgG.[5] The practical significance of these variations is unknown.

In summary, field experience and laboratory data indicate that some gamma globulin preparations may be less effective than others in preventing infectious hepatitis. Whether differences in lots will be important remains to be determined. It is to be hoped, in fact, that no question will need to be raised concerning preparations that meet present produc-

TABLE 6   Lot Variation of Gamma Globulin Preparations with Respect to Titers of Antibodies to Measles Virus[a]

Reciprocal of Neutralizing- Antibody Titer	Lots	
	No.	%
200 or less	5	8
201–400	10	16
401–800	22	34
801–1,200	18	28
1,201–1,400	5	8
1,401–1,600	2	3
1,601–1,800	2	3
Total	64	100

[a]Derived from Meyer *et al.*[7]

TABLE 7 Spectrum of Serologic Results with Selected Lots of Gamma Globulin: Results of Tests at National Communicable Disease Center[a]

Antigen	Test[b]	Reciprocal of Neutralizing-Antibody Titer						
		Lot 1	Lot 2	Lot 3	Lot 4	Lot 5	Lot 6	Lot 7
Measles virus	VN	40	40	>160	>160	>160	>160	160
Measles virus	HI	20	20	320	320	320	640	320
Vaccinia virus	HI	<10	10	160	320	320	320	160
Mumps virus	VN	<10	10	20	80	80	80	80
Rubella virus	HI	160	80	640	1,280	1,280	1,280	1,280
Poliovirus type 1	VN	80	160	640	320	640	640	320
Echovirus 9	VN	20	<20	80	80	160	80	160
Echovirus 11	VN	20	20	20	80	80	20	80
Eastern encephalitis virus	SN	0.1	0.1	0.3	0.2	0.1	0.2	0.3
Western encephalitis virus	SN	2.3	0.9	0.2	2.3	>2.6	>2.6	0.4

[a]Studies carried out by units of Virology Section, Microbiology Branch, Laboratory Division, NCDC, in collaboration with Morris T. Suggs, Diagnostic Reagents Section.
[b]VN=virus neutralization test; SN=serum neutralization test (neutralization index); HI=hemagglutination inhibition test.

242

tion standards. Such assurance, however, can come only from additional field comparisons. Such studies are time-consuming, expensive, and sometimes frustrating. Nevertheless, however inconvenient they may be, they are the only means of assessing the effectiveness of a material being used increasingly for prophylaxis against infectious hepatitis throughout the world.

REFERENCES

1. Cervenka, J. Surveillance of infectious hepatitis: Evaluation of the prophylactic use of gamma globulin. Bull. WHO. (in press)
2. Drake, M. E., and C. Ming. Gamma globulin in epidemic hepatitis. Comparative value of 2 dosage levels, apparently near the minimal effective level. JAMA 155:1302–1305, 1954.
3. Enders, J. F. The concentrations of certain antibodies in globulin fractions derived from human blood plasma. J. Clin. Invest. 23:510–530, 1944.
4. Havens, W. P., Jr., and J. R. Paul. Prevention of infectious hepatitis with gamma globulin. JAMA 129:270–272, 1945.
5. Heiner, D. C., and L. Evans. Immunoglobulins and other proteins in commercial preparations of gamma globulin. J. Pediat. 70:820–827, 1967.
6. Krugman, S., R. Ward, J. P. Giles, and A. M. Jacobs. Infectious hepatitis. Studies on the effect of gamma globulin and on the incidence of inapparent infection. JAMA 174:823–830, 1960.
7. Meyer, H. M., Jr., B. E. Brooks, R. D. Douglas, and N. G. Rogers. Measles serologic standards. Amer. J. Dis. Child. 103:495–502, 1962.
8. Mosley, J. W., D. M. Reisler, D. Brachott, D. Roth, and J. Weiser. Comparison of two lots of immune serum globulin for prophylaxis of infectious hepatitis. Amer. J. Epidem. 87: 539–550, 1968.
9. Painter, R. H., M. J. Walcroft, and J. C. Weber. The efficacy of fragmented immune serum globulin in passive immunization. Canad. J. Biochem. 44:381–387, 1966.
10. Škvařil, F. Changes in outdated human γ-globulin preparations. Nature 185:475–476, 1960.
11. Stokes, J., Jr., J. A. Farquhar, M. E. Drake, R. B. Capps, C. S. Ward, Jr., and A. W. Kitts. Infectious hepatitis. Length of protection by immune serum globulin (gamma globulin) during epidemics. JAMA 147:714–719, 1951.
12. Stokes, J., Jr., and J. R. Neefe. The prevention and attenuation of infectious hepatitis by gamma globulin; preliminary note. JAMA 127:144–145, 1945.

DISCUSSION

DR. JANEWAY: We are assuming that the viruses of hepatitis remain uniform all the time. A great many things have occurred that make one wonder whether that is so. The incidence of hepatitis in epidemic form fluctuates in individual communities in a 7- or 8-year cycle. But we are running into the very disconcerting problem that what we would have considered to be the serum type of hepatitis—which the original human volunteer experiment suggested can be transmitted only by blood or plasma and which is clearly much more resistant to the action of gamma globulin—can probably be transmitted to closely exposed persons by the same routes as the kind of virus that is wild in epidemics in communities. I think everything about these viruses is open to question until someone can isolate them or until many more experiments with human volunteers are allowed to proceed (as I think they should be).

Although we may not be able to measure the fragmentation of gamma globulin in the test tube, we may be dealing with a preparation that is more susceptible to biologic cleavage once it enters the body. In hepatitis, the infectious agent incubates for a long time—much longer than in most infectious diseases—and so the metabolic fate of the antibody transfused is highly important in relation to the duration of its effect in the body. I do not know what to suggest to get at this variable. In the studies being carried on in Israel, obviously the first thing to do is what is being done with Dr. Sgouris's preparation: to compare the two halves of a single batch, one fragmented and the other not. The general characteristics of each have been well documented by us. It is worth considering whether some attempt should be made to follow the catabolism of these two preparations *in vivo*, because, although there may not be obvious fragmentation in the test tube, the linkages may break more easily under the action of the body's own enzymes. Unfortunately, one cannot do this in rabbits, because a rabbit develops antibodies that alter the result. Therefore, one cannot compare the disappearance curves of two preparations in rabbits, although this could be tried as a first approximation; I suspect we will have to go to humans to study this problem adequately.

DR. GOOD: This problem may get us into virologic difficulties, as well as semantic difficulties. We must not equate infection with disease. I think that the observations of Krugman and his colleagues inform us that we are not significantly altering infection, or whatever this agent is. We are altering disease, and that makes it necessary to think of the influence of antibody, not only on the agent, but on the expression of reaction to the agent. For example, with Rh antibodies, one can dramatically alter responses to an antigen by antibody. It may very well be that the influence of the antibody on hepatitis involves an influence not on infection (or at least not significantly), but rather on the expression of the host reaction to that infection.

DR. CONRAD: The age of the host seems to play an important role in his reaction to infection. Infectious hepatitis usually causes a more severe illness in adults than in children. Likewise, gamma globulin therapy seems to be more effective in preventing clinical hepatitis among young children than in older children or adults. Little seems to be known about these host responses and how they are influenced.

DR. LoGRIPPO: In 1961, we studied 87 cases of hepatitis in children 1–15 years old. They were in an institution that had not had an outbreak of hepatitis before the period of study. Immunodepression was found in 10% of these children with icteric hepatitis. Although serum IgM and IgG generally became elevated in this disease, in some the elevation does not always occur. These patients have shown a fourfold or greater loss in specific neutralizing-antibody titers to a variety of enteric viruses present during the acute icteric stage of the disease. This rapid decrease occurred within 4–6 weeks after the jaundice period and did not return within the 6–7 months of the study. Enteric viruses isolated from stools during the acute stage of the disease failed to induce a serum conversion, from negative to positive, against their own virus isolated over the period of study. Similar findings have been demonstrated in adults. The degrees and variations of immunodepression seen in virus hepatitis have not been seen among other clinical entities within the limitations of our tests.

DR. CONRAD: Hepatitis is not only a disease of the liver; it also causes changes in other organs, including the gut, kidneys, and bone marrow. For example, bone marrow aspirates from 30% of soldiers with acute icteric infectious hepatitis showed megaloblastoid changes of erythroid cells and arrest of maturation of granulocytic cells. The generalized nature of this illness makes it a likely cause of functional impairment of a number of organ systems.

DR. WATT: I would like to ask the speakers about the dose levels of gamma globulin used in infectious hepatitis. One wonders what effect repeated uses of gamma globulin may have. We have two programs, one using normal gamma globulin for prophylaxis against rubella in pregnant women, and an anti-D program related to the immediate postpartum period. I am concerned about the possibility that the earlier use of gamma globulin for prophylaxis against rubella will result in formation of antibodies against homologous gamma globulin, with the result that the half-life of the anti-D preparation would be seriously reduced.

DR. MOSLEY: I agree that use of gamma globulin for one purpose may affect its later value for another purpose. Antibodies to heterotypic subclasses may shorten the half-life of administered IgG. The frequency with which such antibodies are induced and their effect on the disappearance of passively acquired immunoglobulins need to be determined, not only in children with hypogammaglobulinemia, but also in normal adults.

Aside from persons with deficiencies in immunoglobulin production, the group most likely to receive relatively large and repeated doses of gamma globulin consists of Americans traveling or living abroad. Protection against infectious hepatitis is certainly needed in some areas for long periods because of persistently high attack rates of icteric disease, especially among adults (Cline *et al.* JAMA 199:551–553, 1967). Whether gamma globulin has progressively less value for this purpose the longer or more often it is used needs to be evaluated in a large group of persons abroad, at sufficiently high risk, and under sufficiently close medical supervision. The Peace Corps is one such population, and it would be helpful to know whether the efficiency of prophylaxis is lowered in the second year in which the volunteers are abroad. Even 2 years may be long enough for lessened effectiveness to become apparent.

DR. ROBBINS: Is there any evidence, Dr. Conrad, that the gamma globulin preparations that did not protect military personnel against hepatitis in Korea and Vietnam work at all?

DR. CONRAD: All I can say is that it is conventional American gamma globulin, prepared from a very diffuse geographic area over the United States.

GEORGE F. GRADY

Use of Immunoglobulins in Preventing Posttransfusion Hepatitis

The preceding two papers recall the remarkable effectiveness of gamma globulin against infectious hepatitis and outline variations in gamma globulin characteristics that might affect potency. One's belief that gamma globulin might also prevent posttransfusion hepatitis is conditioned as much by one's concept of the latter disease as by the available data. A traditional view holds that hepatitis legitimately attributable to transfusions (sometimes called "hepatitis B") has an incubation period of at least 60 days, cannot be transmitted enterically, and does not confer immunity to subsequent challenge with "hepatitis A," the typical infectious hepatitis, which is acquired enterically and has a shorter incubation period. Of those three criteria, the first has been the least useful because most posttransfusion cases have incubation periods of less than 60 days[1,7] and there is no naturally definable division between these and the longer-incubation cases.[6] The possibility of enteric transmission of hepatitis B has never been evaluated extensively,[14] and anecdotal experiences, the study of Mirick and Shank,[11] and the work of Krugman's group at Willowbrook[10] all suggest that such transmission is possible, although it is unusual in normal circumstances.[6]

The failure of hepatitis B to confer cross-immunity (to hepatitis A) is

247

the only original criterion that remains relatively unchallenged.[10] Furthermore, the original studies suggested that even homologous immunity may have been incomplete,[14,18] and more recent experience with addicts, "hippies," and renal-dialysis patients suggests that the same is true of their hepatitis,[6] most of which is presumed to be of parenteral origin, although the incubation periods may not always be long.

In his review in 1960, Stokes[18] stated that, although he favored the hypothesis of antigenic differences between hepatitis A and B as an explanation for the more erratic protection that globulin affords against hepatitis B, he nevertheless felt that possible immunogenic differences between the two types of hepatitis syndromes might account for a number of paradoxes—e.g., maintenance of the carrier state, the noninfectivity of cold-ethanol-fractionated gamma globulin, and the apparent effectiveness against hepatitis B of large doses of gamma globulin, even when given months after transfusion. Other hypotheses have been advanced to explain the various paradoxes, such as protection of latent virus by "blocking antibodies" or by transport and multiplication of virus in leukocytes. Each hypothesis has something to support it, sometimes by virtue of parallel disease models.

About the only theory that has not received much attention is the possibility that hepatitis virus does in fact precipitate along with the "immune" serum globulin fraction. It would have to be assumed that, in the presence of marked antibody excess, the virus would be so attenuated that *it* would contribute to the "active" portion of the active–passive immunization in which the active role is normally attributed to the exogenously introduced infection.[18] Pennell[15] found that marker viruses were recoverable with gamma globulin in Cohn's fraction II. He felt that the techniques used in his study did not differ enough from current ones to explain the evidence that hepatitis virus behaves differently. However, it is reassuring that no evidence of even mild disease was detected in the 10 volunteers whom Murray and Ratner[13] challenged with gamma globulin prepared from known icterogenic plasma, although the evaluation did not include liver biopsy or some of the more sensitive biochemical tests that are now available. Suffice it to say that in neither field trials nor general clinical use has there been evidence of overt hepatitis related to gamma globulin prepared by the cold-ethanol process.[13]

If gamma globulin carries no risk, why is it not more widely used among transfusion recipients in the hope that it might offer some degree of protection, however variable it might be? One reason is the med-icolegal entanglement implicit in selective omissions when one cannot predict which patients are destined to develop hepatitis. From a public-health standpoint, gamma globulin has been considered a limited re-source that should not be diverted from more established uses. The large amounts believed necessary for any possible effectiveness against post-transfusion hepatitis are expensive, and the injection sites can be painful. It is now appreciated that sensitization occurs more often than originally thought[16] and could be worsened by repeated injections, as have been used in various field trials. Overt reactions occur at least once in 1,000 recipients (according to the National Transfusion Hepatitis Study, in progress), and this frequency might offset the potential usefulness if the background incidence of posttransfusion hepatitis had already been minimized by judicious use of blood and careful donor selection.[7] Still, there is a great need to know whether a practical regimen of gamma globulin prophylaxis exists. We need to know for the sake of understand-ing the general immunology of various forms of hepatitis, as well as for protection of specific persons at risk, such as the recipients of blood that is belatedly found to be infectious and possibly the recipients of such high-risk products as fibrinogen.[6] Also, it is reasonable to surmise that any globulin regimen that is effective prophylaxis regarding transfusions would be at least equally effective against the smaller volume of infective material introduced by accidental punctures with contaminated needles.

The data regarding gamma globulin trials are not so much limited as contradictory. The empiric consideration that there might be a vulnerable period during which the virus sheds its protective protein coating led Grossman, Stewart, and Stokes to space two globulin doses a month apart.[18] The more recent availability of disaggregated gamma globulin suitable for intravenous use led Creutzfeldt et al.[3] to report apparent success in using it alone (mixed with the transfused blood) or with sup-plemental intramuscular injections of the more standard preparation.[11] The results were based on very small numbers, and larger studies else-where have yet to be reported in full. The point of this discussion is merely to emphasize the myriad possibilities in doses, timing, gamma globulin composition, and route of administration.

Most studies have been done with standard 16% human serum gamma globulin given intramuscularly. Grossman et al.[8] gave two 10-ml doses to alternate patients at various times after they had received blood, pooled plasma, or both, and again 1 month later; 1.3% of the gamma globulin-treated group developed clinically apparent hepatitis, compared with 8.9% of the controls. A larger study carried out by Duncan et al.,[5] using only one 10-ml dose of gamma globulin, revealed no difference in incidence of hepatitis between treated and untreated patients, although the average incubation period of the gamma globulin-treated patients appeared to be slightly, but significantly, longer.

The results of the trials led Stokes and his co-workers to attempt further definition of gamma globulin prophylaxis by controlled studies of human volunteers challenged with known infectious serum.[19] Gamma globulin in 10-ml doses given several times was not protective, whether administered separately or mixed with the infectious material. It was postulated that the failure to protect against the strain of hepatitis used in the experiments might have been due to a lack of experience with the particular hepatitis virus in the donor population from which the gamma globulin was derived. Accordingly, studies were carried out with presumably hyperimmune gamma globulin derived from other volunteers, who had been infected with the same strain that caused hepatitis 4 months to 6 years earlier; gamma globulin doses of 2–4 ml were tested, but still there was no protection.[4]

Mirick and associates[12] confirmed the results of the first field trial of two 10-ml doses of gamma globulin, which had shown protection. The times of gamma globulin injections were standardized in the major portion of their study to the first and fifth weeks after transfusion. In addition, serial liver-function tests, including SGOT determinations, were performed monthly. Anicteric cases were equally distributed between the treated and control groups, and there was one death in each. At the time these results were published, there was a flurry of enthusiasm for giving gamma globulin. However, shortly thereafter, Holland et al.[9] reported that 10-ml doses of gamma globulin failed to protect patients who had undergone cardiovascular surgery. Holland et al. gave the second injection at about the same time as in the study of Mirick and co-workers, but the first dose was given just before the heavy transfusions. This was similar to the treatment of one subgroup in Mirick's study (which demonstrated no protection but involved numbers that were too small to permit statistical interpretation). One other difference between the Mirick and Holland studies was the average transfusion volume—four and twenty units, respectively. Thus, whenever gamma globulin has appeared to be protective, it has been given in divided doses after low-volume transfusions.

None of these studies was perfect from the standpoint of experimental design, and it is unlikely that any could be, considering the logistic problems necessitated by placebo injections, adequate numbers, complete follow-ups, and so on. However, a large-scale cooperative study, the National Transfusion Hepatitis Study, was begun several years ago, and great attention has been given to these details and to the results of previous studies. The results should be available within a year; it is hoped that they will reconcile differences among the studies mentioned above.

Approximately 10% of patients are being followed by serial transaminase tests in a search for subclinical disease. It was originally thought that approximately 4,000 patients would be studied and that only one common lot of gamma globulin would be used. Fortunately, the study has run enough ahead of schedule that a second lot of gamma globulin is being tested. The large numbers will also aid in the interpretation of potential effects of gamma globulin within study subgroups—according to transfusion volume, incubation period, age, etc. The first lot of gamma globulin was obtained from plasma of American National Red Cross donors selected largely according to the newer criteria, which exclude persons with a history of overt hepatitis. The second lot has been supplied by the Merck Sharp and Dohme Division of Merck and Co., Inc., and was derived from prison donors and professional donors who underwent plasmapheresis. As a sequel to the current cooperative study, it may become feasible to test gamma globulin that is considered "hyperimmune" because of its derivation exclusively from plasma of donors with a history of hepatitis. These variations in donor source may prove interesting, although there is no overt difference among these lots of globulin with regard to standard antibody titrations, fragmentation, and other characteristics.

I am as hopeful as anyone that the newer studies reported by Blumberg et al.[2] and Prince[17] will give us more direct methods of identifying infectious blood and evaluating globulin potency. These properties are being evaluated when possible in the current field trials.

REFERENCES

1. Allen, J. G., and W. A. Sayman. Serum hepatitis from transfusions of blood. Epidemiologic study. JAMA 180:1079–1085, 1962.
2. Blumberg, B. S., B. J. Gerstley, D. A. Hungerford, W. T. London, and A. J. Sutnick. A serum antigen (Australia antigen) in Down's syndrome, leukemia, and hepatitis. Ann. Intern. Med. 66:924–931, 1967.

3. Creutzfeldt, W., H.-J. Severidt, H. Brachmann, G. Schmidt, and U. Tschaepe. The use of gamma-globulin in the prophylaxis of transfusion hepatitis. German Med. Monthly 12: 101–104, 1967.

4. Drake, M. E., J. A. Barondess, W. J. Bashe, Jr., G. Henle, W. Henle, J. Stokes, Jr., and R. B. Pennell. Failure of convalescent gamma globulin to protect against homologous serum hepatitis. JAMA 152:690–693, 1953.

5. Duncan, G. G., H. A. Christian, J. Stokes, Jr., W. F. Rexer, J. T. Nicholson, and A. Edgar. An evaluation of immune serum globulin as a prophylactic agent against homologous serum hepatitis. Amer. J. Med. Sci. 213:53–57, 1947.

6. Grady, G. F. The prevention of (viral) hepatitis. Disease-a-Month, pp. 1–31, July 1968.

7. Grady, G. F., and T. C. Chalmers. Risk of post-transfusion viral hepatitis. New Eng. J. Med. 271:337–342, 1964.

8. Grossman, E. B., S. G. Stewart, and J. Stokes, Jr. Post-transfusion hepatitis in battle casualties and study of its prophylaxis by means of human immune serum globulin. JAMA 129: 991–994, 1945.

9. Holland, P. V., R. M. Rubinson, A. G. Morrow, and P. J. Schmidt. Gamma-globulin in the prophylaxis of posttransfusion hepatitis. JAMA 196:471–474, 1966.

10. Krugman, S., J. P. Giles, and J. Hammond. Infectious hepatitis. Evidence for two distinctive clinical, epidemiological, and immunological types of infection. JAMA 200:365–373, 1967.

11. Mirick, G. S., and R. E. Shank. An epidemic of serum hepatitis studied under controlled conditions. Trans. Amer. Clin. Climat. Assoc. 71:176–190, 1959.

12. Mirick, G. S., R. Ward, and R. W. McCollum. Modification of post-transfusion hepatitis by gamma globulin. New Eng. J. Med. 273:59–65, 1965.

13. Murray, R., and F. Ratner. Safety of immune serum globulin with respect to homologous serum hepatitis. Proc. Soc. Exp. Biol. Med. 83:554–555, 1953.

14. Neefe, J. R., S. S. Gellis, and J. Stokes, Jr. Homologous serum hepatitis and infectious (epidemic) hepatitis; studies in volunteers bearing on immunological and other characteristics of etiological agents. Amer. J. Med. 1:3–22, 1946.

15. Pennell, R. B. The distribution of certain viruses in the fractionation of plasma, pp. 297–310. In F. W. Hartman, G. A. LoGrippo, J. G. Mateer, and J. Barron, Eds. Hepatitis Frontiers. Boston: Little, Brown and Co., 1957.

16. Pretty, H. M., H. H. Fudenberg, H. A. Perkins, and F. Gerbode. Anti-γ globulin antibodies after open heart surgery. Blood 32:205–216, 1968.

17. Prince, A. M. An antigen detected in the blood during the incubation period of serum hepatitis. Proc. Nat. Acad. Sci. USA 60:814–821, 1968.

18. Stokes, J., Jr. Immunization in viral hepatitis. JAMA 172:652–655, 1960.

19. Stokes, J., Jr., M. Blanchard, J. R. Neefe, S. S. Gellis, and G. R. Wade. Methods of protection against homologous serum hepatitis. I. Studies on the protective value of gamma globulin in homologous serum hepatitis SH virus. JAMA 138:336–341, 1948.

DISCUSSION

DR. TERRY: We have heard the word "protection" used with regard to hepatitis, evidently referring to protection from turning yellow. The evidence indicates that anicteric hepatitis occurs with the same frequency. Are the severity and sequelae of hepatitis truly altered by this form of prophylactic treatment?

I would like to comment on the question of whether administration of gamma globulin is a reasonable form of prophylaxis. There have been comments about the compartmentalization of the immune system—the compartmentalization of the humoral system, as well as the IgA secretory system, which also seems to act as a separate compartment. If anicteric hepatitis is truly an enteric infection, then maybe it is not reasonable to attempt prophylaxis by giving an intramuscular or intravenous product. Perhaps what needs to be done is to take secretory IgA from the gut of persons who are convalescing from hepatitis and administer it orally to recipients, in order to achieve prophylaxis against hepatitis.

DR. GRADY: I think your latter suggestions are excellent. I have never felt that it was efficient or practical to give gamma globulin. There are very few who feel that it is. I do think, however, that, like politics, it is the art of the possible.

I am particularly concerned that gamma globulin theoretically can turn an otherwise acute infection into a chronic and smoldering infection; and there is a small amount of evidence that it can. However, the population that we are studying consists of open-heart-surgery patients who average 50 or 60 years of age and have severe limitations of fundamental health. They do not care much about the distant future; they simply do not want to become acutely ill and die on the spot. Although I agree that whether one is yellow or not does not tell the whole story, I do think that there is a broad correlation between the results of liver-function tests (such as transaminase levels and other biochemical indices) and the severity of the disease. We are trying to record not only deaths, but days lost from work, days spent in the hospital, and so on, to try to answer the practical questions. I agree with the disclaimers that perhaps there is a conversion of overt disease to subclinical disease, and I agree that this may not always be good. But, under some circumstances, it is the first, if not the only, concern of the patients at risk. The study serves as a practical stopgap measure. Donor screening and other tests are much more practical, and I think that giving gamma globulin as a third-rate approach to the problem constitutes admission of how unsatisfactory the general field is.

OLOF RINGERTZ

Use of Gamma Globulins in Prophylaxis against Occupational Hepatitis

Studies on the epidemiology of hepatitis and prophylaxis against it are hampered by the lack of virologic or serologic methods to establish a diagnosis. Clinical differences between infectious and serum hepatitis have been reported,[10,25,29] but they are usually based on epidemiologic evidence, which, owing to the long incubation period of the disease, is often incomplete and unclear.

Very little is known of the factors that influence a person's susceptibility to hepatitis. In children, hepatitis is a mild infection[14]; during pregnancy and in women over 45 years old, it is often severe.[2,19] These differences, however, are probably not caused by differences in susceptibility. In serum hepatitis, no age difference has been observed, but the disease may have a high mortality rate in old persons.[1]

Infectious hepatitis is recorded in many countries. Differences in morbidity between countries or groups of people may be explained by differences in living conditions, water supplies, food-handling, and general standard of hygiene. Our knowledge of the morbidity of serum hepatitis has a poor statistical background. Very often, cases are reported as infectious hepatitis. The best source of information on the morbidity of serum hepatitis is supplied by the investigations on frequency of posttransfusion hepatitis.

254

In infectious hepatitis, the route of transmission is usually fecal–oral, but the disease may be transmitted through inoculation. In most cases of serum hepatitis, the disease has been transmitted by blood transfusions, injections, and the like. An exception occurred in Sweden, where over 600 cases of serum hepatitis were reported among Swedish track-finders. Track-finding is a competitive sport that involves running through wooded areas. The disease was transmitted through accidental inoculation of blood into scratches and wounds received during competitions.[26] The epidemic was brought to an end when the competitors were forced to protect themselves against skin lesions.

Around 1950, hepatitis was reported as an occupational hazard of medical personnel. Leibowitz et al.[18] described a case of serum hepatitis in a blood-bank worker. Kuh and Ward[17] reported seven cases of hepatitis among pharmaceutical personnel preparing blood derivatives, and Byrne[3] later described an outbreak of eight cases in the Yale-New Haven Hospital. He also pointed out that the frequency of infectious hepatitis among hospital personnel is directly proportional to its incidence in the general population.

Some authors have compared the risk of contracting hepatitis with the incidence of the infection among hospital personnel. Popper and Raber[22] found the risk for Austrian doctors to be seven times higher than for the general population, and the risk for nurses, four times higher. In Sweden, Strombeck[28] found the incidence of hepatitis to be considerably higher among doctors than among lawyers and nurses.

During the last few years, serum hepatitis has been an increasing problem for personnel in hemodialysis units; outbreaks have been reported from a number of hemodialysis centers.[9,12,15,21,23,24] In a survey conducted by the hepatitis unit of the National Communicable Disease Center in Atlanta,[31] it was found that between October 1, 1966, and October 1, 1967, 5.2% of the hemodialysis patients and 2.8% of the staff had hepatitis. Inasmuch as the survey included 108 hemodialysis units, these figures illustrate an overall risk.

In a large outbreak that included over 100 cases of serum hepatitis among personnel and patients at the hemodialysis centers in Stockholm, the figures were even more striking.[24] One of the hemodialysis departments employed four nurses. During the first 4 months of the outbreak, three of them contracted hepatitis and were replaced. Within 4 months, hepatitis occurred among the new personnel. A total of eight nurses were infected in this little unit during the first year of the outbreak. As may be seen in Table 1, cases also occurred in wards, laboratories, blood banks, and an autopsy department. Five doctors, 22 nurses, 22 nurse's assistants, 21 technicians, 13 technician's assistants, one autopsy attendant, and one office worker contracted hepatitis.

The incidence of hepatitis has also been very high among hemodialysis patients. At present, all patients who have been hemodialyzed for over 3 months at one of the clinics have shown signs of hepatitis. This is probably caused by the fact that the equipment cannot be sterilized after its use. Because the disease is endemic, the personnel of the dialysis unit, the wards, and the laboratories are continuously exposed to serum hepatitis.

Infectious hepatitis may also be an occupational hazard for medical personnel. Some of the outbreaks of hepatitis in hemodialysis units may have involved infectious hepatitis. Capps *et al.*[4] in 1952 reported an outbreak of infectious hepatitis in student nurses, who were infected through contact with unrecognized nonicteric cases among children in an orphanage. Krugman *et al.*[16] reported hepatitis among the attendants at Willowbrook School.

When there is an outbreak of hepatitis, the question arises whether gamma globulin should be given prophylactically. The reason for giving gamma globulin is usually to protect against or modify the disease in persons already exposed to it. There is some evidence that gamma globulin given as late as a week before onset of the disease may be of prophylactic value.[27] It is, however, important that prophylaxis be given as soon as possible. In infectious hepatitis, 0.01 ml of gamma globulin per

TABLE 1 Distribution of 85 Hepatitis Cases in Personnel of a Hemodialysis Center in Stockholm

Place of Employment	No. Cases
Laboratory	33
Dialysis unit	21
Medical ward	13
Intensive-care unit	7
Surgical ward	6
Blood bank	3
X-ray department	1
Autopsy department	1

pound of body weight has been found effective under most conditions of exposure.[16] The effect of the gamma globulin is to change the overt form of hepatitis to a subclinical one. There is little evidence that this change makes the patient less likely to transmit the infection.

The administration of great amounts of gamma globulin has been found to give longer periods of protection than that of small amounts, but not necessarily a higher degree of protection. If the exposure to hepatitis is continued for a long time, a dosage of 0.06 ml/lb of body weight may be given and the administration repeated after 5–6 months. It has been suggested that, if the risk of contracting hepatitis during the first year of gamma globulin protection is very high, further injections might not be necessary, because the exposed person most probably would be immune. Cline et al.[5] and Frame[8] found an increased morbidity in hepatitis among missionaries. The increase in morbidity lasted for several years if the missionaries continued to be exposed. These results suggest that prophylaxis should be continued extensively.

Reports of the effect of prophylaxis with gamma globulins to prevent serum hepatitis are somewhat contradictory.[6,7,11] However, Mirick et al.[20] reported that the frequency of posttransfusion hepatitis with jaundice may be reduced by the administration of 10 ml of gamma globulin with the transfusion and another 10 ml a month later. It may be of epidemiologic significance that prophylaxis probably changes the icteric disease to a nonicteric one.

In the outbreak among hemodialysis personnel in Stockholm, administration of 12 ml or more of a 12% solution of gamma globulin had no prophylactic value.[25] In studies not yet published, we found that the hemodialysis patients had a much milder hepatitis than the personnel. A good correlation was found between the length of the hemodialysis treatment before exposure to hepatitis and the maximal recorded SGPT level (Figure 1). Inasmuch as the hemodialysis treatment often involves administration of many units of transfusion blood, there is also a good correlation between the amounts of blood given and the maximal SGPT level. As can be seen from Figure 2, SGPT values of over 500 units were significantly less common in patients who had received over 40 units of blood before exposure to hepatitis. So far, it has not been possible to establish the reasons for these findings. They may be caused by antibodies present in some blood samples in amounts sufficient to prevent icteric hepatitis.

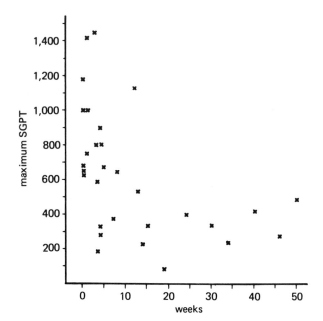

FIGURE 1   Relationship between length of hemodialysis treatment before probable day of exposure to hepatitis and maximal SGPT level.

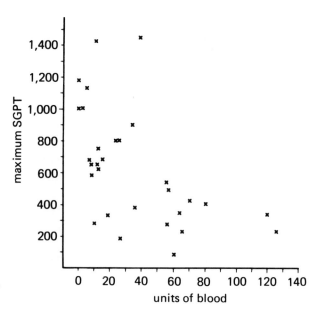

FIGURE 2   Relationship between number of units of transfusion blood received during the 5 months preceding probable day of exposure to hepatitis and maximal SGPT level.

The administration of gamma globulin is rarely followed by any side effects. A few instances of hypersensitivity have been reported, but the risk seems to be extremely small. When given intravenously, however, gamma globulin may cause severe reactions. Antibody production against gamma globulin may occur, but its clinical significance is unknown. These considerations should not prevent the use of gamma globulin when it is indicated as prophylaxis against infectious hepatitis. Prophylaxis by use of gamma globulin is expensive. In our experience, absence from work due to hepatitis often exceeds 100 days. The loss of trained medical personnel for such a period is a far larger problem than the cost of prophylaxis. Nevertheless, because stores of gamma globulin are not unlimited, it should be given only when it is epidemiologically indicated. Circumstances may influence both the decision of whether to give prophylactic gamma globulin and the dosage. It is therefore not possible to suggest any definite rules applicable in all outbreaks. In Table 2, I have outlined a scheme that may be of some practical value.

It is most important to know whether the disease is serum hepatitis or infectious hepatitis. This is often not clear during the early stages of an outbreak. It is my opinion that prophylactic gamma globulin should

TABLE 2 Guidelines for Prophylactic Use of Gamma Globulin (16% Solution) to Prevent Occupational Hepatitis

Type of Hepatitis	Route of Transmission	Exposure	Dosage, ml/lb of Body Weight
Unknown	Unknown	Obvious	0.01–0.02
		Unknown	None
Infectious	Fecal–oral; inoculation	Definite or probable	0.01–0.02
		Possible but not probable	None
		Continuous or repeated	0.03–0.05 every 5–6 months
Serum	Inoculation	Known; obvious instance of exposure	0.07 immediately and 0.07 a month later may be tried
		Continuous or repeated, but without known instance of exposure	None (0.07 immediately and 0.07 a month later may be tried)

be used in all outbreaks to the same extent and in the same dosage as it would be in an outbreak of infectious hepatitis, as long as this diagnosis cannot be excluded. Early in an outbreak, when the source of infection, the routes of transmission, and the type of hepatitis are still unknown, gamma globulin may be given to persons whose risk of exposure has been or still is obvious. Later in the outbreak, when the epidemiologic characteristics of the outbreak have been revealed, a more rational use of gamma globulin is possible. If the outbreak is caused by serum hepatitis, the effect of gamma globulin must be considered doubtful, but it may be tried. During the last few years of the outbreak at the hemodialysis clinics in Stockholm, gamma globulin prophylaxis was restricted to personnel who had a known, obvious exposure, such as by accidental pricking with a needle known to be contaminated with blood from a patient with serum hepatitis. Other personnel continuously exposed but without a definitive instance of exposure were not given gamma globulin.

Hepatitis as an occupational hazard is not a problem exclusively among medical personnel. Several authors[13, 30] have reported cases of infectious hepatitis among chimpanzee handlers, probably due to animal contact. Hepatitis has been reported in pharmaceutical workers preparing blood derivatives. Hepatitis among missionaries, military personnel, and other persons whose work leads them to visit areas with a high risk of hepatitis also may be considered as "occupational." Grounds for prophylactic gamma globulin administration in these groups should be similar to those outlined for medical personnel.

It should be remembered that in most outbreaks gamma globulin is only a complement to other preventive measures. In all work associated with a risk of hepatitis, it is essential to take hygienic measures based on a careful analysis of the possible routes of transmission. Such measures may include change of working routines, wearing of protective gloves, adequate sterilization of equipment, use of disposable equipment, and isolation of the source of infection. These measures are often more important than the use of gamma globulin.

REFERENCES

1. Allen, J. G., and W. A. Sayman. Serum hepatitis from transfusions of blood. Epidemiologic study. JAMA 180:1079–1085, 1962.

2. Bjørneboe, M., M. Jersild, K. Lundbaek, E. Hess Thaysen, and E. Ryssing. Incidence of chronic hepatitis in women in Copenhagen 1944–45. Lancet 1:867–868, 1948.
3. Byrne, E. B. Viral hepatitis: An occupational hazard of medical personnel. Experience of the Yale-New Haven Hospital, 1952 to 1965. JAMA 195:362–364, 1966.
4. Capps, R. B., A. M. Bennett, and J. Stokes, Jr. Endemic infectious hepatitis in an infants' orphanage; epidemiologic studies in student nurses. Arch. Intern. Med. 89:6–23, 1952.
5. Cline, A. L., J. W. Mosley, and F. G. Scovel. Viral hepatitis among American missionaries abroad. A preliminary study. JAMA 199:551–553, 1967.
6. Drake, M. E., J. A. Barondess, W. J. Bashe, Jr., G. Henle, W. Henle, J. Stokes, Jr., and R. B. Pennell. Failure of convalescent gamma globulin to protect against homologous serum hepatitis. JAMA 152:690–693, 1953.
7. Duncan, G. G., H. A. Christian, J. Stokes, Jr., W. F. Rexer, J. T. Nicholson, and A. Edgar. An evaluation of immune serum globulin as a prophylactic agent against homologous serum hepatitis. Amer. J. Med. Sci. 213:53–57, 1947.
8. Frame, J. D. Hepatitis among missionaries in Ethiopia and Sudan. Susceptibles at high risk. JAMA 203:819–826, 1968.
9. Friedman, E. A., and G. E. Thomson. Hepatitis complicating chronic haemodialysis. Lancet 2:675–678, 1966.
10 Gille, G., O. Ringertz, and B. Zetterberg. Serum hepatitis among Swedish track-finders. II. A clinical study. Acta. Med. Scand. 182:129–135, 1967.
11. Grossman, E. B., S. G. Stewart, and J. Stokes, Jr. Post-transfusion hepatitis in battle casualties and study of its prophylaxis by means of human immune serum globulin. JAMA 129:991–994, 1945.
12. Hepatitis and the artificial kidney. Annotation. Lancet 2:1000, 1965.
13. Hillis, W. D. An outbreak of infectious hepatitis among chimpanzee handlers at a United States Air Force Base. Amer. J. Hyg. 73:316–328, 1961.
14. Horstmann, D. M., W. P. Havens, Jr., and J. Deutsch. Infectious hepatitis in childhood; report of 2 institutional outbreaks and comparison of disease in adults and children. J. Pediat. 30:381–387, 1947.
15. Jones, P. O., H. J. Goldsmith, F. K. Wright, C. Roberts, and D. C. Watson. Viral hepatitis. A staff hazard in dialysis units. Lancet 1:835–840, 1967.
16. Krugman, S., R. Ward, J. P. Giles, and A. M. Jacobs. Infectious hepatitis. Studies on the effect of gamma globulin and on the incidence of inapparent infection. JAMA 174:823–830, 1960.
17. Kuh, C., and W. E. Ward. Occupational virus hepatitis: An apparent hazard for medical personnel. JAMA 143:631–635, 1950.
18. Leibowitz, S., L. Greenwald, I. Cohen, and J. Litwins. Serum hepatitis in a blood bank worker. JAMA 140:1331–1333, 1949.
19. Mannbeck, H. The course of infectious hepatitis at varying ages and its spread among different social groups (Stockholm 1948–49). Acta Med. Scand. 155:353–359, 1956.
20. Mirick, G. S., R. Ward, and R. W. McCollum. Modification of posttransfusion hepatitis by gamma globulin. New Eng. J. Med. 273:59–65, 1965.
21. Pendras, J. P., and R. V. Erickson. Hemodialysis: A successful therapy for chronic uremia. Ann. Intern. Med. 64:293–311, 1966.
22. Popper, L., and A. Raber. Die Virushepatitis bei Aerzten und beim Pflegepersonal. Wien. Klin. Wschr. 75:387–389, 1963.
23. Ringertz, O., and B. Melén. Hepatitis and the artificial kidney. Lancet 1:151, 1966.
24. Ringertz, O., and B. Nyström. Viral hepatitis in connection with hemo-dialysis and kidney transplantation. Scand. J. Urol. Nephrol. 1:192–198, 1967.

25. Ringertz, O., B. Nyström, and J. Ström. Clinical aspects on an outbreak of hepatitis among personnel in hemodialysis units. Scand. J. Infect. Dis. 1:51–56, 1969.
26. Ringertz, O., and B. Zetterberg. Serum hepatitis among Swedish trackfinders. An epidemiologic study. New Eng. J. Med. 276:540–546, 1967.
27. Stokes, J., Jr., and J. R. Neefe. The prevention and attenuation of infectious hepatitis by gamma globulin; preliminary note. JAMA 127:144–145, 1945.
28. Strömbeck, J. P. Om risken för hepatitinfektion vid medicinsk yrkesutövning. Svenska Läkartidn. 49:265–273, 1952.
29. Turner, R. H., J. R. Snavely, E. B. Grossman, R. N. Buchanan, and S. O. Foster. Some clinical studies of acute hepatitis occurring in soldiers after inoculation with yellow fever vaccine; with especial consideration of severe attacks. Ann. Intern. Med. 20:193–218, 1944.
30. U.S. Department of Health, Education, and Welfare, Public Health Service, National Communicable Disease Center. Hepatitis Surveillance Report No. 23. 1965.
31. U.S. Department of Health, Education, and Welfare, Public Health Service, National Communicable Disease Center, Hepatitis Surveillance Report No. 28. 1968.

DISCUSSION

DR. CONRAD: In recent years, there have been increasing reports of hepatitis among personnel working in dialysis units. But similar reports among personnel working on wards containing patients with infectious hepatitis have not been forthcoming. Do you think this bespeaks some important difference in either the transmission or the etiology?

DR. RINGERTZ: In Sweden, we have had a large outbreak of hepatitis among hemodialysis patients and personnel. Some of the personnel, when ill, transferred to the infectious-disease hospitals in Stockholm. In these hospitals, newly employed personnel were usually given 1.2 ml of gamma globulin upon arrival, and no additional doses. I do not think that would be very effective in preventing hepatitis in personnel in an infectious-disease hospital. But they did not get hepatitis. When the hemodialysis patients and personnel were taken into the infectious-disease hospitals, cases began to occur among the laboratory personnel there, although in the preceding 10 years no cases of hepatitis had been found. This is a type of hepatitis that differs clearly from the hepatitis that occurred in the Swedish track-finders, and also from the hepatitis that we have seen and know as infectious hepatitis in Sweden.

DR. CONRAD: I have also been most impressed with the low incidence among our personnel who deal with purported infectious hepatitis on the wards, compared with the experience in hemodialysis units.

DR. GOOD: Patients with immunologic deficiency, particularly those with Bruton agammaglobulinemia, do not seem able to resist the hepatitis virus. I know of 12 such patients who had hepatitis; it is a progressive and destructive disease, and

ultimately fatal. Some of these patients developed hepatitis while receiving (by
the standards you are talking about) massive doses of gamma globulin. However,
we do not know what causes the hepatitis. In two instances that we studied in
Minneapolis, the only injections that the patients were receiving were of 0.3–
0.5 ml of gamma globulin per pound of body weight every 3 weeks. There was
nothing in the gamma globulin that protected these patients against whatever the
hepatitis virus was; they were, paradoxically, extraordinarily susceptible. It looks
as though pools of gamma globulin contain very little or no antibody to an agent
that immunoglobulins are believed to neutralize.

DR. BRYAN: As has been mentioned by Dr. Ringertz, the National Communicable
Disease Center has been involved in a cooperative study of hemodialysis-
associated hepatitis in the United States. As of September 1, 1968, 120 dialysis
units were participating in the study. Approximately 41% had experienced hepatitis in dialysis patients at some time during the preceding 11-month period (October 1, 1967, through September 1, 1968). Nearly 20% had experienced hepatitis
in hemodialysis staff (physicians, nurses, technicians) over the same period. These
figures indicate that hemodialysis-associated hepatitis is indeed a widespread problem in the United States and not limited to a few units. A complete report of the
results of this national cooperative study appeared in Hepatitis Surveillance Report 30, April 21, 1969, compiled by the Viral Diseases Branch, Epidemiology
Program, National Communicable Disease Center, Atlanta, Georgia 30333.

S. EDWARD SULKIN *and* ROBERT M. PIKE

Use of Specific Immune Globulin in the Prevention of Laboratory-Acquired Infections

Through accidental exposures to infectious agents in the laboratory, a substantial number of workers contract serious diseases for which there are no adequate therapeutic measures. Until effective vaccines against these agents are developed, the availability of specific immune globulins for prompt use in case of laboratory accidents may prevent many infections or at least limit the severity of the illnesses and reduce the number of fatalities.

The magnitude of the problem of laboratory-acquired infections as it relates to the occupational health of laboratory workers did not become evident until the results of an extensive survey conducted in 1950 became available. Until then, only an occasional report was concerned with the need for protecting personnel who contact disease-producing agents daily. To obtain information regarding the occurrence of all types of laboratory infections and determine where the greatest need for caution existed, the National Institutes of Health sponsored a survey, which revealed over 1,300 instances of overt laboratory-acquired infections, of which 39 were fatal.[21] Since then, a file has been maintained of infections acquired in the laboratory as they have been reported in the literature. In addition, the American Committee on Arthropod-Borne Viruses

in 1963 established a Subcommittee on Laboratory Infections, which
has gathered information concerning experiences with arthropod-borne
viruses and has provided evidence that the arboviruses are of greater
potential hazard to the laboratory worker than any other agents infectious to man.[7] The total number of overt laboratory-acquired infections
now on record is 3,178; 132 were fatal. In addition, numerous inapparent infections have been detected by serologic tests. The distribution
of the overt cases among the principal categories of infectious agents is
shown in Table 1. Brucellosis, typhoid fever, and tularemia constituted
almost half the infections (1,440) and caused almost half the deaths (57).
More than half the 838 infections due to viruses were caused by 36 of
the more than 200 arboviruses. The next most common viral infection
was hepatitis. The highest proportion of fatalities was caused by the
Bedsoniae.

Changes over the years in the kinds of agents involved reflect trends
in areas of research and interest in specific agents.[13] For example, the
typhoid bacillus was high on the list of bacteria responsible for
laboratory-acquired infections before 1950, but between 1950 and
1963, only 2 of 191 bacterial infections acquired in the laboratory were
due to this organism. From 1930 to 1950, bacterial infections in general
predominated over viral infections, whereas since 1950, this order has
been reversed, with close to 40% of the total number of laboratory-

TABLE 1 Recorded Cases of Overt Laboratory-Acquired Infection

Agent	Cases		Deaths	
	No.	% of Total	No.	% of Cases
Bacteria	1,440	45	57	4.0
Viruses	838[a]	26	38	4.5
Rickettsiae	526	17	22	4.2
Fungi	148	5	3	2.0
Bedsoniae	107	3	9	8.4
Parasites	79	2	1	1.3
Unspecified	40	1	2	5.0
Total	3,178	100	132	4.2

[a]Of which 456 were due to arboviruses, with 18 deaths.

TABLE 2 Cases of Overt Laboratory Infection Resulting from Various Accidents

Agent Involved	Accidents Involving Needle and Syringe	Contacts with Infectious Material (Spilling, Spattering, etc.)	Exposures Due to Pipetting	Bites of Animals or Ectoparasites	Injuries with Broken Glass, etc.	Unspecified Cause of Exposure	Totals
Bacteria	73	74	59	28	31	24	289
Viruses[a]	30 (14)	36 (19)	20 (10)	16 (9)	9 (5)	6	117 (57)
Bedsoniae	3	5	1	0	0	3	12
Rickettsiae	12	6	2	5	0	3	28
Parasites	11	7	1	11	0	0	30
Fungi	11	6	0	1	2	1	21
Totals	140	134	83	61	42	37	497

[a]Figures in parentheses refer to arboviruses.

266

acquired infections being due to viruses and only 30% due to bacteria. The limited number of fatal cases among the laboratory-acquired rickettsial and bacterial infections is probably attributable to the effectiveness of active immunization and the use of antibiotics—procedures not yet available for a large number of viruses.

Table 2 categorizes 497 documented laboratory-acquired infections according to the infectious agent involved and the type of accident that resulted in the exposure. Accidents involving needles and syringes were responsible for the greatest number of infections, followed closely by direct contact with infectious material by spilling or spattering. Other infections were attributed to pipetting accidents, bites of animals or ectoparasites, and injuries with broken glass. The final category consists of undescribed accidents.

ACTIVE IMMUNIZATION

The ideal mechanism for protection against the infectious diseases likely to be contracted in the laboratory is the prophylactic production of active immunity by means of vaccines. Vaccines are currently available for only a few of the arboviruses that are prominent causes of laboratory-acquired infections. Limited supplies of formalin-inactivated Eastern equine encephalitis (EEE) and Western equine encephalitis (WEE) virus vaccines are available at the Walter Reed Army Institute of Research for the immunization of technical personnel at high risk. Because formalinized Venezuelan equine encephalitis (VEE) virus vaccines have been known to produce infection and disease in those vaccinated,[18] a preparation made with an attenuated strain of this virus is under investigation and has already been used to limit the occurrence of infection in laboratory personnel.[10] And a vaccine using an attenuated strain of WEE virus is being tested in horses.[8] Hammon and his associates have been attempting to develop a vaccine against Japanese B encephalitis (JBE), using live attenuated strains and formalin-killed virus preparations,[6] and an attenuated Dengue virus vaccine is under study. Most of the arboviruses that have been responsible for laboratory-acquired infections are in group B, and a broad-spectrum immunizing procedure such as that being explored by Price and his associates[15] could make arbovirus laboratory work less hazardous.

RATIONALE OF USING IMMUNE GLOBULINS

There is no evidence that the use of convalescent serum or specific immune globulin is of value once symptoms of a viral infection have appeared, but a rationale for instituting passive immunization immediately after accidental exposure has been developed on the basis of studies in experimental animals. Because specific antibodies can neutralize or inactivate viruses, immune globulin is likely to be effective if given soon after an exposure, when virus is in transit from the primary sites of multiplication to the tissues that will manifest the pathologic effects of the disease. The dose required to limit infection in man is unknown. It has been suggested that levels of antibody that can be detected in the blood for 1–2 weeks might suffice. If available, human immune globulin should be administered after an accident. However, animal sera that contain the appropriate antibodies may be substituted after preliminary skin and ophthalmic tests for sensitivity.[1] There is a risk of transmitting hepatitis when a human blood product is used, but the hazard is virtually eliminated by present methods for processing human serum to obtain gamma globulin. Some laboratories engaged in the processing of blood and blood products administer gamma globulin to personnel periodically with the objective of preventing hepatitis.

INSTANCES OF USE OF IMMUNE GLOBULIN

The incidence of disease among research workers in yellow fever and tick-borne encephalitis (TBE) before the development of vaccines was limited by passive prophylaxis.[1,17]

Human anti-St. Louis encephalitis virus (SLE) immune globulin was supplied by the National Communicable Disease Center (NCDC) to an exposed technician in a laboratory in the South Pacific in 1965; the SLE immune globulin was obtained from laboratory-confirmed cases that occurred during the 1964 St. Louis encephalitis epidemics.

When a severe gas explosion occurred in an arbovirus laboratory in the Far East, producing aerosols from Blake bottles that contained JBE virus, two laboratory workers suffered burns and cuts and other persons were present in the area immediately afterward. Soon after the explosion,

Japanese-made immune globulin was administered to 80% of the exposed persons. No overt cases of encephalitis developed, and no evidence of antibodies to JBE virus was detected in the sera obtained some weeks later from laboratory personnel.

Gamma globulin prepared from the serum of patients convalescing from Bolivian hemorrhagic fever was routinely given to research workers and military personnel in the epidemic area of Bolivia.[19] Each of four investigators who acquired the disease in the field had received prophylactic gamma globulin. The development of hemorrhagic fever in these subjects casts some doubt on the effectiveness of this treatment. It should be emphasized that the titer of Machupo (MAC) virus antibodies in the administered material was not known. Obviously, more information is needed to determine the efficacy of gamma globulin in preventing or modifying the course of this disease.

Instances of the use of passive immunization involve the treatment of laboratory personnel accidentally inoculated through their fingers and hands with EEE or WEE viruses (M. Goldfield *et al.*, unpublished data). Five victims were given fresh human immune plasma or whole blood within 1–4 days of such accidents. In all cases, neutralizing antibodies were detectable in recipients' sera for periods ranging from 22 to 36 days; none of the victims became ill, and none developed serologic evidence that active infection had occurred. In another series of incidents (P. H. Coleman, personal communication), 14 persons were known to have been exposed to SLE, WEE, EEE, or VEE. All received antibody-rich whole blood or plasma, and all remained asymptomatic. In three of four of these persons whose antibody level was followed for 2 months, there was no decrease in antibody titer in 2 months, suggesting slow antibody decay or active immunization due to subclinical infection. Although not conclusive, these data suggest that passive immunity may be effective in preventing human infection after accidental peripheral inoculation with EEE or WEE viruses.

Latent and abortive rabies infections have developed.[2,20] Although we have no proof of a laboratory-acquired case of rabies, exposures continue to occur. Because effective vaccines are available, pre-exposure immunization of high-risk personnel against rabies should be mandatory.[3] However, in cases of severe exposure to known rabid animals, the administration of rabies hyperimmune serum as an adjunct to primary vac-

TABLE 3 Mortality from Arbovirus Infection Resulting from Known Accidents

Outcome	Actively Immunized	Passively Immunized
Died (5[a])	0	0
Recovered (52)	4	9[b]

[a]Three cases of yellow fever, one of TBE, and one of WEE.
[b]Seven with convalescent immune serum, one with immune horse serum, and one with normal human serum.

cination or before a booster dose of vaccine is advocated. The advantage of a source of human rabies immune globulin to replace currently available horse antirabies immune serum is obvious.

If immune globulin is to be effective, one must know when exposure occurred. Of the 453 documented laboratory-acquired arbovirus infections, only 57 were due to known accidents. That 87% of these infections developed as a result of circumstances in the laboratory, with no recognized incident to account for the exposure, emphasizes the importance of developing effective vaccines. Table 3 lists the 57 known cases according to outcome. None of the five persons who died received either previous active immunization or immune serum after the accident, whereas, of the 52 who recovered, four had been actively immunized and nine were given immune or normal serum after exposure.

INTERFERON AS ADJUNCT TO PASSIVE PROPHYLAXIS

The degree of protection likely to be afforded through the use of human immune globulins is directly related to the level of neutralizing antibodies. Interferon, now principally of theoretical interest, might be of value in passive prophylaxis.[22] It is known that interferon exhibits antiviral activity,[5] but useful amounts of this inhibitor have never been available. No synthetic interferon has been developed.[9,11] Field and associates[4] have reported that double-stranded RNA may be an active ingredient in interferon-inducing preparations. Through the administration of seemingly purified double-stranded RNA, it was possible to induce therapeutically active levels of circulating interferon. Park and Baron[12] have demonstrated that synthetic double-stranded complexed polynu-

cleotide RNA (polyinosinic:cytidilic acid) can influence recovery from
severe and fully established herpetic keratoconjunctivitis in rabbits when
administered as late as 3 days after virus inoculation. There are also suggestions that resistance to vesicular stomatitis virus infection in the rabbit eye[14] or in rabbit kidney cultures (A. Billiau *et al.*, unpublished data)
may be mediated by inducers of interferon (bacterial endotoxin, stato-
lon, or complexed polynucleotide RNA). These studies suggest the usefulness of interferon-inducing agents in some situations, especially those
in which immune globulin contains low levels of antibody. Also of interest is information, as yet unpublished, from Russian investigators
(L. L. Fadeeva and associates) suggesting that gamma globulin stimulated the induction of interferon in both tissue cultures and mice and,
in the latter, prevented 87.5% of the mice from becoming infected with
murine hepatitis.

EFFORTS TO STOCKPILE SPECIFIC ANTIVIRAL
IMMUNE GLOBULIN

For most viral diseases, antibodies can be commercially prepared in the
form of immune globulin from persons recovering from the illness or
experiencing inapparent infections or from those actively immunized.
Human gamma globulin from some geographic areas in which a given
disease is known to occur repeatedly (e.g., Japanese encephalitis in the
Far East) is likely to contain antibodies for which a demand exists elsewhere. Stockpiling of such human immune globulin would be desirable.

The increasing incidence of laboratory-acquired infections prompted
the American Committee on Arboviruses to concern itself with the
procurement, processing, and use of immune globulin for emergency
treatment of exposed workers and to collaborate with the World Health
Organization, which has prepared an inventory of the type, quantity,
and location of viral and specific immune globulins available in different
laboratories (A. C. Saenz, personal communication).

The procurement of immune sera, the production of immune globulin
from them on a commercial scale, and their assay for potency constitute
a formidable undertaking. Efforts are being made by the National Communicable Disease Center, the World Health Organization, and other
agencies to process gamma globulin from normal human plasma in areas

in which the population has been subjected to multiple infections with numerous arboviruses and in which the gamma globulin of the population contains antibodies with a high titer. Sera from those convalescing from arbovirus infections are also being collected. The gamma globulins that have been prepared from plasma from persons with antibodies to SLE, WEE, VEE, California encephalitis, and MAC viruses and that will eventually be available on a restricted basis for use after some types of laboratory accidents are as follows:

Anti-JBE gamma globulin processed at National Institute of Health, Tokyo, Japan (Dr. Masami Kitaoka): Plasma (120 liters) from healthy donors from JBE endemic areas. Gamma globulin available in 3.0-ml ampuls. Protects monkeys and mice up to 24 hr after challenge.

Anti-central European tick-borne encephalitis (TBE) gamma globulin processed at Institute of Epidemiology and Microbiology, Prague, Czechoslovakia (Dr. K. Zacek): Plasma from 22 donors who had had proven TBE within 3 years of being bled. Gamma globulin in 16% solution available in 1.9-ml ampuls. Low potency due to time interval. Recent convalescents scarce.

Anti-EEE gamma globulin processed at NCDC, Atlanta, Georgia (Dr. Morris T. Suggs): Plasma from volunteers immunized against EEE. Gamma globulin available in 10.0-ml ampuls. Potency data not available.

Human-origin rabies gamma globulin (HRIG) processed at NCDC, Atlanta, Georgia[16] : Plasma from volunteers (mostly veterinarians) immunized against rabies. Biologic containing 165 IU/ml. Apparently as effective as equine antirabies serum in protecting experimental animals challenged with street virus.

To our knowledge, the anti-JBE and anti-TBE products have not yet been tested in emergency situations.

The mechanisms for the exchange and distribution of specific human immune globulins and for honoring requests in emergency situations are under study. It had previously been recommended[1] that stocks of specific arboviral vaccines be made available to the World Health Organization as they are developed, for distribution through cooperating laboratories. Human gamma globulin may be distributed in a similar way.

We are grateful to Drs. William McD. Hammon, Arturo C. Saenz, Morris T. Suggs, and Telford H. Work and others for providing information contained in this report.

REFERENCES

1. Arboviruses and Human Disease. Report of a WHO Scientific Group. WHO Tech. Report Series No. 369. Geneva: World Health Organization, 1967. 84 pp.
2. Bell, J. F. Abortive rabies infection. I. Experimental production in white mice and general discussion. J. Infect. Dis. 114:249–257, 1964.
3. Fenje, P., I. M. Cass, and R. J. Wilson. Pre-exposure immunization against rabies in high risk personnel. Canad. J. Public Health 56:325–328, 1965.
4. Field, A. K., A. A. Tytell, G. P. Lampson, and M. R. Hilleman. Inducers of interferon and host resistance. II. Multistranded synthetic polynucleotide complexes. Proc. Nat. Acad. Sci. USA 58:1004–1010, 1967.
5. Finter, N. B., Ed. Interferons. Philadelphia: W. B. Saunders Co., 1966. 340 pp.
6. Hammon, W. McD. Arboviruses. Present and future of killed and live arbovirus vaccines, pp. 252–259. In First International Conference on Vaccines Against Viral and Rickettsial Diseases of Man. Scientific Publ. No. 147. Washington, D.C.: Pan American Health Organization, World Health Organization, 1967.
7. Hanson, R. P., S. E. Sulkin, E. L. Buescher, W. McD. Hammon, R. W. McKinney, and T. H. Work. Arbovirus infections of laboratory workers. Extent of problem emphasizes the need for more effective measures to reduce hazards. Science 158:1283–1286, 1967.
8. Johnson, H. N. Selection of a variant of Western encephalitis virus of low pathogenicity for study as a live virus vaccine. Amer. J. Trop. Med. Hyg. 12:604–610, 1963.
9. Lampson, G. P., A. A. Tytell, M. M. Nemes, and M. R. Hilleman. Purification and characterization of chick embryo interferon. Proc. Soc. Exp. Biol. Med. 112:468–478, 1963.
10. McKinney, R. W., T. O. Berge, W. D. Sawyer, W. D. Tigertt, and D. Crozier. Use of an attenuated strain of Venezuelan equine encephalomyelitis virus for immunization in man. Amer. J. Trop. Med. Hyg. 12:597–603, 1963.
11. Meyer, H. M., Jr. The control of viral diseases. Problems and prospects viewed in perspective. J. Pediat. 73:653–675, 1968.
12. Park, J. H., and S. Baron. Herpetic keratoconjunctivitis: Therapy with synthetic double-stranded RNA. Science 162:811–813, 1968.
13. Pike, R. M., S. E. Sulkin, and M. L. Schulze. Continuing importance of laboratory-acquired infections. Amer. J. Public Health 55:190–199, 1965.
14. Pollikoff, R., A. DiPuppo, and P. Cannavale. Vesicular stomatitis virus (VSV) infection in rabbit eye: Role of antibody and interferon. Invest. Ophthal. 8:488–496, 1969.
15. Price, W. H., J. Parks, J. Ganaway, R. Lee, and W. O'Leary. A sequential immunization procedure against certain group B arboviruses. Amer. J. Trop. Med. Hyg. 12:624–638, 1963.
16. Sikes, R. K. Human rabies immune globulin. Progress Report. Public Health Rep. 84:797–801, 1969.
17. Silber, L. A., and V. D. Soloviev. Far Eastern tick-borne spring-summer (spring) encephalitis. Amer. Rev. Soviet Med. 5 (Special Suppl.):6–80, 1947–1948.
18. Smith, D. G., H. K. Mamay, R. G. Marshall, and J. C. Wagner. Venezuelan equine encephalomyelitis. Laboratory aspects of 14 human cases following vaccination and attempts to isolate the virus from the vaccine. Amer. J. Hyg. 63:150–164, 1956.

19. Stinebaugh, B. J., F. X. Schloeder, K. M. Johnson, R. B. Mackenzie, G. Entwisle, and E. De Alba. Bolivian hemorrhagic fever. A report of four cases. Amer. J. Med. 40:217–230, 1966.
20. Sulkin, S. E. The bat as a reservoir of viruses in nature. Progr. Med. Virol. 4:157–207, 1962.
21. Sulkin, S. E., and R. M. Pike. Survey of laboratory-acquired infections. Amer. J. Public Health 41:769–781, 1951.
22. Wagner, R. R. Interferon. A review and analysis of recent observations. Amer. J. Med. 38:726–737, 1965.

L. K. DIAMOND

Use of Immune Globulin in Prevention of Rh Sensitization in Pregnancy

In the last year, a gamma globulin concentrate of anti-Rh serum has become commercially available. After some 5 years of clinical trial, it has proved almost unbelievably successful in preventing Rh sensitization of Rh-negative women recently delivered of Rh-positive infants. The development of this protective treatment might have occurred several years earlier, inasmuch as it has long been recognized that the passage of Rh-positive erythrocytes from an infant to its mother caused her sensitization. But it was believed that such cells leaked across the placenta during pregnancy and that therefore nothing could be done after the infant was delivered. In support of this concept of sensitization during pregnancy, the studies of Cohen et al.[4] had shown, by fluorescent-antibody tagging techniques, that fetal cells could be found in the maternal circulation early as well as late in pregnancy. Other investigators, however, particularly Fear and Queenan,[5] had evidence that sensitization of an Rh-negative woman was much more likely to take place during or after delivery, particularly abnormal delivery—such as cesarean section, manual removal of the placenta, and other operative and potentially traumatic types—which probably permitted greater admixture of maternal and fetal blood. If it had been recognized that sensitization of

275

TABLE 1   Fetal-Cell Counts in Maternal Blood after Delivery in Fetomaternal ABO Compatibility and Incompatibility[a]

Fetal Cells in Maternal Blood, ml (Kleihauer count)	ABO-Compatible		ABO-Incompatible	
	No.	%	No.	%
0	320	39.7	138	71.1
<0.25	331	41.1	48	24.7
>0.25	155	19.2	8	4.1

[a]Derived from Clarke.[2]

the Rh-negative woman commonly occurred during or after delivery of her Rh-positive infant, attempts to block such antibody production might have been considered feasible.

An interesting observation, first made by Levine in 1943 and confirmed later,[7] was that a pregnancy involving an Rh-positive infant that was incompatible with its Rh-negative mother by ABO blood groups was much less likely to produce Rh sensitization in her than if infant and mother were ABO-compatible. That suggested that circulating antibodies—anti-A, anti-B, and so on—against the fetal erythrocytes protected the woman from sensitization.

In Liverpool, England, Clarke *et al.*[3] accumulated definitive data on the number of fetal cells in the maternal circulation after delivery and compared the cases of ABO incompatibility between mother and child with those of ABO compatibility. As shown in Table 1, the fetal-cell count in ABO incompatibility was much smaller than in ABO compatibility; that, of course, was independent of the Rh type of the infant. The fetal-cell count was done by the Kleihauer technique (or a modification of it) in which advantage is taken of the alkali or acid resistance of fetal hemoglobin, compared with adult hemoglobin. These data confirmed that there was a blocking or destruction of the A- or B-incompatible fetal cells by the anti-A or anti-B of the maternal serum.

The next step in this train of evidence is shown in Table 2. Clarke and his associates showed that the larger the number of Rh-positive fetal cells in the circulation of the Rh-negative woman shortly after delivery, the greater the chance of her becoming sensitized. Even when

no fetal cells were demonstrable, there was still a 2% risk of sensitization; such cells might have escaped the counting process or become
sequestered in various organs or tissue spaces, or, if there was a delay
between delivery and blood examination, they might already have been
taken out of the circulation by the reticuloendothelial system.

Reasoning that an Rh antibody might equally well block initiation of
sensitization by Rh-positive cells entering the mother's circulation after
delivery, the Liverpool group began the intravenous use of relatively
large amounts of high-titer anti-Rh plasma from known sensitized
women in Rh-negative unsensitized mothers of recently delivered Rh-
positive infants. The results were encouraging in a small series of cases,
but there were some handicaps to this mode of treatment. It required
fairly large volumes of anti-Rh plasma; the antibody had to have a high
titer to be effective after dilution by the much larger plasma volume of
the recipient; and, most hazardous, there was an unpredictable danger
of serum hepatitis in the recipient. These problems were resolved by
following the lead offered by Freda et al.,[6] who, starting at about the
same time but from a different theoretical approach, had developed a
successful method of preventing Rh sensitization through the use, not
of anti-Rh serum, but of a gamma globulin concentrate prepared from
pools of plasma obtained from known sensitized persons. They decided
to apply the principles developed through the well-known work of
Theobald Smith, who showed in 1909 that the injection of an antitoxin
combined with an excess of toxin stimulated antibody production, but
that immunization was prevented if there were a surplus of antitoxin to
toxin. Applying this to the problem of Rh sensitization, Freda and his

TABLE 2 Rh Immunization 6 Months after Delivery Related to Fetal-Cell Count in Maternal
Blood at Delivery (Rh-Negative Primiparas with Rh-Positive ABO-Compatible Babies)[a]

No. Fetal Cells in Maternal Blood	Women Immunized		No. Women Not Immunized
	No.	%	
0	5	3	186
1–4	11	8	121
5–60	9	17	44
>60	3	50	3

[a]Derived from Brit. Med. J.[8]

associates decided to inject protective amounts of anti-Rh plasma with
Rh-positive cells into Rh-negative male volunteers. To avoid the use of
large-volume infusions of raw plasma and particularly the risk of infection with the virus of serum hepatitis, they prepared an anti-Rh gamma
globulin extract of plasma containing a high titer of Rh antibody. This
concentrate could be given intramuscularly in relatively small volume
and carried no hepatitis risk. When the trial with male volunteers
proved eminently successful, Freda and his associates started injecting
anti-Rh gamma globulin into Rh-negative unsensitized women who had
recently delivered Rh-positive infants. As seen in Table 3, the results in
both the male volunteers and the recently delivered women were completely successful. A large field trial in dozens of obstetric centers
could then be set up.

The Ortho Research Foundation of Raritan, New Jersey, arranged
for the collection of large pools of plasma from Rh-negative sensitized
donors who were shown to have high-titer anti-Rh antibodies. The
plasma was fractionated. The immune globulin fraction, over a period
of about 5 years, was distributed and tried in more than 40 obstetric
centers in this country and others; the controls were comparable cases
either not treated or given gamma globulin without Rh antibodies. The
criteria for the use of the anti-Rh immune globulin were as follows:
The women, either at delivery or shortly thereafter, were retested to
verify their Rh-negative typing and the absence of any Rh antibodies.
After delivery, the cord blood of the infant was tested for its Rh type
and the direct Coombs test was done to ensure again the complete
absence of Rh antibodies. Initially, immune globulin was given only to

TABLE 3 Trial Protection against Rh Sensitization in Rh-Negative Men Given Anti-Rh Plasma
and Rh-Positive Erythrocytes (Intravenously) and Rh-Negative Women Given Anti-Rh Gamma
Globulin after Rh-Positive Pregnancy[a]

	Men		Women	
Group	No.	No. with Rh Antibodies	No.	No. with Rh Antibodies
Control (no protection)	18	12	59	7
Protected (gamma globulin injection)	18	0	48	0

[a]Derived from Freda *et al.*[6]

TABLE 4   Rh Immunization 6 Months after Delivery in ABO-Compatible Mothers Who Received
1 ml of Immune Globulin at Delivery[a]

Group	No.	Immunized	
		No.	%[b]
Treated	1,534	2	0.1
Control	815	54	6.6

[a]Derived from Ascari et al.[1]
[b]$p < 0.001$.

women who were also ABO-compatible with their infants, because the
risk in ABO incompatible cases was relatively slight and the immune
globulin was scarce. In addition, in some centers, Kleihauer counts of
fetal cells were done on each woman and the injection was given only
if an estimated 0.25 ml or more of fetal cells could be found. Table 4
shows the results of this field trial as reported by Ascari et al.[1] They
confirmed the almost uniform protection against Rh immunization in
all recipients of the anti-Rh immune globulin. It is of interest to note
that only two women were immunized, probably because of an inadequate dose of immune globulin.

In the Liverpool study, there were also two failures of protection by
the anti-Rh immune globulin in some 1,500 cases. One occurred in a
woman who, through repeated injections of gamma globulin to protect
her against hepatitis in a foreign country in which the disease is endemic,
had developed sensitivity to this plasma fraction. When she received the
anti-Rh immune globulin after the birth of her infant, a large local reaction occurred and presumably interfered with the rapid or adequate
absorption of the gamma globulin, thereby leaving her unprotected. The
other case involved a woman whose infant had bled a large amount into
her circulation; the relatively small regular dose of anti-Rh immune
globulin was inadequate to protect her from immunization by the
large volume of Rh-positive fetal erythrocytes.

A further concern was that the anti-Rh immune globulin injected
after the first pregnancy might only suppress antibody production, and
that a minimal amount or a very weak antibody might not be detected
by standard testing methods, only to appear during a second pregnancy.

It was necessary, therefore, to delay final judgment on the efficacy of this treatment until a number of the supposedly protected women had passed through a second pregnancy, had once more been given anti-Rh immune globulin, and were proved still unsensitized some 6 months later. As seen in Table 5, the concern has been dispelled, and proof of the efficacy of the protective injection has been obtained in a sufficient number of cases to be completely convincing.

Because of the recognized difficulties of judging the potency of an antibody by titer measurements based on agglutination of susceptible erythrocytes, it seemed desirable to have a quantitative measurement of the antibody concentration in the gamma globulin. This was done by Hughes-Jones of London with radioactive tagging methods. It has been shown that 300 μg of antibody per milliliter of gamma globulin is sufficient to protect most Rh-negative unsensitized women. The injection is given intramuscularly within 72 hr of the delivery of an Rh-positive infant. Now that the anti-Rh immune globulin is freely available commercially, even mothers of ABO-incompatible infants should be considered as candidates for treatment, although the risk of sensitization is much smaller in such cases. It may be as low as 2%, compared with the average of 10% in Rh-negative women delivering ABO-compatible Rh-positive infants, but even this slight risk can now be avoided. Finally, if the newborn infant is carefully observed for the first 24 hr and shows evidence of anemia from blood loss into the mother, or if the Kleihauer count on the mother's blood smear shows large amounts of fetal cells, the standard dose of 1 ml of anti-Rh

TABLE 5   Rh Immunization 6 Months after Delivery of a Second Rh-Incompatible Fetus of Mothers Twice Protected by Anti-Rh Immune Globulin[a]

	Control			Treated	
	No.	Immunized No.	%	No.	No. Immunized
U.S. centers	39	12	30.8	44	0
European centers	33	7	21.2	30	0
Totals	72	19	26.4	74	0

[a]Derived from Freda *et al.*[6] and Clarke *et al.*[3]

immune globulin containing 300–400 μg of anti-Rh antibody should be increased to an amount estimated to be protective in the individual situation.

There are possible uses for the anti-Rh immune globulin in addition to those described. If an Rh-negative woman has a miscarriage beyond the third month of gestation, when the fetal erythrocytes can already possess the Rh antigen, and particularly if the father of the child is known to be Rh-positive, the use of the anti-Rh immune globulin would be indicated, especially if a Kleihauer fetal-cell count on the woman's blood were positive. There is considerable evidence that such a miscarriage can be the sensitizing episode that produces hemolytic disease of the fetus and the newborn in a firstborn Rh-positive infant—an occurrence that may be anticipated by the finding of anti-Rh antibodies in such a woman during pregnancy.

Chown and his associates in Winnipeg, Canada, have also tried the injection of small amounts of anti-Rh immune globulin during the latter stages of pregnancy of Rh-negative unsensitized women bearing Rh-positive infants (presumably predictable because the father is found to be homozygous Rh-positive). These investigators believe that they can prevent the occasional sensitization from taking place during pregnancy without harming the infant, even though a relatively small amount of anti-Rh antibody crosses the placenta and may produce a mild hemolytic anemia.

In accidental transfusions of incompatible blood, as sometimes occur through laboratory or secretarial errors, the timely use of anti-Rh immune globulin in carefully graded amounts (so as not to produce a sudden and severe kidney-damaging destruction of the donor's Rh-positive cells) may keep the recipient from developing Rh antibodies later. Reports of such use of the material are too few to permit a clear statement of how often, how much, and what strength antibody concentrate should be given in these unfortunate circumstances. Undoubtedly, the literature on this subject will soon be augmented, and criteria for the safe use of anti-Rh immune globulin to protect against Rh sensitization by transfusion will be developed.

Another corollary of the development of antibody concentrates in the form of immune globulins may be used to take care of the rare instances of possible sensitization against unusual blood factors—Kell, the subtypes of Rh, such as C, E, c, e, and others. One could readily produce immune globulins against the other clinically important blood-group antigens that can cause hemolytic disease of the fetus and the newborn in the maternal–fetal incompatibilities involving these factors.

It should be possible to eradicate erythroblastosis fetalis, a disease that can afflict over 35,000 infants each year in this country alone. A generation from now, this hemolytic disease of the fetus and the newborn should be of only historical interest.

REFERENCES

1. Ascari, W. Q., P. Levine, and W. Pollack. Incidence of maternal Rh immunization by ABO compatible and incompatible pregnancies. Brit. Med. J. 1:399–401, 1969.
2. Clarke, C. A. Prevention of Rh-haemolytic disease. Brit. Med. J. 4:7–12, 1967.
3. Clarke, C. A., R. Finn, D. Lehane, R. B. McConnell, P. M. Sheppard, and J. C. Woodrow. Dose of anti-D gamma-globulin in prevention of Rh-haemolytic disease of the newborn. Brit. Med. J. 1:213–214, 1966.
4. Cohen, F., W. W. Zuelzer, D. C. Gustafson, and M. M. Evans. Mechanisms of isoimmunization. I. The transplacental passage of fetal erythrocytes in homospecific pregnancies. Blood 23:621–646, 1964.
5. Fear, R. E., and J. T. Queenan. Factors affecting the transplacental passage of fetal erythrocytes. Obstet. Gynec. 29:444–445, 1967. (abstract)
6. Freda, V. J., J. G. Gorman, and W. Pollack. Rh factor: Prevention of isoimmunization and clinical trial on mothers. Science 151:828–830, 1966.
7. Levine, P. The influence of the ABO system on Rh hemolytic disease. Hum. Biol. 30:14–28, 1958.
8. Prevention of Rh-haemolytic disease: Results of the clinical trial. A combined study from centres in England and Baltimore. Brit. Med. J. 2:907–914, 1966.

E. H. SADUN, R. L. HICKMAN, *and*
N. T. BRIGGS

Use of Immune Globulin in the Prevention and Therapy of Malaria

The role of circulating antibodies in malarial immunity has been the object of numerous investigations since the initial demonstration that immune serum exerted a protective activity in rhesus monkeys infected with *Plasmodium knowlesi*.[4] A humoral factor was demonstrated in the blood of subjects living in hyperendemic areas of West Africa. When passively transferred, it was capable of markedly reducing *P. falciparum* parasitemia in the recipients. This factor was separated with IgG and was transmitted transplacentally from immune mother to offspring.[5,6,10,14] It was observed that immune serum from West Africa was also effective against East African strains, and it was suggested that no marked antigenic differences were attributable to geographic separation of strains of this parasite. Adult rats also acquire an immunity to infection with rodent malaria and produce an antiserum that modifies the course of infection in young animals.[3,7,11,13,16]

These reports have led to a series of investigations in chimpanzees infected with *P. falciparum* and in mice and rats infected with *P. berghei* to determine the role of humoral factors in immunity, to evaluate the suppressive efficacy of immune globulin, and to assess the degree of specificity of this immunity.[1,2,12,15]

283

IMMUNE GLOBULINS IN CHIMPANZEES INFECTED WITH *P. FALCIPARUM*

A West African strain of *P. falciparum* (WA) that is chloroquine-sensitive
and a Malayan (Camp) strain (SEA) that is drug-resistant were used.
Immune globulin was extracted from plasma obtained from adult
Nigerians living in a malaria hyperendemic area and from American men
who had acquired the infection in Southeast Asia. Nonimmune American globulin was used as a control. The globulin was given intramuscularly in the total amount of 440 mg/kg of body weight for a period of
4 days. Plasma clearance of ^{131}I-labeled human globulin in chimpanzees
showed that the half-life was 11.5 days in the uninfected animals and 9
days in the infected animals. The therapeutic effect of West African
human immune globulin was studied in six chimpanzees infected with
the WA strain and in 16 chimpanzees infected with the SEA strain of

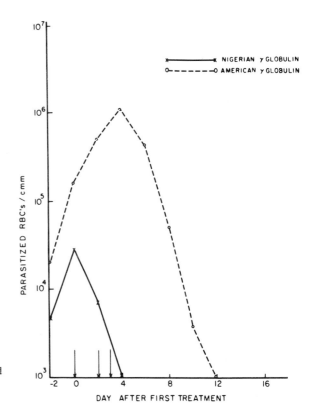

FIGURE 1 Immunosuppressive effect
of WA human gamma globulin in paired
chimpanzees infected with a WA strain
of *P. falciparum.*

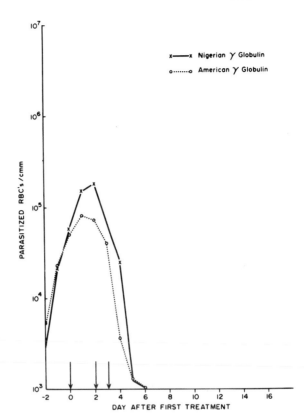

FIGURE 2 Immunosuppressive effect
of WA human gamma globulin in paired
chimpanzees infected with an SEA
strain of *P. falciparum*.

P. falciparum. The animals were paired according to their parasitemia
levels at the time of the first gamma globulin injection. As indicated in
Figures 1 and 2, the immune globulin had a significant suppressive
effect in the animals infected with falciparum malaria from the same
geographic area, but not in those from a different strain isolated from a
different geographic area.

IMMUNE GLOBULINS IN RODENTS INFECTED WITH
P. BERGHEI

Other studies on the passive transfer of immunity were carried out in
mice infected with *P. berghei* by injecting immune globulin obtained
from either immunized rats or mice. Figure 3 shows the normal course

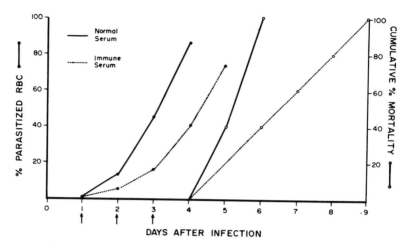

FIGURE 3   Effects of rat antiserum (from repeatedly infected white rats) on the course of parasitemia and survival time of mice infected with 2×10^7 parasitized erythrocytes. Three injections of serum (0.5 ml/injection) were given, on days 1, 2, and 3.

of infection for mice that received 2×10^7 parasitized erythrocytes intravenously. As expected, the parasites multiplied very rapidly, and, by the fourth day after inoculation, approximately 80% of the circulating erythrocytes were infected. Mortalities occurred after the fourth day of infection, and all the mice were dead approximately a week after infection. Immune globulin from infected rats modified the course of infection. Parasitemia was held down for a day or so but eventually began to increase very rapidly. Essentially the same results have been obtained with immune globulin from immunized mice—i.e., a delay in the course of parasitemia followed by a very rapid increase in the number of parasites. This delay, which could represent destruction of almost 90% of the parasites injected, was essentially the same whether single or multiple injections of immune globulin were given (Figure 4). That suggests that the parasites increasing so rapidly after the third day were variants resistant to the antiserum used.

Additional experiments were done to determine whether this assumption was correct. As indicated in Figure 5, when mice infected with the stock strain were treated with a rat antiserum, the same delay in parasitemia resulted. On the fourth day after infection, the rapidly increasing parasites (of the suspected derived strain) were subinoculated

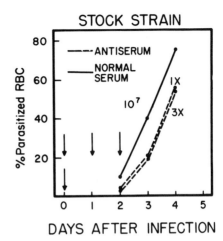

FIGURE 4 Effects of single versus multiple
injections of rat antiserum (0.5 ml/injection)
on the course of parasitemia in mice.

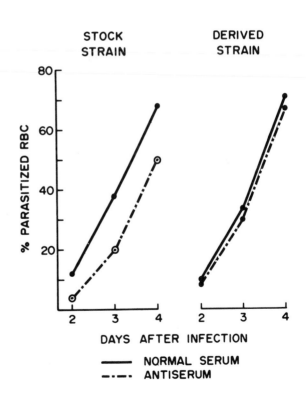

FIGURE 5 Effects of rat antiserum
on the course of parasitemia produced
by inoculation of 2 X 10^7 parasites of
the stock strain and the derived or
variant strain. One injection of antiserum (0.5 ml) on the day of
infection.

into two groups of normal mice, which were then treated with either the same rat antiserum or normal serum. The antiserum effective against the stock strain had no significant effect against the derived or variant strain. In other words, exposure to immune globulin probably produced some immunologic change in the parasite.

Work to date has not demonstrated any change in virulence in populations of variant parasites. As can be seen in Figure 5, control animals infected with the two strains showed the same course of infection and rate of parasite increase. Similar results were obtained in four additional experiments with a smaller inoculum (2×10^3); during the first or second passage in normal untreated mice, variant strains showed a rate of parasite increase almost identical with that for the stock strain.

Variant parasites have also been detected in other experimental situations. Mice can be actively immunized against our stock strain of parasites by repeated injections of x-irradiated, infected erythrocytes. When these mice were challenged with the same stock strain (Figure 6), parasitemia appeared later, increased more slowly, and reached lower

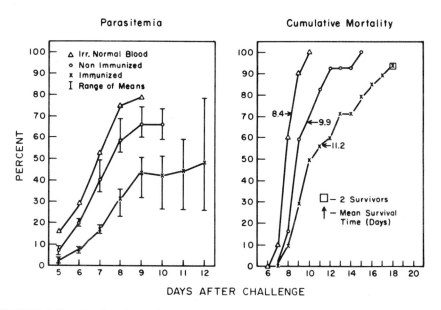

FIGURE 6 Parasitemia and cumulative mortality in mice immunized three times (twice weekly) by injections of 10^8 parasitized erythrocytes exposed to 20,000 r. All animals were challenged with 2×10^4 parasitized erythrocytes a week after the last immunizing injection.

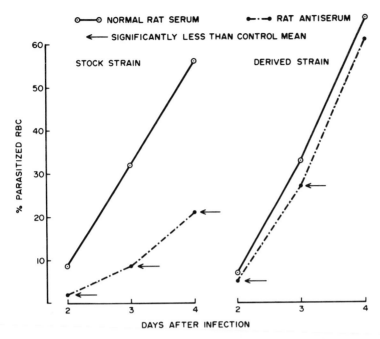

FIGURE 7   Effects of rat antiserum on the course of parasitemia produced by inoculation of 2×10^7 parasites of the stock strain and the derived or variant strain. The latter strain was originally isolated from mice immunized against the stock strain.

peak levels than in the controls. Thus, immunity is often not completely protective against the stock strain, and it was thought that parasites relapsing and persisting in immunized mice may have been altered in some way. To test this assumption, suspected variant strain parasites were isolated from immune mice that had "relapsed" infections. Suspected variant-strain parasites and stock-strain parasites were then tested for sensitivity to the same antiserum. Figure 7 shows that the rat antiserum used had markedly different effects on the two strains, indicating that parasites relapsing in immunized mice were different from the stock strain; i.e., they had changed during their exposure to the immune serum.

Later work showed that repeated injections into mice of irradiated parasites of the stock strain stimulated the formation of antibodies, some of which were protective in passive-transfer studies and showed effects similar to those obtained with the rat antiserum.

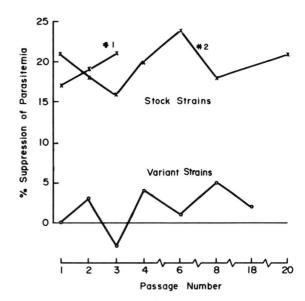

FIGURE 8 Resistance of variant
strains to rat antiserum during
repeated passage.

The resistance of variant strains to antiserum persisted during repeated passages of the strains through normal mice (Figure 8). A variant
strain was isolated from immunized and challenged mice in an experiment similar to the previous ones; this strain was passed biweekly
for over 10 weeks and tested repeatedly during this interval for sensitivity to the same rat antiserum. This variant showed no sensitivity to
antiserum at the time it was isolated (first passage), and it remained
about the same for over 20 passages. In contrast, the stock strains (isolated in the same experiment from two control groups) showed consistently high sensitivity to the same antiserum during the same interval.

Preliminary work has been done in fractionating some rat antisera
with demonstrated protective activity in the passive-transfer system.
Protective activity has been found in the 7S fractions of antiserum obtained after either single or multiple immunizing infections. Fractionation of the 7S component indicated that the greatest activity was in a
fraction that contained both IgG and IgA. No activity was detected in
the IgM from hyperimmunized rats, and only equivocal activity was
found in the IgM fraction from rats infected for only a short time.

A quantitative assay of the protective effect of serum on the course

SADUN *and others*: Use of Immune Globulin in the
Prevention and Therapy of Malaria
291

and outcome of *P. berghei* infection in rats has been developed recently.[8,9] It was found that the protective activity of hyperimmune serum is primarily associated with a 7S fraction and persists in the circulation for more than 6 months after infection.

CONCLUSIONS

Whole serum and fractions thereof, obtained from humans and rodents repeatedly infected with human or rodent malarias, respectively, can modify the course of experimentally induced blood infections in chimpanzees, rats, and mice. The resistance is manifested immunosuppressively and appears to be strain-specific. The effectiveness of immune serum is limited by the multiplication of variant parasites resistant to immunity that was acquired before parasite relapse. There is a great need for improvement of methodology for studying and classifying malarial antigens that elicit protective antibodies.

REFERENCES

1. Briggs, N. T., B. T. Wellde, and E. H. Sadun. Effects of rat antiserum on the course of *Plasmodium berghei* infection in mice. Milit. Med. 131 (Suppl.):1243-1249, 1966.
2. Briggs, N. T., B. T. Wellde, and E. H. Sadun. Variants of *Plasmodium berghei* resistant to passive transfer of immune serum. Exp. Parasit. 22:338-345, 1968.
3. Bruce-Chwatt, L. J., and F. D. Gibson. Transplacental passage of *Plasmodium berghei* and passive transfer of immunity in rats and mice. Trans. Roy. Soc. Trop. Med. Hyg. 50:47-53, 1956.
4. Coggeshall, L. T., and H. W. Kumm. Demonstration of passive immunity in experimental monkey malaria. J. Exp. Med. 66:177-190, 1937.
5. Cohen, S., and I. A. McGregor. Gamma globulin and acquired immunity to malaria, pp. 123-159. In P. C. Garnham, A. E. Pierce, and I. M. Riott, Eds. Immunity to Protozoa. Philadelphia: F. A. Davis Co., 1963.
6. Cohen, S., I. A. McGregor, and S. Carrington. Gammaglobulin and acquired immunity to human malaria. Nature 192:733-737, 1961.
7. Corradetti, A. Particolari fenomeni immunitari nell'infezione da *Plasmodium berghei*. Riv. Parassit. 11:201-210, 1950.
8. Diggs, C. L., and A. G. Osler. Humoral immunity in rodent malaria. I. Estimation of parasitemia by electronic particle counting. J. Immun. 102:292-297, 1969.
9. Diggs, C. L., and A. G. Osler. Humoral immunity in rodent malaria. II. Inhibition of parasitemia by serum antibody. J. Immun. 102:298-305, 1969.

10. Edozien, J. C., H. M. Gillse, and I. O. Udeozo. Adult and cord-blood gamma-globulin and immunity to malaria in Nigerians. Lancet:2:951–955, 1962.
11. Fabiani, G., and G. Fulchiron. Démonstration *in vivo* de l'existence d'un pouvoir protecteur dans le sérum de rats guéris de paludisme expérimental. C.R. Soc. Biol. 147:99–103, 1953.
12. Hickman, R. L. The use of subhuman primates for experimental studies of human malaria. Milit. Med. 134(Suppl.):741–756, 1969.
13. Isfan, T. Evaluation du processus immunogène dans l'infection à *Plasmodium berghei* par le test de séroprotection. Arch. Roum. Path. Exp. Microbiol. 25:65–76, 1966.
14. McGregor, I. A. Studies in the acquisition of immunity of *Plasmodium falciparum* infections in Africa. Trans. Roy. Soc. Trop. Med. Hyg. 58:80–92, 1964.
15. Sadun, E. H., R. L. Hickman, B. T. Wellde, A. P. Moon, and I. O. Udeozo. Active and passive immunization of chimpanzees infected with West African and Southeast Asian strains of *Plasmodium falciparum*. Milit. Med. 131(Suppl.):1250–1262, 1966.
16. Terry, R. J. Transmission of antimalarial immunity (*Plasmodium berghei*) from mother rats to their young during lactation. Trans. Roy. Soc. Trop. Med. Hyg. 50:41–46, 1956.

GEOFFREY EDSALL

Use of Newly Available Hyperimmune Serum Globulin Preparations

This presentation will deal with several hyperimmune globulin preparations that are applicable to infectious-disease control and are of newly increased interest or availability. Some are derived from convalescent sera, others from high-titer sera induced by artificial immunization. It is neither possible nor appropriate to discuss fully here the background information on these preparations, but Kabat published a splendid review a few years ago.[13] I would like to comment on tetanus immune globulin, vaccinia immune globulin, rabies immune globulin, varicella-zoster immune globulin, and what I will take the liberty of calling rubella immune globulin. It is also warranted at least to mention mumps immune globulin, pertussis immune globulin, and some others that should be considered for development.

TETANUS IMMUNE GLOBULIN

At the time of Kabat's review,[13] tetanus immune globulin (TIG) was available in limited supply as a substitute for the classical equine tetanus antitoxin, but the prophylactic dose had not yet become stabilized.

293

Reports like that of Rubbo and Suri,[27] which supported the use of a
400-unit dose, nevertheless suggested that considerably smaller doses
would be adequate. Rubinstein,[28] McComb and Dwyer,[20] McComb,[19]
and Levine et al.[15] all showed that a 250-unit dose given intramuscularly would produce an antitoxin level of at least 0.01 unit/ml of serum
in the circulating blood of the recipient within 2 or 3 days; this level is
generally accepted as the threshold of protection.[19] For the last few
years, the National Institutes of Health (NIH) has authorized the distribution of a prophylactic package of this amount, whose usefulness
has been described by the American Medical Association Council on
Drugs.[1] The product is now available from several manufacturers, the
plasma generally being derived from hyperimmunized donors. The
feasibility of selecting high-titer pools of plasma, from routine salvage
programs in cooperation with blood banks, for the preparation of this
product has also been established.[16] Studies by Mahoney et al.[18] have
suggested the possibility that smaller doses might be considered, but
larger-scale observations along these lines have not yet appeared. Four
groups[3,17,25,37] have reported the use of TIG in the therapy of tetanus.
Nation et al.[25] gave doses of 3,000–6,000 antitoxin units; 14 of 20
patients treated in this fashion survived, and the six who died were all
past the age of 45. Whether the ones who lived were saved by TIG
therapy or by their relative youth is an unanswered question. The 71%
case–fatality rate reported by Young et al.,[37] contrasted with the 29%
in the series collected by Ashley and Bell,[3] may reflect the great difference between these two studies in the techniques used for case
finding.

As might be expected, passive prophylaxis with 250 units of human
antitoxin has not proved to be a perfect measure. In February 1968, a
tetanus surveillance report from the National Communicable Disease
Center[35] noted seven cases of tetanus (with three deaths) that were reported to have occurred despite prophylaxis with 250–500 units of TIG,
and an eighth such case has recently been reported.[12] In all but the last
case, the TIG was given more than 48 hr after injury. One must conclude tentatively that either the 250-unit dose is not adequate in all
cases, or (as has often been suggested since equine tetanus antitoxin was
first used for this purpose) passive prophylaxis is of uncertain value. In
the absence of more detailed information concerning the failures, it is
reasonable to assume that successful prophylaxis with TIG may depend

on adjustment of the dose to the circumstances, that the 250-unit dose is adequate for what appear to be routine cases, but that larger doses should be used if treatment has been delayed or if extensive growth of the tetanus bacillus is likely.

VACCINIA IMMUNE GLOBULIN

As illustrated in the review by Kabat,[13] vaccinia immune globulin (VIG) has been used with apparent efficacy in the prevention and treatment of all complications of vaccinial infection except postvaccinial encephalitis, and it has apparently been effective prophylactically in the mitigation of even that most serious complication.[24] It has also proved of value in reducing the incidence of smallpox in susceptible contacts.[14] Until very recently, however, it has in the United States been an experimental product, distributed under the procedures prescribed for new-drug investigations. In 1969, it was licensed by the NIH, a step that now places it under the control of a standard of minimal potency, which will do much to ensure its efficacy in the various uses to which it is applied. The preparation was derived originally from plasma obtained from military recruits a few weeks after they had undergone primary smallpox vaccination. However, as Cadigan and Bellanti[6] pointed out, the neutralizing-antibody titer of any recently revaccinated person with a major reaction after the second injection may well be at least as high as that seen after primary vaccination. Thus, the potential source of donors is greatly broadened, and the availability of the product should therefore be improved. Although definitive information on the value of VIG in the prevention or therapy of each of the various complications of vaccinia is difficult to obtain, it must be regarded, until proved otherwise, as of primary importance in the handling of these complications.

RABIES IMMUNE GLOBULIN

It has been 10 years since Hosty et al.[11] reported on their pioneer attempts to prepare a human antirabies gamma globulin. The long delay in producing an effective, available preparation has been due largely to the great difficulty in obtaining sufficient human hyperimmune serum with a titer high enough to yield a globulin that does not require the injection of enormous volumes. Sikes[32] recently described such a globulin prepared from carefully selected hyperimmunized donors with exceptionally high titers of neutralizing antibody. The preparation has a titer equal or superior to that of the standard equine preparations that have been on the market for over a decade, in contrast with the low titer of material made from unselected bleedings from hyperimmunized human groups, such as veterinarians.

This leaves another major problem to be solved: Will the human immune globulin, accepted as it is by the host recipient as a native protein, persist so long in the circulation that it will blanket the immunizing effect of rabies vaccine given at the same time? The experimental studies of Habel[9] suggested that this need not be a problem, but the recently reported studies of Archer and Dierks[2] demonstrate that the problem can be significant. However, they clearly showed (using animal models) that the problem can be surmounted with a very-high-titer rabies vaccine. As Sikes has pointed out, the next step is to determine the interrelationships between gamma globulin dosage, type of vaccine, vaccine schedules, and the production of an effective active immune response—using a potent vaccine according to an accepted schedule. Experiments pointing to some of the guidelines for development of effective schedules have recently been reported.[36]

VARICELLA-ZOSTER IMMUNE GLOBULIN

Several years ago, Ross[26] published evidence strongly suggesting that normal gamma globulin, given in very large doses, could modify clinical varicella to some extent. However, the doses, 0.1–0.6 ml/lb of body weight, were massive by any ordinary standards, and the degree of reduction of the disease was moderate at best. Brunell *et al.*[5] have now obtained an immune globulin with a titer 64–128 times higher than that of normal gamma globulin, by bleeding persons who have recently recovered from herpes zoster. In a very small series of cases, this preparation has completely suppressed varicella infection in susceptible contacts. The controls, inoculated with gamma globulin, developed classical varicella. Much more work remains to be done before the use of such a product can be standardized, the dose established, the indications clearly defined, and so on. But these results support the hope that a genuinely effective hyperimmune globulin against varicella is in sight. As Brunell *et al.* point out, such a preparation would be of particular value after exposure of children with malignant disease, children under steroid or antimetabolite therapy, newborn infants of susceptible mothers, and adults susceptible to the disease.

RUBELLA IMMUNE GLOBULIN

No product deserving of the title "rubella immune globulin" is yet available. Normal gamma globulin has been extensively used for years in attempts to prevent rubella, particularly in exposed pregnant women, with various and conflicting results. The studies of Green *et al.*[8] indicated that gamma globulin in ordinary doses did not prevent experimental infection in human volunteers challenged with rubella virus, although it appeared to have some marginal capability of reducing the incidence of clinical disease. But McDonald and Peckham's epidemiologic study in Great Britain[22] suggested that significant reduction of the incidence of congenital anomalies occurred when pregnant women exposed to rubella were given the relatively small doses of gamma globulin generally used in the United Kingdom. By contrast, a more recent study[34] from the same area suggested that the reduction in the incidence of actual rubella infection, as confirmed by laboratory tests, was minor; again, the dose of gamma globulin used was only about one fourth of the dose that is customary in the United States. It appeared significant in McDonald's review[21] of this subject that the relatively few reports of epidemiologic failure to protect with gamma globulin had been found to be associated with the use of outdated preparations, which might have been subject to the fragmentation that has been shown to occur in some gamma globulin preparations.[33] Indeed, the literature on rubella and gamma globulin is so vast and so inconsistent that one can conclude only that, although there appears to be some evidence that gamma globulin produces at least some degree of protection against clinical rubella, there is almost no evidence that gamma globulin can be depended on to prevent infection of the fetus.

Therefore, it is of special interest that Schiff has recently reported[29,30] success, with a high-titer preparation, in completely suppressing rubella infection in five persons, whereas five controls who received low-titer immune globulin all showed evidence of infection. The completeness of the suppression in those receiving the high-titer material was confirmed by subsequent challenge of three of the five subjects, who responded with complete susceptibility. The prospect of securing any large quantity of high-titer material is uncertain, but at least these findings suggest that the principle of passive prevention by human rubella antibody is valid. That in itself provides sufficient reason to hope that useful preparations of this type will become available for administration to women who remain susceptible and who become exposed to the disease in early pregnancy. It should be pointed out, particularly in this connection, that the technique of preparing high-titer immune globulins by specific immunoadsorption and re-elution is still in its infancy, from the point of view of application to preparations for human use. When this technique becomes generally applicable, it may make possible the preparation of selected antibodies, with a potency beyond that of any present procedure.

OTHER HYPERIMMUNE HUMAN GLOBULINS

Despite the continuing paucity of evidence regarding the efficacy of mumps immune globulin, at least one study[4] has shown that repeated injections of gamma globulin (given in a study of the effect of such injections on the general incidence of infections) apparently reduced the incidence of clinical mumps by 70%. Although the p value for this observation was only 0.06 and the total incidence of infection was not reduced, the results suggest that mumps immune globulin might have some immunologic effect on the clinical disease, if the proper timing and the dose can be established.

Pertussis immune globulin is still considered to have a place in the prevention and treatment of this disease in young infants, in whom the case–fatality rate from pertussis is highest and the likelihood of permanent damage is greatest. However, the marginal and conflicting observations on the value of this preparation have not changed since the Kabat review,[13] and there is nothing new to add now.

There are several other areas in which there is hope for the development of an effective immune globulin. One that deserves some attention is the control of bacterial infections, especially infection with Pseudomonas in severely burned patients. The apparently beneficial effect of gamma globulin on such complications, noted in man and animals over a decade ago,[10,23] has led to the trial of more potent and specific preparations,[7] so that the preparation of concentrated solutions of immunologically selected antibodies should soon provide an unequivocal basis for evaluating immunotherapy of bacterial infections.

Finally, immunoprophylaxis and immunotherapy of diphtheria deserve attention, because, as with tetanus, the incidence of untoward reactions from administration of the equine antitoxin is tolerable only until a better preparation can be provided. Because the supplies of equine diphtheria antitoxin in this country are running low, the time is ripe for the development of a human diphtheria immune globulin; indeed, its preparation and preliminary testing have been reported.[31]

SUMMARY

The very widespread and growing use of tetanus immune globulin, the continuing need for vaccinia immune globulin, the promising developments in rabies immune globulin production, and the new studies on varicella-zoster immune globulin and high-titer rubella immune globulin all indicate the importance of continued pursuit of the possibility of using the antibodies in human plasma—either normal or specifically stimulated with appropriate antigens—to control infectious and other diseases. The fundamental studies in progress in this field will unquestionably provide the basis for improving the quantity, quality, and variety of applications of immune globulins derived from man.

REFERENCES

1. A new agent for prophylaxis of tetanus. Tetanus immune globulin. (Hyper-Tet). Council on Drugs. JAMA 192:471, 1965.
2. Archer, B. G., and R. E. Dierks. Effects of homologous or heterologous antiserum on neutralizing-antibody response to rabies vaccine. Bull. WHO 39:407–417, 1968.
3. Ashley, M. J., and J. S. Bell. Tetanus in Ontario: A review of the epidemiological and clinical features of 102 cases occurring in the 10-year period 1958–1967. Canad. Med. Assoc. J. 100:798–805, 1969.

4. Baron, S., E. V. Barnet, R. S. Goldsmith, S. Silbergeld, W. R. Ehrmantraut, J. E. Boyland, and B. L. Burch. Prophylaxis of infections by gamma globulin. Amer. J. Hyg. 79:186–195, 1964.

5. Brunell, P. A., A. Ross, L. H. Miller, and B. Kuo. Prevention of varicella by zoster immune globulin. New Eng. J. Med. 280:1191–1194, 1969.

6. Cadigan, F. C., Jr., and J. A. Bellanti. Increase in source of vaccinia immune globulins. J. Pediat. 69:815–816, 1966.

7. Feller, I., and C. Pierson. Pseudomonas vaccine and hyperimmune plasma for burned patients. Arch. Surg. 97:225–229, 1968.

8. Green, R. H., M. R. Balsamo, J. P. Giles, S. Krugman, and G. S. Mirick. Studies of the natural history and prevention of rubella. Amer. J. Dis. Child. 110:348–365, 1965.

9. Habel, K. Isogeneic versus allogeneic antiserum in the prophylaxis of experimental rabies. Bull. WHO 38:383–387, 1968.

10. Harris, J. R., and B. Schick. Use of gamma globulin in infection refractory to antibiotics. J. Mount Sinai Hosp. N.Y. 21:148–161, 1954.

11. Hosty, T. S., R. E. Kissling, M. Schaeffer, G. A. Wallace, and E. H. Dibble. Human antirabies gamma globulin. Bull. WHO 20:1111–1119, 1959.

12. Johnson, D. M. Fatal tetanus after prophylaxis with human tetanus immune globulin. Letter to the editor. JAMA 207:1519, 1969.

13. Kabat, E. A. Uses of hyperimmune human gamma globulin. New Eng. J. Med. 269:247–254, 1963.

14. Kempe, C. H., C. Bowles, G. Meiklejohn, T. O. Berge, L. St. Vincent, B. V. Babu, S. Govindarajan, N. R. Ratnakannan, A. W. Downie, and V. R. Murthy. The use of vaccinia hyperimmune gamma-globulin in the prophylaxis of smallpox. Bull. WHO 25:41–48, 1961.

15. Levine, L., J. A. McComb, R. C. Dwyer, and W. C. Latham. Active-passive tetanus immunization. Choice of toxoid, dose of tetanus immune globulin and timing of injections. New Eng. J. Med. 274:186–190, 1966.

16. Levine, L., L. Wyman, and J. A. McComb. Tetanus immune globulin from selected human plasmas. Six years of experience with a screening method. JAMA 200:341–344, 1967.

17. Lundstrom, R., O. Ramgren, C. Thoren, and K. Ullberg-Olsson. Immune globulin against tetanus. Acta Paediat. (Suppl. 40):100–102, 1963.

18. Mahoney, L. J., M. A. Aprile, and P. J. Moloney. Combined active-passive immunization against tetanus in man. Canad. Med. Assoc. J. 96:1401–1404, 1967.

19. McComb, J. A. The prophylactic dose of homologous tetanus antitoxin. New Eng. J. Med. 270:175–178, 1964.

20. McComb, J. A., and R. C. Dwyer. Passive-active immunization with tetanus immune globulin (human). New Eng. J. Med. 268:857–862, 1963.

21. McDonald, J. C. Gamma globulin prophylaxis of rubella, pp. 371–377. In First International Conference on Vaccines against Viral and Rickettsial Diseases of Man. Scientific Publication No. 147. Washington, D.C.: Pan American Health Organization, World Health Organization, 1967.

22. McDonald, J. C., and C. S. Peckham. Gammaglobulin in prevention of rubella and congenital defect: A study of 30,000 pregnancies. Brit. Med. J. 3:633–637, 1967.

23. Millican, R. C., J. Rust, and S. M. Rosenthal. Gamma globulin factors protective against infections from Pseudomonas and other organisms. Science 126:509–511, 1957.

24. Nanning, W. Prophylactic effect of antivaccinia gamma-globulin against post-vaccinal encephalitis. Bull. WHO 27:317–324, 1962.

25. Nation, N. S., N. F. Pierce, S. J. Adler, R. F. Chinnock, and P. F. Wehrle. Tetanus; the use of human hyperimmune globulin in treatment. Calif. Med. 98:305–307, 1963.

26. Ross, A. H. Modification of chicken pox in family contacts by administration of gamma globulin. New Eng. J. Med. 267:369–376, 1962.

27. Rubbo, S. D., and J. C. Suri. Passive immunization against tetanus with human immune globulin. Brit. Med. J. 2:79–81, 1962.

28. Rubinstein, H. M. Studies on human tetanus antitoxin. Amer. J. Hyg. 76:276–292, 1962.

29. Schiff, G. M. The efficacy of titered lots of immune globulin (IG) in preventing rubella in human volunteers. Clin. Res. 17:40, 1969. (abstract)

30. Schiff, G. M. Titered lots of immune globulin: Efficacy in the prevention of rubella. Amer. J. Dis. Child. 118:322–327, 1969.

31. Sgouris, J. T., V. K. Volk, F. Angela, L. Portwood, and R. Y. Gottschall. Studies on diphtheria immune globulin prepared from outdated human blood. Vox Sang. 16:491–495, 1969.

32. Sikes, R. K. Human rabies immune globulin. Progress report. Public Health Rep. 84:797–801, 1969.

33. Škvařil, F. Changes in outdated human γ-globulin preparations. Nature 185:475–476, 1960.

34. Studies on rubella in pregnancy. Report of the Public Health Laboratory Service Working Party on Rubella. Brit. Med. J. 3:203–206, 1968.

35. Tetanus Surveillance Report No. 1. National Communicable Disease Center, U.S. Public Health Service. Feb. 1968.

36. Winkler, M. G., R. C. Schmidt, and R. K. Sikes. Evaluation of human rabies immune globulin and homologous and heterologous antibody. J. Immunol. 102:1314–1321, 1969.

37. Young, L. S., F. M. LaForce, and J. V. Bennett. An evaluation of serologic and antimicrobial therapy in the treatment of tetanus in the United States. J. Infect. Dis. 120:153–159, 1969.

ROBERT O. PECKINPAUGH

Hyperimmune Globulin in the Control of Acute Respiratory Disease*

Immune globulin has been used successfully to provide passive protection from or modification of a variety of infectious diseases.[5,8,11] However, when it has been used against respiratory disease, the results have been inconsistent.[1-3,7] Antibody titers in preparations of gamma globulin vary, depending on the source of plasma; the antibodies may not be specific for the infectious agent causing disease in the recipients.

In 1962–1963, a unique opportunity was offered by a program sponsored by the American National Red Cross to obtain hyperimmune vaccinia globulin from recently vaccinated naval recruits at Great Lakes, Illinois. This hyperimmune globulin was expected to contain antibodies to the agents causing the acute respiratory disease (ARD) endemic in this population.[12] On each of two occasions, approximately 1,000 recruits, most of whom had experienced ARD during their training, donated blood from which gamma globulin was separated. The purpose of the two studies reported here was to evaluate the effectiveness of immune globulin in preventing ARD, including nonbacterial pneumonia.

The immunization procedures have been described elsewhere.[10] Fig-

*From research project MF 022.03.07-4007. The opinions and assertions expressed herein are those of the author and cannot be construed as reflecting the views of the Navy Department or of the naval service at large. Usage of a commercially available product in connection with this study cannot be construed as an endorsement of such product.

302

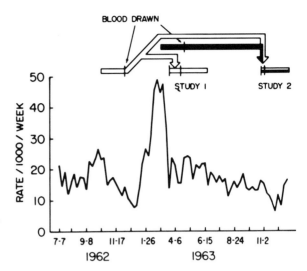

FIGURE 1 Admission rate for acute
respiratory disease among naval recruits
at Great Lakes, Illinois, 1962–1963,
and overall pattern of blood donations
and study periods.

ure 1 shows the ARD admission rates of the recruits during the period
covered in this report. The overall pattern of blood donations and study
periods is also shown. The immune globulin from blood drawn in the
fall of 1962 and the spring of 1963 was processed by E. R. Squibb &
Sons, New Brunswick, New Jersey, and processing costs were paid by
the American National Red Cross.

Normal gamma globulin was obtained from the Red Cross. Inactivated
trivalent (types 3, 4, and 7) adenovirus vaccine was obtained from commercial sources. Normal saline was used as a placebo.

In the first study, 2,600 persons were randomly assigned to eight
treatment groups, as follows:

Number of Volunteers	Treatment
212	1 ml fall 1962 immune globulin
209	5 ml fall 1962 immune globulin
194	5 ml fall 1962 immune globulin plus 1 ml adenovirus vaccine
207	1 ml gamma globulin
194	5 ml gamma globulin
200	5 ml gamma globulin plus 1 ml adenovirus vaccine
409	1 ml adenovirus vaccine
975	5 ml normal saline

In the second study, 1,067 persons were randomly assigned to four treatment groups, as follows:

Number of Volunteers	Treatment
207	10 ml fall 1962 immune globulin
152	10 ml spring 1963 immune globulin
204	10 ml gamma globulin
504	10 ml normal saline

In this second study, all received 1 ml of adenovirus vaccine and one of the above treatments 1 week later.

Table 1 shows the percentage of serologically positive sera in patients with ARD. The most prevalent seroconversion is to adenovirus 4, but other seroconversions are also present. Table 2 shows the antibody titers in the immune globulin and gamma globulin preparations.

In the first study (Figure 2), the 5-ml doses of immune globulin and gamma globulin, with or without adenovirus vaccine, resulted in partial control of ARD; however, the only group statistically different from the placebo group was the one that received 5 ml of gamma globulin plus

TABLE 1　Etiologic Agents Detected Serologically in Naval Recruits Admitted for Inpatient Care with Acute Respiratory Illness, as Manifested by Fourfold Rise in Titer between Acute and 3-Week-Convalescent Sera

Etiologic Agent	Method of Detection	Sept.–Oct. 1962 No. Tested	% Positive	Jan.–Apr. 1963 No. Tested	% Positive
Adenovirus	Complement fixation	159	82	60	83
Adenovirus type 3	Virus neutralization	164	29	58	9
Adenovirus type 4	Virus neutralization	164	84	58	81
Adenovirus type 7	Virus neutralization	163	40	57	28
Influenza C	Complement fixation	261	2	71	10
Parainfluenza 1	Complement fixation	261	0	77	3
Parainfluenza 2	Complement fixation	261	1	77	0
Parainfluenza 3	Complement fixation	261	<1	77	0
Respiratory syncytial virus	Complement fixation	261	<1	77	5
Rhinovirus 1A	Virus neutralization	261	2	35	9
Mycoplasma pneumoniae	Complement fixation	261	9	77	8

TABLE 2 Viral-Antibody Titers of Serum Gamma Globulins Used

| | | Neutralizing-Antibody Titers against Various Viruses[b] | | | | | | | | | HAI[d] Titer |
| | | Adenoviruses | | | Rhinoviruses | | Coxsackie | | Para- | | |
Source of Gamma Globulin[a]	Vaccinia	3	4	7	1A	2	A-21	REO 3	influenza 1	RSV[c]	Rubella
Standard gamma globulin	4	16	16	128	<16	64	16	<20	192	256	160
Fall 1962 immune globulin	12	96	96	128	192	192	<16	<20	192	256	640
Spring 1963 immune globulin	8	48	64	256	192	384	<16	–	192	256	320

[a]Prepared by American National Red Cross.
[b]Reciprocals of initial dilutions.
[c]Respiratory syncytial virus.
[d]Hemagglutination inhibition antibody.

305

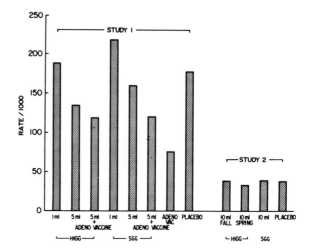

FIGURE 2   Admission rates for acute respiratory disease in each study period among naval recruits at Great Lakes, Illinois, 1963.

1 ml of adenovirus vaccine ($p \leqslant 0.05$). All groups are statistically different from the vaccine-only group at the 1–5% level, except for the group that received 5 ml of immune globulin plus 1 ml of adenovirus vaccine ($p = 0.07$). The 1-ml dose of gamma globulin had no effect. Similarly, the second study showed no effect of either immune or gamma globulin, compared with the placebo. Although it is not shown in Figure 2, the larger doses of immune globulin protected against clinical rubella, as reported by Miller *et al.*[9]

The immune globulin preparations contained antibodies specific for the ARD agents, but passive protection was only partial, even against adenovirus. This study confirms those of Rytel *et al.*,[13] Houser,[6] and Chin *et al.*[4]

Appreciation is expressed to Dr. James H. Pert for supplying the gamma globulin preparation, and to the investigators of studies reported herein: Dr. Michael W. Rytel, Dr. John M. Dowd, Earl A. Edwards, Willard E. Pierce, Ralph I. Lytle, and Capt. Lloyd F. Miller.

REFERENCES

1. Abernathy, R. S., E. L. Strem, and R. A. Good. Chronic asthma in childhood: double-blind controlled study of treatment with gamma-globulin. Pediatrics 21:980–983, 1958.

2. Baron, S., E. V. Barnet, R. S. Goldsmith, S. Silbergeld, W. R. Ehrmantraut, J. E. Boyland, and B. L. Burch. Prophylaxis of infections by gamma globulin. Amer. J. Hyg. 79:186–195, 1964.

3. Botstein, A., and E. B. Brown. Gamma globulin in the prevention of upper respiratory infections in children. New York J. Med. 62:1799–1803, 1962.

4. Chin, J., R. A. Stallones, and E. D. Lennette. The effect of gamma globulin on acute respiratory illness in military recruits. Amer. J. Epidem. 86:193–198, 1967.

5. Gross, P. A., D. Gitlin, and C. A. Janeway. The gamma globulins and their clinical significance. IV. Therapeutic uses of gamma globulins. New Eng. J. Med. 260:170–178, 1959.

6. Houser, H. B. Gamma globulin prevention of severe respiratory illness caused by adenovirus types 4 and 7. Clin. Res. 7:270–271, 1959. (abstract)

7. Jackson, G. G., H. F. Dowling, and T. O. Anderson. Neutralization of common cold agents in volunteers by pooled human globulin. Science 128:27–28, 1958.

8. Krugman, S. The clinical use of gamma globulin. New Eng. J. Med. 269:195–201, 1963.

9. Miller, C. H., J. M. Dowd, M. W. Rytel, L. F. Miller, and W. E. Pierce. Prevention of rubella with gamma globulin. JAMA 201:560–561, 1967.

10. Miller, L. F., M. Rytel, W. E. Pierce, and M. J. Rosenbaum. Epidemiology of nonbacterial pneumonia among naval recruits. JAMA 185:92–99, 1963.

11. Roantree, R. J. The uses of gamma globulin in prophylaxis and treatment. Med. Clin. N. Amer. 49:1745–1756, 1965.

12. Rosenbaum, M. J., E. A. Edwards, P. F. Frank, W. E. Pierce, Y. E. Crawford, and L. F. Miller. Epidemiology and prevention of acute respiratory disease in naval recruits. I. Ten years' experience with microbial agents isolated from naval recruits with acute respiratory disease. Amer. J. Public Health 55:38–46, 1965.

13. Rytel, M. W., J. M. Dowd, E. A. Edwards, W. E. Pierce, and J. H. Pert. Prophylaxis of acute viral respiratory diseases with gamma globulin. Dis. Chest 54:499–503, 1968.

THOMAS G. AKERS *and*
CATHERINE M. PRATO

Response of Mice to Airborne Encephalomyocarditis Viruses

In studies on aerogenic immunization at the Naval Biological Laboratory, we have used attenuated strains of the encephalomyocarditis (EMC) group of viruses for these reasons:

1. Viruses in this group are antigenically similar and highly pathogenic in mice.

2. Virulent strains form large plaques (Lpf), and avirulent strains, small plaques (Spf). Lpf aerosols of the Columbia-SK (Col-SK) or mengovirus strains are lethal for mice, whereas Spf aerosols of mengovirus-37A are avirulent and induce immunity to otherwise lethal Lpf strains.

3. After inhalation of an immunogenic dose, serum antibodies can be titered serologically and characterized physically.

4. EMC viruses replicate and can be assayed readily in L-cell monolayers. Thus, one has available a means to study aerosols both qualitatively and quantitatively.

The purpose of this report is to present our current studies on the immune response of mice exposed to aerosols of mengovirus-37A and the response of immunized mice later exposed to lethal Lpf aerosol doses of either Col-SK or infectious mengoviral RNA.

Pools of Col-SK and mengovirus-37A were prepared in L-cells (L-929) and assayed.[1] Infectious mengoviral RNA was extracted as previously described[2] and assayed according to the method of Pagano and Vaheri.[3] The equipment and procedures used for exposure and the methods of collecting tissues for virus assay, histologic examination, hemagglutination inhibition (HAI), complement fixation (CF), neutralizing-antibody or plaque-reduction tests, and immunoglobulin characterization have been described.[2,4]

The aerosol exposure of mice to Spf strains (mengovirus-37A) resulted in recovery of virus from the lungs, spleen, liver, blood, and intestines (Figure 1). Brain, lymph nodes, heart, kidney, and pancreas were free from viruses. Mice exposed to mengovirus-37A aerosol exhibited pathologic but nonfatal changes in heart and lung tissues. The

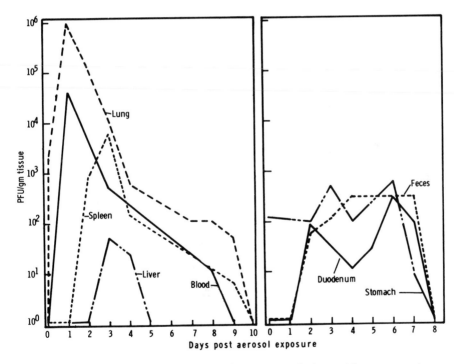

FIGURE 1 Virus content of selected tissues after exposure of mice to airborne mengovirus-37A. [Reprinted with permission from Akers et al.[2] © (1968) The Williams & Wilkins Co., Baltimore, Md. 21202, U.S.A.]

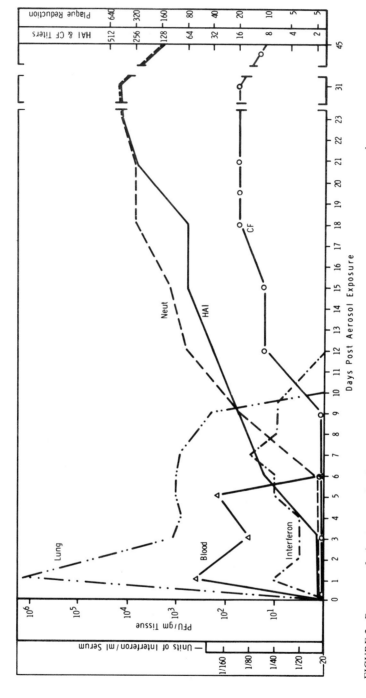

FIGURE 2   Response of mice to aerosols of mengovirus-37A. [Reprinted with permission from Prato and Akers.[4] © (1969) The Williams & Wilkins Co., Baltimore, Md. 21202, U.S.A.]

syndrome may be described as a mild myocarditis with marked
pneumonitis.

The serum-antibody response in mice exposed to mengovirus-37A
aerosol followed a course that was essentially similar to that observed
after parenteral administration of various antigens. However, the first
appearance of circulating antibody was slightly delayed. As Figure 2
shows, antibody was detected by hemagglutination on the sixth day
after aerosol exposure. By the ninth day, the HAI titer had increased
significantly, and neutralization by the 50% plaque-reduction method
was clearly evident.

Both HAI and neutralizing-antibody titers increased steadily until
they reached a peak at day 31; a decline was then noted until day 45,
the last day of the study. Complement-fixing antibodies were slow to
appear (day 12) and attained relatively low titers.

Early antibodies (days 6 and 9) were sensitive to 2-mercaptoethanol
(Table 1). Antibodies resistant to 2-mercaptoethanol (2-ME) treatment
appeared by day 12 and were the predominant type from day 15 on.

Serum globulins separated by means of DEAE-column chromatography and gel filtration with Sephadex G-200 showed some correlations
with the antibody's ultracentrifugal and immunoelectrophoretic properties, as well as with diminished activity after 2-ME treatment. HAI and
neutralizing antibodies were found in both the IgG and IgM fractions.
The fractions were not tested by complement fixation. Early antibodies
were IgM and were sensitive to 2-ME. The IgG globulins resistant to
2-ME appeared by day 12 and thereafter became the major immune
globulin component.

When, 21 days after exposure to mengovirus-37A aerosol, the mice
were challenged with lethal aerosol doses of Lpf Col-SK virus, no
deaths occurred, although virus could be recovered for a period of 96
hr from the lungs, liver, spleen, blood, and intestines. Histologically,
the lungs showed signs of acute inflammation. In contrast, normal control mice simultaneously exposed to Col-SK aerosol succumbed within
96–120 hr. Virus could be isolated from the same tissues as in the immunized mice and, in addition, from the brain, lymph nodes, kidney,
and pancreas. Virus titers were consistently higher in the nonimmune
animals.

Mice that were immunized to mengovirus-37A when exposed to
aerosols of infectious mengoviral RNA also survived. However, virus

TABLE 1 Humoral-Antibody Response in Mice Exposed to Mengovirus-37A Aerosols[a]

Days after Aerosol Exposure	Neutralizing Antibodies			HAI Antibodies		
	Titer of Whole Sera[b]	Titer after 0.2M 2-ME Treatment[b]	Predominant Type of Antibody[c]	Titer of Whole Sera	Titer after 0.2M 2-ME Treatment	Predominant Type of Antibody[c]
0	<5	—	—	<2	—	—
3	<5	—	—	<2	—	—
6	<5	<5	—	8	<2	19S
9	30	20	19S	16	2	19S
12	40	160	7S	32	16	7S
15	160	320	7S	64	32	7S
18	320	320	7S	64	64	7S
21	320	320	7S	256	128	7S
31	320	160	7S	512	256	7S
45	160	160	7S	128	64	7S

[a] Adapted from Prato and Akers.[4]
[b] Reciprocal dilution of serum that resulted in 50% reduction in number of plaque-forming units of virus.
[c] Based on results of 2-ME treatment, ultracentrifugation, and immunoelectrophoresis of whole serum and DEAE or Sephadex G-200 fractions.

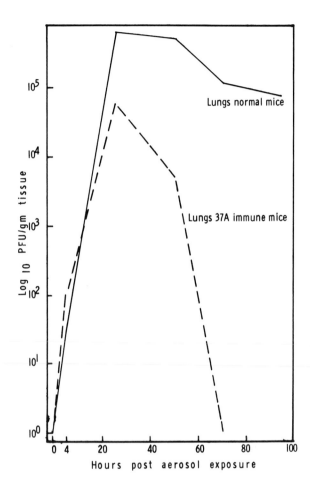

FIGURE 3 Virus content of lung
tissues of normal mice and mice im-
munized to mengovirus-37A after
aerosol exposure to mengoviral RNA.
[Reprinted with permission from
Akers *et al.* [2] © (1968) The Williams
& Wilkins Co., Baltimore, Md. 21202,
U.S.A.]

was isolated from lung tissue only (Figure 3), and titers peaked in this
tissue 24 hr after exposure. All exposed normal control mice died. The
inferences are that neutralizing antibodies were sufficient to limit
viral-RNA–initiated viral infection to lung tissue only and that viral
RNA did not retain its infectivity through gastrointestinal passage.

In conclusion, the EMC model system offers a unique potential for
studying aerogenic immunization against either intact virus or infectious
viral nucleic acids. The role of IgA in this model system will be the subject of a future endeavor.

The work reported here was supported by the Office of Naval Research and the Bureau of Medicine and Surgery, United States Navy, under a contract between the Office of Naval Research and the Regents of the University of California. Reproduction in whole or in part is permitted for any purpose of the United States Government.

REFERENCES

1. Akers, T. G., S. B. Bond, C. Papke, and W. R. Leif. Virulence and immunogenicity in mice of airborne encephalomyocarditis viruses and their infectious nucleic acids. J. Immun. 97:379–385, 1966.
2. Akers, T. G., S. H. Madin, and F. L. Schaffer. The pathogenicity in mice of aerosols of encephalomyocarditis group viruses or their infectious nucleic acids. J. Immun. 100:120–127, 1968.
3. Pagano, J. S., and A. Vaheri. Enhancement of infectivity of poliovirus RNA with diethylaminoethyl-dextran (DEAE-D). Arch. Ges. Virusforsch. 17:456–464, 1965.
4. Prato, C. M., and T. G. Akers. The immunologic response of the mouse to aerosols of an attenuated encephalomyocarditis virus strain. J. Immun. 103:79–86, 1969.

VI
FRACTIONATION
OF SERUM AND
PREPARATION OF
IMMUNOGLOBULINS

H. F. DEUTSCH

Problems and Perspectives in the Preparation of Human Immunoglobulin Fractions

Commercial methods of fractionating plasma proteins on a large scale have undergone little change in the United States since their introduction about 25 years ago.[11] That is due to the utility of the ethanol fractionation procedure for the separation of clinically suitable forms of the three major protein fractions—IgG, fibrinogen, and albumin—from large volumes of plasma and of IgG and albumin from placental extracts or retroplacental blood. With the exception of antihemophilia A concentrates, no new human plasma-protein fractions have been introduced into clinical practice. A major block in the application of new fractionation methods for the isolation of IgG, albumin, and other protein fractions for clinical use is the danger that they may be contaminated with the virus of hepatitis. The extensive clinical testing required has undoubtedly acted as a deterrent in the United States to the probing that might lead to the introduction of new methods. The value of a test to establish whether individual units of plasma or pools thereof possess hepatitis virus and whether the isolated fractions are free of the virus is apparent.

Any deviations from the present methods used for preparing gamma globulin concentrates must also take cognizance of their possible effects on the separation of other plasma proteins in the overall fractionation scheme. A rather wide variety of fractionation approaches that have been used in the research laboratory would find application to the fractionation of human plasma on a commercial scale. All the remarks on some probable future directions of gamma globulin separation are made in the context of the probability that the hepatitis problem will be overcome. Several recent promising leads for detecting hepatitis virus in plasma or serum are of interest in this respect.[21,30]

The commercial low-temperature ethanol fractionation procedure used by most large-scale fractionators, which is based on the variables of pH, ionic strength, ethanol concentration, and temperature, is so well known that it will not be discussed here in any detail.[11,24] It is applicable to large volumes, and it inhibits bacterial growth and thus diminishes the likelihood of the formation of pyrogens. The ease of removing the ethanol by lyophilization is an important characteristic of the method. The bulk of the IgG of higher isoelectric point separates in fraction II, and the other forms of immunoglobulins separate largely in fraction III. Laboratory-scale preparations of gamma globulin concentrates recognized as mixtures of IgA, IgM, and IgG were separated from fraction III over 20 years ago by ethanol fractionation.[12] Such material has not, however, been subjected to further studies in terms of its large-scale preparation or to clinical evaluation. It does contain some of the antibody activities found in pooled human plasma.[13]

The lowering of the dielectric constant of solutions by the addition of various water-soluble substances, with consequent selective precipitation of proteins, is the basic step in most large-scale plasma-fractionation methods. Substances other than ethanol whose effects also depend on lowering the dielectric constant of the medium have received some use. Methanol has somewhat similar dielectric properties, is completely miscible with water, and, like ethanol, can be used to precipitate proteins out of solution selectively. Methanol is inherently toxic and could impose hazardous working conditions if the atmosphere in the fractionation laboratory were not exchanged sufficiently. Residual methanol in the final products could also be a problem. These have not, however, proved to be hazardous in large-scale fractionation conditions, and methanol is being used for the large-scale fractionation of plasma proteins for clinical use (A. Koehler, personal communication). Its advantage over ethanol is that it distills at 64.6 C, which is considerably lower than the 78 C of the constant-boiling azeotropic water–ethanol mixture. If the pressure is lowered substantially, the methanol can be removed by thin-film evaporation at temperatures so low that there is little danger of protein denaturation, and the protein solution may be obtained in a form suitable for sterile filtration. Such processing circumvents the expensive and tedious procedures of shell freezing, lyophilization, and reconstitution of ethanol precipitates. It is perhaps somewhat surprising that methanol has not found its way into more general use in the fractionation of plasma proteins.

A method for fractionating plasma protein that uses diethyl ether as the precipitant has been developed.[18] Ether has several limitations, among which are its flammability and its relatively low solubility. The latter requires exact temperature control when the ether is near its solubility limits; small rises in temperature readily lead to separation of two phases.

Some use has been made of water-soluble, high-molecular-weight polymers in the fractionation of plasma proteins. Their precipitation effects are also related to the lowering of the dielectric constant of protein solutions. These polymers are asymmetric molecules, and at higher concentrations viscous solutions make centrifugation and filtration difficult. Such polymers as 1,4-nonylphenylethylene oxide, polypropylene glycol, polyvinyl alcohol, and polyvinylpyrrolidone tend to denature some proteins. Polyethylene glycol (PEG) has found some application in plasma-protein fractionation. It was first used by Polson et al.[26] on a laboratory scale. They found that PEG with an average molecular weight of nearly 4,000 was a more effective protein precipitant than lower-molecular-weight fractions. It is important to use fractions with maximal precipitating activity that have the lowest viscosities. PEG has also been used recently by Chun et al.[9] to prepare immunoglobulin concentrates from human serum and to refractionate Cohn's fraction II. The IgG fractions isolated from those sources lacked the 8S-10S component that is commonly associated with stored fraction II and is presumed to consist mostly of dimerized 7S IgG molecules. The authors did not indicate whether the IgG separated with PEG tended to form the 8S-10S material with aging or whether the spontaneous plasmin-catalyzed degradations found to occur in some Cohn's fraction II preparations[23,32,33] also occurred with the IgG separated with PEG. PEG has been used in commercial operations for the preparation of factor VIII (antihemophilic factor) concentrates (A. J. Johnson *et al.*, unpublished data); the starting material in this case is a cryofibrinogen fraction prepared from fresh-frozen plasma.[27] However, in this case, PEG is not introduced into the general fractionation procedure. The supernatant plasma from the cryoprecipitate is used for the preparation of the usual protein fractions.

A departure from the usual fractionation procedures has been the introduction of a method that uses Rivanol (2-ethoxy-6,9-diaminoacridine) in conjunction with ammonium sulfate.[14,16] The use of Rivanol is based on its ability to form relatively insoluble complexes with proteins in their anion forms.[17] In contradistinction to the ethanol fractionation procedure, the first precipitation in this method removes proteins of lower isoelectric point and leaves the IgG in solution. The Behringwerke in Marburg, Germany, uses such methods on a large commercial scale and has adopted a vacuum-ultrafiltration apparatus to remove salt and simultaneously concentrate the protein solutions.[14] Some apparent advantages of this type of fractionation are operation at room temperature, removal of some precipitates by relatively rapid filtration procedures, and simultaneous dialysis of the salts used to precipitate the protein and concentration of some protein solutions sufficiently to obviate lyophilization and subsequent reconstitution. Some trace protein components of plasma may be more stable in the ammonium sulfate fractionation conditions than in the ethanol type, thus making their separation from crude fractions more feasible.

Other complexing agents may be found useful in the fractionation of plasma proteins. An example is the use of caprylate by Steinbuch[34] and by Audran and Steinbuch[3] in the isolation of IgA from Cohn's fraction III. The contaminating a_2-macroglobulins in the final stages of purification are precipitated by the addition of caprylate. The mode of action of this substance is not apparent.

In the light of existing problems, it does not appear likely that any major innovation will be introduced into immunoglobulin fractionation methods in the United States in the immediate future. The application of newer fractionation procedures will probably be at the level of reworking fractions that are now being discarded but that contain desired clinical entities. The rate at which newer methods will be introduced will probably be related to the demands for a wider variety of discrete fractions for specific-component therapy. Let us consider briefly some of the problems in the immunoglobulin area that may exert pressure to exploit available methods or to develop newer methods for the isolation of desired components.

Immunoglobulins of the IgG class are currently being separated and used clinically. These proteins are electrophoretically heterogeneous[2,10] with a range of isoelectric points from pH 5 to 9. This is attested to by the extensive area of specific precipitation of the IgG immunoglobulins when they are studied by immunoelectrophoresis. Cohn's fraction II separates the more basic molecules of this class of immunoglobulins. The role of the more acidic types has not been probed. It is known that Rh-blocking antibodies are IgG immunoglobulins and that some sensitized persons have considerable amounts of these antibodies with electrophoretic mobilities characteristic of β- and a_2-globulins.[7,8] The present standards for Rh antibody preparations stipulates a mobility range such that IgM immunoglobulins will not be present. However, if we desire greater yields of Rh-blocking antibodies and if the more acidic members of this class of antibodies are found to have a unique use, we will have to develop methods for their separation. As more Rh-blocking antibody is used clinically in the prevention of erythroblastosis, there will be fewer natural immunizations and the source of the donor material will shift to hyperimmunized persons. If prolonged immunization tends to produce more acidic IgG antibodies, as in the response of horses to tetanus and diphtheria antigens, we may face the problem of low antibody yields of this important clinical entity, unless different methods of separation are developed.

Concentrates of IgA and IgM immunoglobulins have not yet been isolated in this country on a large scale, although various preparations are undergoing clinical trial in Europe (personal communications from H. G. Schwick and M. Steinbuch). Because the IgM of humans may be the major source of antibodies to various gram-negative antigens, particular interest is directed to this immunoglobulin fraction.

Related to these problems are present-day organ-transplantation programs. The immune response in the recipients is held in abeyance by various means, and the patient often experiences severe infections. The need for large amounts of homologous immune globulins for these patients is obvious. The amounts needed are such as to require their intravenous administration, and preparations with a long *in vivo* half-life are desired. IgG that has been subjected to mild digestion with pepsin, papain, and plasmin appears to be better tolerated than undigested fraction II when given by the intravenous route, but has a much shorter half-life.[19,22] In addition, there may be a danger of exposing patients to new antigenic groups in fractions prepared by proteolytic methods, with consequent sensitization of the recipients. The problem of preparing IgG suitable for intravenous use appears to have been met in part; some undigested IgG preparations are being routinely given by this route.[35]

Our knowledge of the complexities of IgG in terms of there being at least 30 different allotypic species (Gm and Inv factors) and the roles of some of them in discrete biologic phenomena is growing. Some clinical conditions might create a demand for immunoglobulins of a particular serotype. Inasmuch as there appears to be no way, at present, to separate allotypes of a given class of immunoglobulins, such a demand would be met by fractionating plasmas that had been pooled according to their individual serologic properties.

Hyperimmunization of various persons to provide particular relatively high-titered antisera is also being carried out. Some of the antibodies that are being produced by direct immunization are present in the normal population in small amounts. The specific isolation of these antibodies from the so-called normal immunoglobulins would obviate the involved and expensive approaches that are now necessary to generate hyperimmune IgG fractions.

These are some of the projections that the fractionation laboratories are facing at present. Solutions to some of the problems may be found within the framework of present fractionation methods; others will necessitate the introduction of new methods and detailed investigations. The following are some fractionation approaches that may have future utility in the separation of immunoglobulins on a large scale.

Solubility Techniques   The present precipitation methods used to fractionate large volumes of plasma or serum most likely will continue to be used for some time. Further studies of ion complexes that greatly modify the solubility of some plasma proteins may result in the modification of specific procedures. The utility of Rivanol and of caprylate has already been mentioned.

A most likely direction will be toward automation of fractionation processes. Some variation in the precipitants used at present or in the introduction of combinations of precipitants may ensue. Efforts toward automation of the ethanol fractionation method have been made at the Scottish Blood Transfusion Service in Edinburgh. A module that effects a continuous mixing of ethanol solutions and of plasma with continuous monitoring of temperature and pH has been developed for some of the precipitation steps (J. Watt, personal communication): the suspensions of precipitated protein are fed continuously into a Sharples centrifuge while additional protein is being precipitated.

The introduction of some type of centrifuge, such as those* which permit periodic discharge (i.e., "desludging" of precipitates accumulating during centrifugation), will be necessary to the true automation of any fractionation scheme. Such centrifuges are not refrigerated and would not find utility in their present form in low-temperature fractionation methods. It is also questionable whether they could discharge precipitates of the consistency of those formed in the usual ethanol fractionation.

Two-Phase Systems The utility of linear polymers as precipitants and the specific use of PEG in the preparation of antihemophilic concentrates has been mentioned. Solutions of various hydrophilic polymers that form liquid two-phase systems may be readily prepared. For example, dextrans form liquid two-phase systems with PEG's of molecular weights greater than 1,000. In this case, both polymers are uncharged. It is possible, however, to use a neutral polymer with either an anionic or a cationic polymer and two-phase systems with a cationic polymer (i.e., diethylaminoethyldextran–HCl) in one phase and an anionic polymer (i.e., dextran sulfate–Na) in the other. The latter would be essentially a liquid ion exchanger. A detailed description of different polymer systems that can be used in two-phase separations of proteins has been given by Albertsson,[1] with many results of their use. The distribution of a given protein between the two phases of such a system can be controlled in considerable degree by the ionic strength of the systems. Variations in pH do not usually introduce distribution effects of the magnitude of those given by ionic-strength variations. Combinations of different polymers, variations in their concentrations, and the use of

*Available from Centrico, Inc., 75 W. Forest Ave., Englewood, N.J.

different pH's and ionic strengths can be used to offer a wide range of conditions to effect distribution of the proteins of a mixture in selectively removing one or two of them into one of the phases.

Applications of this method might have utility in separating various classes of immunoglobulins from crude fractions, but detailed investigations would be necessary. Considerable flexibility might result from the use of polymer mixtures, including one that may have denaturating effects on proteins. Some polymer components used in the two-phase systems might ameliorate the deleterious effects of others.

Separations of the two-phase systems giving adequate distributions of desired components could be effected by a Sharples or zonal centrifuge. If an adequate partition coefficient were not obtained, both the separated light and heavy phases could be remixed to reconstitute the original phase composition. This could be again separated. Such a process would be analogous to a large-scale countercurrent distribution.

One of the limitations of the use of the hydrophilic polymers in plasma-protein separations of any type is removal of the polymer from the purified or concentrated protein. A second fractionation must be instituted to separate proteins and polymers. This could pose extensive problems.

Electric-Transport Methods   At a given pH, the various immunoglobulins possess considerable charge differences, but they are usually present with other proteins of similar charge. It would appear that only the more basic IgG immunoglobulins could be separated from whole plasma or from partially purified fractions in highly purified form by electrophoretic convection,[7] electrodecantation,[6,25] or the carrier-free-flow electrophoretic method of Hannig.[15] In many cases, the protein solution requires dialysis to adjust the pH and ionic strength to the range needed for separation. It does not appear that these methods could compete with the relatively simple fractionation process now used for separation of IgG, unless the products were vastly superior—e.g., possessed greater stability and could be administered intravenously. Because IgA and IgM appear to have overlapping isoelectric points, their separation by such methods does not appear feasible. Some resolution of Cohn's fraction II to give fractions richer in antibodies to more basic and more acidic antigens might be achieved by electrophoretic methods. Robbins *et al.*[31] have reported that in rabbits the antibodies to acidic antigens are present in greatest amount in the IgG of highest isoelectric point; the reverse is true for basic antigens.

Ion-Exchange Methods   Ion-exchange materials find their best utility in removing from protein mixtures either the most acidic or the most basic components or in permitting an isoelectric component, or one with a net charge that is the same as that of the ion exchanger, to pass through the column with retention of charged impurities. On a laboratory scale, DEAE–cellulose or DEAE–Sephadex can be used for the rapid preparation of IgG fractions of good purity from plasma or globulin fractions.[5,20] Problems found in electric-transport separations present themselves in separations based on ion exchange. It does not appear that practical methods that use this principle will be developed for the large-scale separation of human serum immunoglobulins.

Molecular Sieving   A rather large variety of gel-filtration agents are available, and they permit separation of proteins in the size ranges of those found in plasma. Such methods—i.e., separations of proteins based on size—would appear to find utility in the separation of IgM and IgA polymers from 7S/IgG and IgA. The Institute of Biochemistry of the University of Uppsala and the laboratories of Pharmacia Fine Chemicals, Inc., have pioneered the development of gel-separation apparatus with bed volumes of over 1,000 liters. These can be operated on an automatic cycling system. These systems are more useful with "hard" gels, i.e., highly cross-linked gels that permit separation of molecules of molecular weight below 50,000. Different apparatus would be required for the "softer" gels whose use is necessary in the separation of proteins in the size ranges of the immunoglobulins.

Solid-Phase Systems   A most attractive method for purifying specific plasma antibodies is based on their reactions with antigens coupled to hydrophilic supporting media. Cellulose, agarose, and cross-linked dextrans (Sephadex) on treatment with cyanogen bromide are converted to derivatives that couple with compounds containing amino groups.[4,28,29] Thus, a column to which an antigen is coupled will selectively remove the antibodies from a plasma or serum sample passed over it. After the uncombined proteins are washed away, the absorbed antibodies are eluted. The columns may be reused for long periods. An example of the applicability of the method is seen in the work of Kristiansen, Sundberg, and Porath.[28] Partially deacylated blood substance A was coupled to agarose, and a human plasma sample containing a-isoagglutinins was passed over the column. The antibody could be eluted quantitatively and purified more than 25,000-fold in a single step. Antibody purified by this method will be a mixture of various immunoglobulins. If necessary, the IgM components could be separated from the IgG and IgA by gel filtration. Separation of the more basic IgG from the IgA in the resulting fraction could be effected by ion exchange or by electrophoretic decantation methods.

The work on a-isoagglutinins described above is a unique example of the utility of the solid-phase absorption method for purifying antibodies. However, we must ask whether this method can be applied to the separation of specific antibodies found in normal human plasma in small amounts. The present approach to provide potent antibody preparations for specific clinical use is to separate the usual fraction II from the plasma of persons immunized against such agents as tetanus toxoid, Rh_D antigen, and vaccinia and rabies viruses. It would appear that of these antigens only tetanus toxin (toxoid) is presently available in a form suitable for the preparations of the solid-phase material required for the separation of the specific antibody. The separation of antibodies to gram-negative bacteria by this method will require some definition of which antigens in a given organism are important and the ability to separate them in a form suitable for coupling to hydrophilic supporting media. The main problem in this area appears to involve basic research directed to the isolation of antigens to the antibodies desired. Secondary problems—e.g., whether the adsorbed antibodies eluted from such columns by the rather drastic methods required will have suitable *in vivo* activity and survival time—will most likely be encountered.

In summary, we can state that there is a need to exploit existing knowledge for the preparation of fractions of human plasma that contain antibodies that are essentially absent from the usual fraction II. It is imperative that more stable preparations of IgG be made and that the more electronegative species of this class of immunoglobulins be isolated. In such endeavors, a variety of hitherto unexploited methods must be introduced into general, large-scale fractionation work. The problems of separating highly purified specific antibodies of different classes and of definitive serotypes will raise many technologic questions.

REFERENCES

1. Albertsson, P. A. Partition of Cell Particles and Macromolecules. New York: John Wiley & Sons, Inc., 1961. 231 pp.
2. Anderson, E. A., and R. A. Alberty. Homogeneity and the electrophoretic behavior of some proteins. II. Reversible spreading and steady-state boundary criteria. J. Phys. Colloid. Chem. 52:1345–1364, 1948.
3. Audran, R., and M. Steinbuch. Proceedings of the 10th Congress of the European Society of Haematology, p. 922. Part II. Strasbourg, 1965.
4. Axén, R., J. Porath, and S. Ernback. Chemical coupling of peptides and proteins to polysaccharides by means of cyanogen halides. Nature 214:1302–1304, 1967.
5. Baumstark, J. S., R. J. Laffin, and W. A. Bardawil. A preparative method for the separation of 7S gamma globulin from human serum. Arch. Biochem. Biophys. 108:514–522, 1964.
6. Bier, M., Ed. Electrophoresis; Theory, Methods, and Applications. New York: Academic Press Inc., 1959. 563 pp.
7. Cann, J. R., J. G. Kirkwood, R. A. Brown, and O. J. Plescia. The fractionation of proteins by electrophoresis-convection. An improved apparatus and its use in fractionating diphtheria antitoxin. J. Amer. Chem. Soc. 71:1603–1608, 1949.
8. Chan, P. C., and H. F. Deutsch. Immunochemical studies of human serum Rh agglutinins. J. Immun. 85:37–45, 1960.
9. Chun, P. W., M. Fried, and E. F. Ellis. Use of water-soluble polymers for the isolation and purification of human immunoglobulins. Anal. Biochem. 19:481–497, 1967.
10. Cohn, M., H. F. Deutsch, and L. R. Wetter. Biophysical studies on blood plasma proteins; analysis of immunological heterogeneity of human gamma globulin fractions. J. Immun. 64:381–395, 1950.
11. Cohn, E. J., L. E. Strong, W. L. Hughes, Jr., D. J. Mulford, J. N. Ashworth, M. Melin, and H. L. Taylor. Preparation and properties of serum and plasma proteins. IV. A system for the separation into fractions of the protein and lipoprotein components of biological tissues and fluids. J. Amer. Chem. Soc. 68:459–475, 1946.
12. Deutsch, H. F., R. A. Alberty, and L. J. Gosting. Biophysical studies of blood plasma proteins; separation and purification of new globulin from normal human plasma. J. Biol. Chem. 165:21–35, 1946.
13. Deutsch, H. F., R. A. Alberty, L. J. Gosting, and J. W. Williams. Biophysical studies of blood plasma proteins; immunological properties of γ_1-globulin from plasma of normal humans. J. Immun. 56:183–194, 1947.
14. Dietzel, E., and H. Geiger. Gewinnung und Eigenschaften therapeutisch wichtiger Human-Plasma-proteine. Behringwerk-Mitteilungen 43:129–159, 1964.
15. Hannig, K. Eine Neuentwicklung der trägerfreien kontinuierlichen Elektrophorese. Zur Trennung hochmolekularer und grobdisperser Ieilchen. Hoppe Seyler Z. Physiol. Chem. 338:211–227, 1964.
16. Heide, K., and H. Haupt. Darstellung noch nicht therapeutisch angewandter Plasmaproteine. Behringwerk-Mitteilungen 43:161–193, 1964.
17. Horejsi, J., and R. Smetana. Isolation of gamma globulin from blood-serum by rivanol. Acta Med. Scand. 155:65–70, 1956.
18. Kekwick, R. A., and M. E. Mackay. The Separation of Protein Fractions from Human Plasma with Ether. Medical Research Council Special Report Series No. 286. London: Her Majesty's Stationery Office, 1954, 75 pp.
19. Koblet, H., S. Barandun, and H. Diggelmann. Turnover of standard-gammaglobulin, pH-4-gammaglobulin and pepsin desaggregated gammaglobulin and clinical implications. Vox Sang. 13:93–102, 1967.

20. Levy, H. B., and H. A. Sober. A simple chromatographic method for preparation of gamma globulin. Proc. Soc. Exp. Biol. Med. 103:250–252, 1960.
21. Mella, B., and D. J. Lang. Leukocyte mytosis: suppression in vitro associated with acute infectious hepatitis. Science 155:80–81, 1967.
22. Merler, E., F. S. Rosen, S. Salmon, J. D. Crain, and C. A. Janeway. Studies with intravenous gamma globulin. Vox Sang. 13:102–103, 1967.
23. Painter, R. H., and G. E. Connell. Instability of immune serum globulin preparations. Vox Sang. 10:355–356, 1965.
24. Pennell, R. B. Fractionation and isolation of purified components by precipitation methods, pp. 9–50. In F. W. Putnam, Ed. The Plasma Proteins. Vol. I. Isolation, Characterization, and Function. New York: Academic Press Inc. 1960.
25. Polson, A. Multi-membrane electrodecantation and its application to isolation and purification of proteins and viruses. Biochem. Biophys. Acta 11:315–325, 1953.
26. Polson, A., G. M. Potgieter, J. F. Largier, G. E. Mears, and F. J. Joubert. The fractionation of protein mixtures by linear polymers of high molecular weight. Biochim. Biophys. Acta 82:463–475, 1964.
27. Pool, J. G., E. J. Gershgold, and A. R. Pappenhagen. High-potency antihaemophilic factor concentrate prepared from cryoglobulin precipitate. Nature 203:312, 1965.
28. Porath, J. Molecular sieving and adsorption. Nature 218:834–838, 1968.
29. Porath, J., R. Axén, and S. Ernback. Chemical coupling of proteins to agarose. Nature 215:1491–1492, 1967.
30. Prince, A. M. An antigen detected in the blood during the incubation period of serum hepatitis. Proc. Nat. Acad. Sci. USA 60:814–821, 1968.
31. Robbins, J. B., E. Mozes, A. Rimon, and M. Sela. Correlation between net charge of antigens and electrophoretic mobility of immunoglobulin M antibodies. Nature 213:1013–1014, 1967.
32. Škvařil, F. Changes in outdated human γ-globulin preparations. Nature 185:475–476, 1960.
33. Škvařil, F., and D. Grünberger. Inhibition of spontaneous splitting of γ-globulin preparations with epsilon-aminocaproic acid. Nature 196:481–482, 1962.
34. Steinbuch, M. Isolation of gamma-A globulin as by-product of large-scale fractionation. Bibl. Haemat. 23:1196, 1965.
35. Steinbuch, M., R. Audran, P. Amouch, and C. Blatrix. The preparation of γ-globulin for intravenous use in Paris. Vox Sang. 13:103–106, 1967.

DISCUSSION

DR. WATT: We have designed two machines that we use in the fractionation of plasma. One, an earlier version (Figure 1), was based on a continuous small-volume mixing process in which plasma adjusted in terms of pH and ionic strength was passed through a jet into a chamber along with a similar jet of alcohol. The conditions of flow were arranged so that the jets produced no pulses. Mixing of the liquid streams was achieved with a magnetic stirring bar, and the mixed liquid was decanted into a cooling column for secondary cooling.

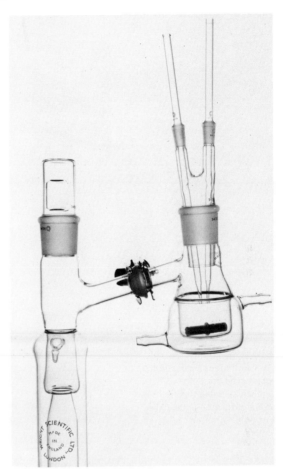

FIGURE 1 Continuous small-volume mixing process. An early design of the mixing chamber, showing the jets for introduction of plasma and alcohol.

This apparatus was effective in small-scale experimentation but completely ineffective for large-scale production techniques.

In the second version (Figure 2), we continued to use the jet system, but directed the jets at the top of a column of concentric coils at the junction of three coils that run in opposing spirals. Mixing is achieved by the flow of opposing liquid streams down the coils, where they can mix and remix thoroughly. Such an apparatus is capable of working at a plasma input of 15 liters/hr, processing all fractions of the Cohn method (J. Amer. Chem. Soc. 68:459–475, 1946) or any similar fractionation system, such as those of Kistler and Nitschmann (Vox Sang. 7:414–424, 1962) and Hink (Vox Sang. 2:174–186, 1957), or methods using polyethylene glycol.

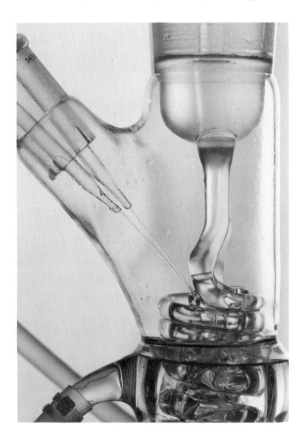

FIGURE 2   Continuous small-volume mixing process. The present version of mixing chamber, showing the liquid jets meeting on the surface of chilled glass coils at their point of union.

Professor Deutsch also has alluded to several points related to large-scale automatic fractionation processes, on some of which we have had experience. He spoke about the possibility of using a precipitate-recovery system other than the batch-wise Sharples centrifuge, which has, among others, the disadvantage that it must be stopped periodically for cleaning. We have investigated the manufactures of three different companies in a search for an effective self-cleaning centrifuge. These have several disadvantages, in my opinion. There are problems of temperature control, but one model of Westphalia centrifuge may be adapted to give better control of cooling of the spinning bowl. However, one realizes that there is likely to be some difficulty in persuading the company to make major adaptation of the machine for such a small market. The Florida citrus growers bought more Westphalia centrifuges last year than, possibly, the whole world's plasma-fractionation industry would require.

The precipitate discharged from these centrifuges contains a large portion of

entrained liquid. The Sharples centrifuge, even run at low flow rates, produces a
paste containing approximately 60% of its mass as entrained liquid. This is not
easily removed without further centrifugation.

The effect of low temperature must also be considered. Because of the need
to control pyrogens, we are probably faced with always working at relatively low
temperatures. Low temperature has a deleterious effect on the valve mechanism
that opens and closes the bowl on the centrifuge. It is possible to use glycol solutions or alcohol to operate the valves, instead of water, which is recommended
by the manufacturer; but these solutions, to a greater or lesser degree, tend to
cause stickiness of the valve components and corrosion of the metal parts.

Two adaptations of the Sharples centrifuge have been devised. In Holland, Dr.
Krijnen and his co-workers have developed a plastic tube liner for the bowl. This
can be simply removed and pressed clean by a hydraulic plunger system. It reduces the bowl capacity and introduces a further barrier for effective temperature
control of the liquid passing through the machine. The Sharples company itself
has developed a paper liner for the bowl. This, however, tears very easily. Teflon
or fiberglass sheets can be used; they work extremely well and make recovery of
the precipitated paste fairly easy.

I do not consider the periodic shutdown of a centrifuge a great disadvantage in automatic fractionation processes. In a completely automated plant, it
would be necessary to stop each centrifuge once every 4–5 hr. This brings staff
into contact with the operational plant at regular intervals. If this were not necessary, there might be a tendency to neglect this point and rely completely on
the automatic control system. This can be expected to deal only with foreseeable
plant failures and should never be trusted completely.

Finally, I wish to comment on the electrodecantation process referred to
by Dr. Deutsch. The force-flow electrophoresis system developed by Bier
(Science 125:1084–1085, 1957) is capable of very-large-scale fractionation at
various levels of pH and ionic strength. We are currently examining this process
for the subfractionation of fraction II + III, with encouraging results, although
preliminary. I consider that this process offers tremendous scope for exploitation
in this field.

DR. ASHWORTH: Dr. Watt, how do you separate the precipitate? It is known
that, when alcohol and plasma are brought together and instantaneously precipitated, the precipitate is so finely divided that it cannot be centrifuged.

DR. WATT: We have introduced between the mixing shell and the centrifuge an
aging column into which the mixed liquid is decanted. This column is fairly tall,
so that the effect of mixing near the point of addition can be discounted. The
aged liquid is removed from the bottom of the column.

H. W. KRIJNEN, H. G. J. BRUMMELHUIS, *and*
S. P. BEENTJES

Production of Specific Antibody Concentrates

During the last 10 years, normal human gamma globulin preparations have been partly replaced in clinical use by specific immune globulins. This development has been caused not only by the acquisition of more knowledge in the clinical use and effectiveness of these specific antibody concentrates, but also by the availability of more precise determinations of antibody activity. Whereas normal gamma globulin is isolated from the plasma of nonselected donors, the preparation of immune globulins requires the collection of blood either from selected donors with high natural titers against specific antigens or from donors who have been hyperimmunized against specific antigens.

This presentation discusses the production of several specific immune globulins: the antivaccinia, antirubella, antitetanus, and anti-D immune globulins.

However, before going into the details of the production of these immune globulins, it is important to discuss the cold-ethanol fractionation method, because it is used most frequently for the isolation of both gamma globulin and specific immune globulin concentrates. Figures 1 and 2 show the method in use in the Central Laboratory of the Netherlands Red Cross Blood Transfusion Service. It consists mainly of Cohn's

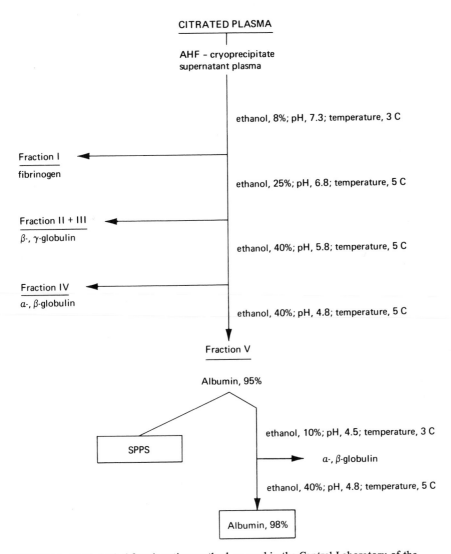

FIGURE 1   Cold-alcohol fractionation method, as used in the Central Laboratory of the Netherlands Red Cross Blood Transfusion Service, Amsterdam. SPPS = soluble plasma-protein solution.

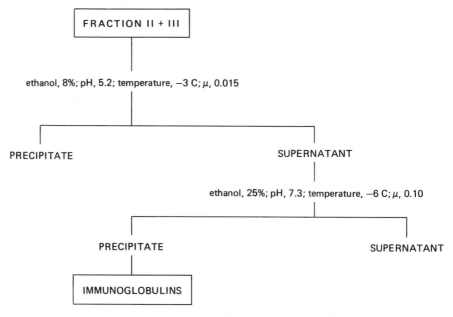

FIGURE 2   Isolation of immune globulin concentrates from fraction II + III.

method 6, with modifications in the isolation of the antibody concentrate in fraction II + III—modifications inspired by the work of Deutsch *et al.*[2] After the dissolved gamma globulin paste is freeze-dried, the protein powder is dissolved in 0.3M glycine solution containing 1:10,000 thimerosal, to a final protein concentration of 10–16% with a pH of 6.9. The sterile filtration is through asbestos sheets. Depending on the quantity of plasma that is available, the batch size varies between 100 and 1,000 liters of plasma; in the isolation of normal gamma globulin, each batch contains plasma obtained from approximately 4,000 donors.

This gamma globulin preparation is shown by moving-boundary electrophoresis to be over 95% gamma globulin and by ultracentrifugal analysis to be 85% 7S and 15% 10S. Assuming that 11% of the proteins in citrated plasma are gamma globulins, the overall yield of gamma globulin on a protein basis is approximately 85%. The antibody activity in the final product is theoretically 25 times higher than that of the starting plasma.

We turn now to the preparation of the specific immune globulins mentioned earlier.

Antivaccinia Immune Globulin (WHO definition: an immunoglobulin preparation containing at least 500 IU of vaccinia antibody per milliliter of final solution): Plasma intended for the preparation of antivaccinia immune globulin is usually obtained from the blood of donors taken 4–6 weeks after a successful primary vaccination or 3–4 weeks after a revaccination. It is the experience in the Netherlands that the vaccinia antibody titer in the pool of plasma obtained from military personnel usually ranges between 30 and 80 IU/ml. Although the yield of gamma globulin is about 85%, our main concern in recent years has been in antibody recovery. It seems that, even taking into account the inaccuracy of some of the methods used to determine the antibody concentration in the starting plasma and the final preparation, there is no reliable correlation between the protein and antibody yields. It is our experience that the vaccinia-antibody yield varies between 50% and 60% when the quantity of vaccinia antibody is determined by a 50% plaque-reduction neutralization test. The final 16% antivaccinia immune globulin solution has a potency between 500 and 1,000 IU/ml.

Antirubella Immune Globulin (WHO definition: none available): Prophylaxis against fetal damage caused by rubella is carried out with either a high dose of normal gamma globulin or a lower dose or rubella convalescent immune globulin. In the Netherlands, the general source of plasma for the preparation of rubella convalescent immune globulin has been blood taken from rubella convalescents at least 4 weeks after the onset of rash. The isolation of an antibody concentrate from this convalescent plasma has usually resulted in a 16% gamma globulin preparation with a neutralizing titer between 128 and 256. Since the introduction of faster tests for the determination of the antibody content of individual plasma samples, we have started a screening program that permits preselection of high-titered plasma from convalescents or from normal donors. In this way, it is possible, starting with a plasma pool whose titer is 512, to obtain a titer greater than 12,288 (measured by inhibition of hemagglutination).

Antitetanus Immune Globulin (WHO definition: an immune globulin preparation containing at least 50 IU of tetanus antibody per milliliter of final solution): High-titered plasma intended for the preparation of antitetanus immune globulin can be obtained from the blood of donors taken 3–4 weeks after the third booster injection. Because of practical problems in relation to such a specific donor program, a preselection of the plasma obtained from normal donors is generally used to acquire sufficient plasma for the production of antitetanus immune globulin. In the Netherlands, the main source of antitetanus plasma is blood from military donors screened by a precipitation test in agar, set at a sensitivity of 7 IU/ml of plasma. As a result of this fast (overnight) screening procedure, it is possible to salvage 25–30% of all blood donated by military personnel for the isolation of antitetanus immune globulin. It is our experience with plasma batches of 1,000 liters that this selection procedure results in a starting plasma containing approximately 12–14 IU of tetanus antitoxin per milliliter of plasma. The final 16% antitetanus immune globulin has a mean potency of 200 IU/ml, as determined by a neutralization protection test in animals. The concentration factor of the antitoxin activity in the immune globulin solution compared with the activity in the plasma pool is 15, giving an antibody yield of 60% of the theoretical expected 25-fold concentration. In this respect, our findings are in close correlation with those of Levine et al.[3] and Billaudelle et al.[1]

Anti-D Immune Globulin (WHO definition: none available): High-titered incomplete anti-Rh donor plasma can be obtained by collecting blood from mothers who have recently had a child with hemolytic disease or from volunteers immunized by injection of Rh-positive cells. It would be inappropriate to discuss extensively the different immunization schemes that are in use to promote antibody formation. But we should mention that, for protecting volunteers against the hazards of the transmission of serum hepatitis, Rh-positive erythrocytes should be preserved in the frozen state. By this method, large quantities of erythrocytes can be maintained without the uncertainty that exists after each separate donation of Rh-positive cells that will be used as an antigen in volunteers. Thus far, not much information has been made available by publications on experience in the production of anti-D immune globulin. Our own experience is that it is possible to isolate from anti-D plasma pools, varying from 20 to 400 liters and having an indirect Coombs test between 1:600 and 1:800, a 16% anti-D immune globulin preparation with a specific activity between 210 and 260 μg/ml (determined by Dr. Hughes-Jones). Yields of approximately 50% have been obtained in the preparation of this specific immune globulin.

We hope that this summary of some aspects of the production of specific antibody concentrates has created a sufficient basis for discussion on the subject. The following questions should be raised: How can antibody yield be improved (by revision of the alcohol fractionation method or by introducing other methods for large-scale production, including the use of ammonium sulfate, gel filtration, preparative electrophoretic methods as developed by Bier, electrodecantation, and immunoadsorbents)? In which IgG fraction does the antibody activity reside? Does it change during the course of immunization, during the period thereafter, and during exposure to plasmapheresis? What happens to stability during isolation and storage, as measured by potency tests?

REFERENCES

1. Billaudelle, H., G. Lundblad, L.-G. Falksveden, and K. Ullberg-Olsson. Fractionation of human immune serum anti tetanus by gel filtration. Z. Immunitaetsforsch. 131:170–183, 1966.
2. Deutsch, H. F., L. J. Gosting, R. A. Alberty, and J. W. Williams. Biophysical studies of blood plasma proteins. III. Recovery of γ-globulin from human blood protein mixtures. J. Biol. Chem. 164:109–118, 1946.
3. Levine, L., L. Wyman, and J. A. McComb. Tetanus immune globulin from selected human plasmas. Six years of experience with a screening method. JAMA 200:341–344, 1967.

DISCUSSION

DR. MANNIK: I would like to add a note of enthusiasm to the use of immunoadsorbents. The coupling of purified antigens to cross-linked dextrans by the cyanogen bromide activation method is simple. We have used this technique in our laboratory to isolate specific rabbit antibodies for animal experimentation. Individual columns have been used for over a year, with continued reproducibility. I think this technique might be applicable to the isolation of specific human antibodies. We have done some animal experiments with isolated antibodies. Their biologic half-life (after removal of aggregates by gel filtration) appears to be the same as that of unaltered IgG. We have used low pH, as well as various ions for dissociation of antibodies from the immunoadsorbent. With low pH, however (that is, in 0.01M hydrochloric acid in physiologic saline at a pH slightly above 2), there is aggregation of the resulting pure antibodies.

DR. DEUTSCH: I think there are differences in the stability of animal and human gamma globulins. When human Cohn's fraction II (or myeloma proteins) is treated at pH 4, there is a shift in sedimentation constant. This is interpreted as being caused by unfolding of the polypeptide chain. When subjected to papain digestion, molecules so treated never form an Fc fragment, because it gets digested to small peptides. Papain acts like pepsin on such materials. I think we have to look for better dissociation methods for human proteins. Dr. Schwick indicated that plasmin can be removed very effectively from plasma by coupling lysyl-lysine to columns. Removal of antibodies by passing serum over columns to which antigen is complexed allows small amounts of antigen to elute with the antibodies. Clinical use of these materials may lead to immunization of the patient to the residual antigen. The adsorbing columns cannot be completely eluted, and one has to prepare new columns often. The eluted antibodies may be partially denatured. These are limitations of the methods. Columns are wonderful for the research laboratory, but not necessarily for commercial production of clinically useful materials.

DR. JOHNSON: I was interested in Dr. Krijnen's experience in producing a rubella immune globulin apparently by selection from a normal donor population. We have had similar experience recently in this country. We have titered our entire population of professional donors, and find approximately 15% with a hemagglutination-inhibition titer of 512 or above. By selecting those with titers of 512 or above, we can obtain a plasma pool that titers at about 1,200, and from this we obtain a rubella immune globulin titering at about 16,000, all without any artificial hyperimmunization.

DR. KRIJNEN: It is our experience in screening that about 20% of the donors have titers higher than 256.

DR. PENNELL: Dr. Krijnen, in your screening procedures, you select 25–30% of the donors from the armed services. Do you get from this pool enough tetanus antibody to supply the needs of the Netherlands?

DR. KRIJNEN: It is sufficient so that in the coming year the equine antitoxin will be completely replaced by the use of this tetanus immune globulin.

DR. PAINTER: I wanted to correct the impression that more stable preparations of gamma globulin result if fresh plasma is used. Our experience has been that gamma globulin prepared from fresh plasma—for example, for the preparation of tetanus immune globulin—has been just as prone to fragmentation as that prepared from outdated plasma.

LEONARD G. DAUBER, LOUIS J. REED,
H. PHILIP FORTWENGLER, JR., *and* FRANK R. CAMP, JR.

Placental versus Nonplacental Sources of Gamma Globulins: The Hazard of Blood Groups A and B Sensitization*

Materials used for the immunization of humans have been known to be contaminated with A and B blood-group-like substances. Diphtheria and tetanus toxoids prepared from material grown on hog peptones have caused isoantibody-titer rises in recipients of these vaccines; plague vaccine† similarly obtained has been likewise contaminated. These vaccines may render group O recipients "dangerous" universal donors, as defined by the *in vitro* serologic criteria. Because the need for universal donor blood is great in the military, the U.S. Army Medical Research Laboratory at Fort Knox, Kentucky, has been screening vaccines for the presence of blood-group-like substances. This study is concerned with the results of *in vitro* and *in vivo* studies on placental and nonplacentally derived gamma globulin preparations used in prophylaxis against infectious hepatitis and rubella.

Various lots of gamma globulin preparations of placental origin from Pitman-Moore and Lederle Laboratories, as well as gamma globulin de-

---

*Presented by H. Philip Fortwengler, Jr., at the 21st Annual Meeting of the American Association of Blood Banks, Washington, D.C., October 27–31, 1968, under the title "The Occurrence of Blood Group Substances A and B in Proprietary Gamma Globulin of Placental Origin."
†Current plague vaccine is satisfactory.

339

rived from pooled plasma prepared at Hyland Laboratories, were examined for A and B blood-group substance by hemolysin and hemagglutination inhibition.

Figure 1 shows the results of hemagglutination-inhibition assays on the commercial gamma globulin preparations. Because of the presence of isoagglutinins in all the preparations and cold agglutinins in the placental gamma globulin, these materials were adsorbed with the appropriate cells at 4 C. An inhibition curve is obtained when the percent of expected agglutination is plotted against the reciprocal of the dilution. These curves show the isoagglutinin inhibition obtained by Lederle and Pitman-Moore gamma globulin before and after adsorption of pre-existing agglutinins. The curve undergoes a shift to the right after adsorption, showing increased activity. The nonplacental gamma globulin preparations showed no inhibition before or after adsorption. By comparison with a National Institutes of Health (NIH) reference standard, there is marked B substance activity (the approximate equivalent of 167 μg/ml) and far smaller A substance activity (approximately 20 μg/ml). Only placental gamma globulin preparations were found to contain blood-group substance activity.

The hemolysin-inhibition assay was ineffective in measuring this activity in gamma globulin, because all specimens tested contained significant anticomplementary activity that could not be overcome by increasing the amount of adsorbed group O serum used in the assay as a source of complement. Inasmuch as the hemolysin reaction is complement-dependent, the results were consistently false positive. Attempts to separate blood-group substance activity by ultracentrifugation or starch-block electrophoresis were unsuccessful.

To confirm the results of the *in vitro* assay, the gamma globulin preparations were administered to volunteers as an *in vivo* test for the presence of group-specific antigens.

Two base-line specimens were obtained before immunizations; they were in all cases essentially identical in antibody content and have been averaged. They have been designated the "pre" specimens in Table 1 and are seen in the first column under each type of antibody. The hemolysins are reported as CH_{50} values—that is, the reciprocal of the dilution of serum that, in the presence of a standard amount of excess complement, causes lysis of 50% of the standard cell suspension. Isoagglutinins and immune agglutinins are given as the reciprocals of the end dilutions.

DAUBER *and others*: Placental versus Nonplacental Sources of Gamma Globulins: The Hazard of Blood Groups A and B Sensitization

341

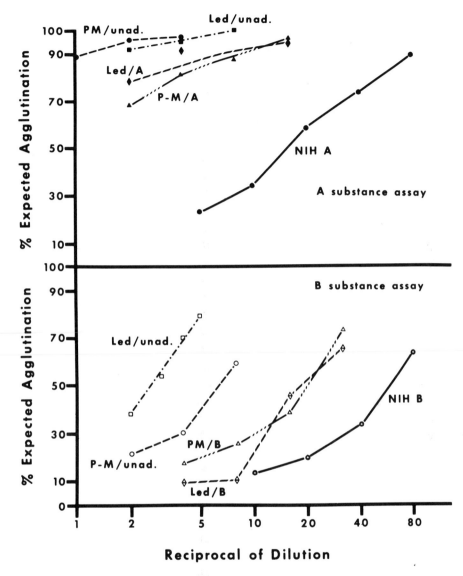

FIGURE 1 Isoagglutinin-inhibition assays of placental gamma globulin preparations. Led = Lederle Laboratories Immune Serum Globulin, lot 107-572. P-M = Pitman-Moore Immune Serum Globulin, lot 172-311. The preparations were assayed unadsorbed and after adsorption with packed, washed group A_1 or B erythrocytes by standard agglutinin reagents (anti-A and anti-B typing serum, in dilution of 1:4, Spectra Biological, Inc., lots A-34 and B-34). NIH reference standard, containing 500 μg of each A and B substance per milliliter, was assayed for comparison.

TABLE 1 Mean Isoantibody Responses in Volunteers Given Porcine A and/or Equine B Blood-Group Substances (Charles Pfizer and Co.)

Blood-Group Type	No. Subjects	Antibodies Measured	Antibody Type							
			Hemolysin[a]		Isoagglutinin[b]		Immune Agglutinin[b]		Saliva Agglutinin[c]	
			Pre	Post	Pre	Post	Pre	Post	Pre	Post
O	{ 5	Anti-A	0.6	5.6	4.0	6.2	0.2	2.8	0.6	1.4
		Anti-B	0.2	12.1	1.7	7.0	0	5.5	1.0	4.0
A	4	Anti-B	0.9	11.3	2.8	5.5	0	1.8	0	0
B	4	Anti-A	0.2	6.9	3.9	6.5	0	0.3	0	0

[a]Given as CH_{50} values.
[b]Given as end-titer tube numbers.
[c]Given as end titers.

342

Table 1 shows the mean isoantibody titers of reference groups that had been stimulated with porcine A and equine B substance. The most dramatic rises are seen in the anti-B isoantibodies. For example, the five type O subjects had a mean anti-B hemolysin activity of 0.2 units before immunization and 12.1 units after administration of the soluble blood-group substance. Their anti-A response was generally less. And the saliva agglutinins were increased only in the type O subjects.

Table 2 indicates that the volunteers who received nonplacental gamma globulin showed no substantial change in isoantibodies, compared with preimmunization sera. The volunteers who received placental gamma globulin, however, showed distinct serologic changes, as can be seen in the mean titers of Table 3. In the three groups of volunteers receiving Lederle material, all displayed rises in isoantibody titers. This change, again, was greatest in the anti-B antibodies and, as in the reference group, only type O subjects produced detectable saliva agglutinins. Volunteers receiving Pitman-Moore material showed similar rises in iso-antibody titers.

Because there is contamination of gamma globulin derived from placental materials only, and because it has been demonstrated by immunofluorescent techniques that the mature placental trophoblast is devoid of blood-group antigens, the release of blood-group substances from erythrocytes sequestered in the placenta may occur during processing manipulations, such as freezing and thawing.

Hemolysin- and hemagglutination-inhibition assays both clearly indicate the presence of measurable amounts of group-specific substance in the hemolysates derived from A_1 or B cells after freezing, thawing, and passage through Millipore filters. Indeed, in materials derived from equal volumes of packed cells, five to seven times as much B substance as A substance appeared in the hemolysate after passage through an 0.22-μ filter (Figure 2). It is likely that the greater concentration of B substance in the commercial gamma globulin preparations, as demonstrated by *in vitro* and *in vivo* testing, reflects the results obtained from these freeze–thaw experiments.

The volunteers who made saliva agglutinins were group O subjects who had the more dramatic increases in their hemolytic antibodies in response to either porcine A and equine B or human A and B substance contained in placental gamma globulin. These data are thought to represent the first direct demonstration of the stimulation of saliva agglutinins by blood-group-specific substances.

TABLE 2 Mean Isoantibody Responses in Volunteers Given Nonplacental (Serum) Gamma Globulin (Hyland Laboratories)

Blood-Group Type	No. Subjects	Antibodies Measured	Antibody Type								
			Hemolysin[a]		Isoagglutinin[b]		Immune Agglutinin[b]		Saliva Agglutinin[c]	
			Pre	Post	Pre	Post	Pre	Post	Pre	Post
O	5	{ Anti-A	1.0	1.0	4.6	4.4	3.0	2.8	0	0
		{ Anti-B	0.5	0.7	4.2	3.8	2.1	2.4	0.2	0.2
A	5	Anti-B	0.1	0	1.7	1.0	0	0	0.2	0.2
B	3	Anti-A	0.4	1.0	4.7	4.3	0	0	0.7	0.7

[a]Given as CH$_{50}$ values.
[b]Given as end-titer tube numbers.
[c]Given as end titers.

TABLE 3 Mean Isoantibody Responses in Volunteers Given Placental Gamma Globulin (Lederle Laboratories)

Blood-Group Type	No. Subjects	Antibodies Measured	Antibody Type											
			Hemolysin[a]		Isoagglutinin[b]		Immune Agglutinin[b]		Saliva Agglutinin[c]	
			Pre	Post	Pre	Post	Pre	Post	Pre	Post
O	5	{ Anti-A	1.0	2.0	2.6	6.0	1.2	3.6	0.2	1.0
		Anti-B	0.1	7.0	1.9	6.8	0.8	7.0	0.2	2.2
A	5	Anti-B	0.4	37.7	2.1	6.8	0.4	3.3	0	0
B	3	Anti-A	0.5	2.1	4.7	5.3	0	0	0	0

[a]Given as CH_{50} values.
[b]Given as end-titer tube numbers.
[c]Given as end titers.

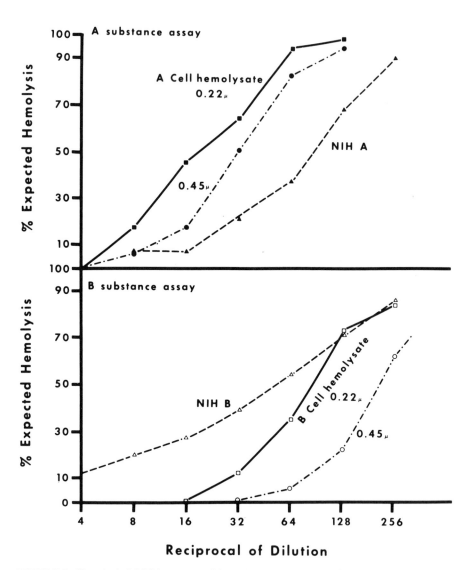

FIGURE 2   Hemolysin-inhibition assays of hemolysates derived from frozen, thawed, washed erythrocytes and passed through successively smaller Millipore filters (0.45-μ, 0.22-μ pore size). Assays of NIH reference standards A and B are included for comparison. Hemolysin reagents were obtained from a single group A (anti-B) and a single group B (anti-A) volunteer who had been immunized with porcine A or equine B substances.

DISCUSSION

DR. KABAT: It seems that one should consider the desirability of giving serum gamma globulin, and not placental gamma globulin, to women of childbearing age. That should be an important consideration with respect to subsequent production of hemolytic disease due to anti-A and anti-B antibodies.

VII
STANDARDIZATION AND
SURVEILLANCE OF
THE USE OF
IMMUNOGLOBULINS

D. S. ROWE, S. G. ANDERSON, *and* JOYCE SKEGG

Standardization of Quantitative Measurements of Human Immunoglobulins G, A, and M

The measurement of the concentration of the serum immunoglobulins is now a common clinical and research practice. The frequency with which these measurements are carried out reflects the current awareness of immunologic phenomena in disease and has been made possible by the development of simple gel-diffusion methods, notably that of Mancini et al.[4] and its modifications.

Such methods offer reasonable precision. For example, in our hands the standard error of replicates carried out on different days, using the modification of Fahey and McKelvey,[1] is around 10%. There is, however, much less certainty when comparisons are made between results obtained in different laboratories using different reagents; it is not yet possible to decide with what confidence results obtained in different laboratories can be compared.

How important is this? As long as only major differences of concentration must be recognized, measurement does not present great problems. It is not difficult to decide, for example, that a serum is grossly deficient in IgG and has an excess of IgM when the amounts of these proteins differ from the normal means by a factor of 10 or more. In addition, the ranges of plasma concentration of immunoglobulin found

351

in health are wide. At first sight, it may appear that great precision of measurement is not called for, at least for clinical purposes. However, when groups of individuals are being compared, greater precision of measurement becomes much more important. Figure 1 demonstrates differences in serum IgG concentrations in postpartum mothers in Lausanne, Switzerland; Ibadan, Nigeria; and Bathurst, The Gambia. Mothers with malarial parasitemia in The Gambia had the highest values, followed by nonparasitemic Gambian and Nigerian mothers. Lausanne mothers had the lowest values. The differences between these groups, especially between parasitemic and nonparasitemic Africans, could not have been

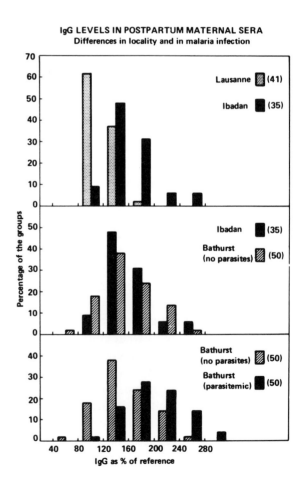

FIGURE 1   Serum IgG concentrations in postpartum African and European mothers, expressed as percentage of the "reference preparation for human immunoglobulins" reconstituted to 1 ml with water. The number of individuals in each group is indicated in parentheses. Data from unpublished work of Rowe, McGregor, and Gautier.

inferred with confidence if measurements had been made in different laboratories without the use of standards. The use of standards in measurement will be necessary for the full significance of immunoglobulin changes in health and disease to be appreciated.

Specific antisera are the only reagents now available that possess the selectivity necessary to distinguish the different immunoglobulin classes from each other and from other plasma proteins. In the foreseeable future, therefore, measurements of immunoglobulin concentrations will be carried out with immunochemical techniques. These methods are essentially comparative: the reactivity of a sample under test is compared with that of a "working" standard or reference reagent, using antiserum specific for the class in question; the result is a ratio of activity—i.e., the ratio of the activity of the test sample to the activity of the standard; if the activity of the standard is known, that of the test sample can be calculated. Methods therefore require a suitable standard and an appropriate antiserum. We shall devote this discussion to a consideration of standards and antisera, with some mention of different techniques.

STANDARDS

Three qualities are required of a standard for immunoglobulins: the immunoglobulins in it must be stable; the immunoglobulins must be comparable with immunoglobulins in test sera; and the activity of the immunoglobulins must be defined.

It is an objective of our laboratories to investigate materials with regard to their suitability as standards for immunoglobulins so that scientifically evaluated and reliable standards may be made generally available. Three proposed standards for human immunoglobulins have been prepared and freeze-dried. Their examination in collaborative studies has been arranged with Dr. John L. Fahey. These studies are being carried out at the World Health Organization (WHO) Regional Reference Centre for the Human Immunoglobulins in Springfield, Virginia, and in numerous other collaborating laboratories, as well as in ours.

Ideally, standards for immunoglobulins might consist of the highly purified immunoglobulins themselves. Indeed, if these proteins were generally available in a homogeneous and stable form, there would be little need for standardization. However, purified immunoglobulins other than IgG are difficult to prepare in large quantity, and probably immunoglobulins of all classes are unstable in the purified state. It was considered that pooled human serum from healthy donors, lyophilized and stored at low temperature, would be a preparation in which immunoglobulins would be more likely to be stable.

To assess this, a pilot accelerated-degradation study was carried out. This is the classical method of assessing the stability of biologic materials.[3] Aliquots of the preparation under test are held at different temperatures for a suitable period. The activities of the material held at different temperatures are compared. Characteristically, material stored at high temperatures suffers more loss of activity than that stored at low temperatures. The rate of degradation at lower temperature is inferred from the slope of the temperature-degradation plot. For the pilot test, human serum was lyophilized, and aliquots were stored at –20 C and +37 C in all-glass ampuls containing nitrogen. After 6 months of storage, the ampul contents were reconstituted with water, and the characteristics of immunoglobulins G, A, and M of the various aliquots were compared with the quantitative single-radial-diffusion method, to provide an index of the "relative potency" of the immunoglobulins. Log dose-response curves were obtained for each of the reconstituted materials from measurements of ring diameters produced in antibody in agar plates by a series of dilutions. The relative potencies were calculated by transformation of the data to parallel-line assays. The results, shown in Table 1, indicate some loss of potency (smaller ring diameters

TABLE 1   Pilot Accelerated Degradation of Potency of Immunoglobulins[a]

Immunoglobulin	Potency of Material Stored for 6 Months at +37 C Relative to That of Material Stored for 6 Months at –20 C	95% Confidence Limits of Relative Potency
IgG	0.85	0.82–0.89
IgA	0.93	0.87–1.00
IgM	1.00	0.92–1.08
IgD	0.89	0.77–1.03

[a]Potency determined from statistical analyses of dose-response lines obtained by single-radial-diffusion method.

for the same dilution) on storage at the higher temperature. Further
analyses have indicated that this may be due to aggregation of immunoglobulins. The changes of potency were sufficiently small to suggest that
these immunoglobulins in serum stored in this way would be likely to
be stable at –20 C for a number of years.

Accordingly, a large amount of serum was prepared as a possible
standard for human immunoglobulins. Plasma was obtained from healthy
adult male donors in England. Cryoprecipitate was removed from most
samples. Samples that contained increased IgD and rheumatoid factor
were discarded; 465 samples were pooled, calcified, and clotted. They
were then filtered through membranes down to 0.45 μ, and the material
was placed in ampuls in 1-ml quantities. These were freeze-dried, flooded
with nitrogen, sealed by glass fusion, and stored at –20 C. The total
number of ampuls was approximately 70,000. It was not possible to
lyophilize all this material in one machine and on one occasion. Accordingly, it was divided into portions that were processed in different
machines and at different times.

International collaborative assays are in progress on this material to
assess its suitability for use as a quantitative reference reagent for IgG,
IgA, and IgM. These studies are concerned with the stability of these
immunoglobulins, with their comparability with the immunoglobulins
of fresh-frozen serum, and with the material's weight content of
immunoglobulins. The stability experiments are being carried out as
described for the pilot study. The comparability studies involve the
comparison of dose-response curves of the reconstituted reference preparation with those of fresh-frozen human samples. These curves are being
analyzed statistically to determine the precision of estimation of the
relative activities of immunoglobulins in the reference and serum preparations and to test linearity and parallelism. The weight content of immunoglobulins is being assessed by similar assay, comparing the reference
preparations with known concentrations of isolated, purified immunoglobulins, which have been assessed by immunochemical and physicochemical criteria. Several laboratories in Europe and the United States
are collaborating in this work, and their data are now being analyzed.
Preliminary results have indicated that this material is suitable for use
as a reference reagent for quantitative analyses.

Because of the immediate need for a reference preparation, it was
decided to make this material generally available before the full analysis

was complete. Accordingly, an announcement was published recently in various journals of immunology and immunochemistry, which contained a preliminary description of this material (for example, Bull. WHO 39:992–993, 1968). It should be noted that this material is not now a WHO standard preparation. It is correctly referred to as a "reference preparation for human serum immunoglobulins IgG, IgA, and IgM." When the full analysis is complete, this reagent will be submitted for consideration as a WHO standard and as a national standard in individual countries. If it is acceptable, a unitage of immunoglobulins would be assigned. An announcement would then appear in appropriate journals.

Meanwhile, it is suggested that measurements of the concentrations of immunoglobulins G, A, and M in a serum sample be expressed as a percentage of their concentrations in the reconstituted reference preparation. In this way, valid comparisons between results obtained in different laboratories should be possible.*

ANTISERA

Antisera should be monospecific. A corollary of this characteristic is that the same ratio of concentrations of test sample to reference sample should be given by a number of different specific antisera, and there is some evidence that at least rabbit antisera to human immunoglobulins react in this way.

To assess this, comparisons have been made between measurements of concentrations of IgA, IgM, and IgD in approximately 50 serum samples, with two antisera for each class. Sera were selected to show a broad range of concentrations of immunoglobulins, but samples containing myeloma proteins were excluded. Antisera to IgA and IgD were prepared for two different myeloma proteins of each class. For IgM, one antiserum was prepared for a Waldenström macroglobulin, the other† to an antibody of the somatic antigen of *Salmonella typhosa*. No difference greater than that expected due to the error inherent in the method was observed between measurements using the two antisera to each class. Antisera prepared in the rabbit are satisfactory reagents

---

*The WHO recommendations for the use of the reference preparations are included as an appendix to this paper.—Ed.
†Kindly provided by Prof. J. F. Soothill.

for the estimation of immunoglobulins in serum. Other experiments are
in progress with antisera to normal and "monoclonal" proteins of various classes prepared in various species to obtain further evidence on this
point.

TECHNIQUES

There are a great variety of methods in which antisera can be used as
quantitative reagents. These range from the classical quantitative precipitin techniques through many gel-diffusion methods to the highly
sensitive inhibition techniques that use isotopically labeled antigen. A
principle of the use of biologic standards is that the same relative activities of test sample and standard should be obtained, regardless of
technique.

Heterogeneity of molecular size is important in relation to technique.
It is known that some gel-diffusion techniques are sensitive to the diffusion constant of antigen. This has been shown by Fahey and McKelvey[1]
in measurements of κ and λ concentrations in solutions of immunoglobulin molecules of different sizes. Smaller molecules gave propor-
tionately larger diameters of zones of precipitation. It is also possible
that monomers and polymers differ both qualitatively and quantitatively with respect to their antigenic determinants. Of the serum immunoglobulins, IgA shows size heterogeneity and IgM may occur both as
macroglobulin and as smaller subunits. Measurements of the concentrations of these proteins in serum may on occasion be invalidated because
of differences in molecular size between the immunoglobulins in the
serum sample and in the standard. A simple test of assay validity is to
compare the log dose-response curves of a series of dilutions of the
standard and the sample. Nonparallelism indicates that the comparison
is invalid. However, parallelism in itself does not necessarily validate the
measurements. Ideally, the size distribution of the immunoglobulin
should be determined, for example, by chromatography on Sephadex
G-200. These reservations concerning the measurement of serum immunoglobulins apply also to measurements of those proteins in body
fluids. In particular, secretory IgA differs from serum IgA in size and in
its possession of an extra distinctive polypeptide chain. IgG in normal
urine is present both as the intact molecule and as fragments. Fragments
of immunoglobulins may also occur in stools. Due regard must there-

fore be paid to the size and antigenic characteristics of immunoglobulins in these and other body fluids in the interpretation of quantitative results.

There is one further point with regard to techniques, which has been made by Heremans[2]: rheumatoid factor in the serum sample may interact with the heated rabbit IgG present in the agar. Under these circumstances, IgM measurements are not possible and the measurements of other serum immunoglobulins may be affected.

This section of this presentation has necessarily been concerned with some of the difficulties and limitations of quantitative immunochemical techniques. We would like to end on a more positive note. We believe that such measurements of serum immunoglobulins will continue to be of value in the study of the immune status of individuals and that they will find an application in the study of populations. We have described our efforts to date in relation to standardization for IgG, IgA, and IgM. A similar reference reagent for IgD is now being studied and should soon be available. A reference reagent for IgE is also available for limited distribution. This material is pooled, lyophilized serum of relatively high IgE content obtained from Africans. Its use as a quantitative reagent has not yet been validated, but IgE may be more positively identified by its use in conjunction with specific antiserum.

We are optimistic that the provision of standards for human immunoglobulins of the kinds described here will remove some of the present anomalies of quantitative measurements of these proteins. As new knowledge and techniques become available, we expect that reference reagents for qualitative and quantitative purposes will be provided for further classes and subclasses and for the L chains of human immunoglobulins. We also recognize a need for such reagents for the immunoglobulins of various animal species.

REFERENCES

1. Fahey, J. L., and E. M. McKelvey. Quantitative determination of serum immunoglobulins in antibody-agar plates. J. Immun. 94:84–90, 1965.
2. Heremans, J. F. Immunologic deficiency diseases in man. Birth Defects, Original Article Series 4:339, 1968.
3. Jerne, N. K., and W. L. Perry. The stability of biological standards. Bull. WHO 14:167–182, 1956.

4. Mancini, G., A. O. Carbonara, and J. F. Heremans. Immunochemical quantitation of antigens by single radial immunodiffusion. Int. J. Immunochem. 2:235–254, 1965.

APPENDIX: RECOMMENDATIONS FOR THE USE OF THE
REFERENCE PREPARATIONS*

1. On receipt the reference preparation should be stored at –20°C.

2. One ampoule of the reference preparation should be reconstituted by the addition of 1 ml of distilled water. The powder should dissolve readily on standing for 1 hour at room temperature to give a slightly turbid solution. An appropriate series of dilutions of this solution should be prepared and used on the same day as the material was reconstituted.

3. The total volume of the solution of this preparation made in this way will exceed 1 ml. It has been calculated from the wet and dry weights of the ampoule contents and from specific gravity measurements that the average volume of this solution will be 1.06 ml; this solution will, therefore, contain the number of units of immunoglobulin in the standard in 1.06 ml. . . .

4. The concentration of each immunoglobulin in the solution under test should be compared with that of the standard, by using techniques which have been validated statistically. The potencies of immunoglobulins in the test solutions in relation to the standard should be estimated by a valid statistical analysis of the results of the comparative experiments.

5. The relative potency should be expressed as units of activity of each immunoglobulin per ml of solution.

DISCUSSION

DR. BUCKLEY: I would like to identify another problem related to the standardization of serum immunoglobulin concentrations. I am referring to the independent sources of biologic variation that can be observed in apparently healthy persons. Once standardized reagents become available, our ability to identify ab-

*From D. S. Rowe, S. G. Anderson, and B. Graf. A research standard for human serum immunoglobulin IgG, IgA, and IgM. Bull. WHO 42:535–552, 1970.

normal sera will become more meaningful. Adequate controls are important. Recent studies have identified an additional important source of variation in normal serum immunoglobulin concentrations. Major changes in concentration can be related to the aging of apparently healthy adults (Figure 1).

The data in the figure are not presented as a percentage of the WHO reference standard, but the figure shows the extent to which the serum concentrations of IgG, IgA, and IgM vary throughout life. Age (in years) is presented on the abscissa of the figure. Geometric mean serum concentrations of IgG, IgA, and IgM are shown on a logarithmic scale on the ordinate. The oldest of the 630 persons of all ages who were studied was 91 years old. The more than 200 persons older than 60 represented in this figure became available for our study through the Center for the Study of the Aging at the Duke University Medical Center.

A dramatic and consistent fall in the average concentrations of IgG and IgM occurs from about the age of 35. A period of physiologic hypogammaglobulinemia can be observed near the end of the life of man, as well as very soon after birth. In contrast, serum IgA concentrations are well maintained. The average fractional concentration of IgA (not shown) in the serum of older persons increases with age. This change in IgA may be a part of the hyperglobulinemia that can be identified by paper electrophoresis of the serum of older persons. Differences related to race and sex can also be identified in older persons. These changes primarily involve IgG and IgA and are small in comparison with the striking effect of aging itself.

Finally, there is a first-order interaction effect of sex on race, which is represented as the crossover in the concentrations of IgG and IgM between the sexes in each race. This event occurs before adulthood. It can be identified as a first-order interaction in the multivariate form of statistical analysis used to evaluate these data. These changes also represent a statistically significant source of biologic variation.

In summary, I think it is important to begin work on another aspect of standardization. I refer to the identification of the confidence intervals of serum immunoglobulin concentrations in healthy persons. It is clear that age, as well as race and sex, contributes significant sources of biologic variation. It is necessary to define our estimates of normal confidence intervals as functions of age, as well as of race and sex. Otherwise, many of our comparisons made in disease states may be hazardous and difficult to interpret.

DR. ROWE: I agree with Dr. Buckley's comments. However, the changes with age in one country may not take place in other countries. Our data from Africa suggest that the levels of IgG change very little with age, at least up to the age of 55 or so. Levels of IgA and IgM, on the other hand, tend to vary among individuals.

It is very important to know the normal range of values at any particular age

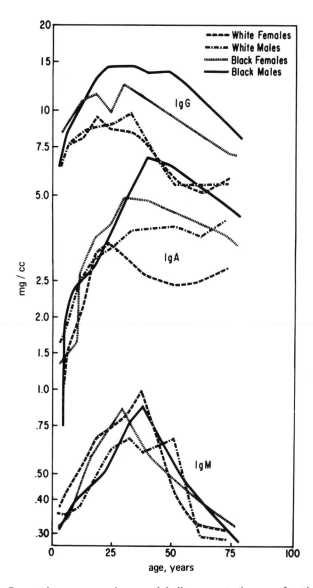

FIGURE 1   Geometric mean serum immunoglobulin concentrations as a function of age.

or in a particular sex. The comparison of values from one person with the mean value may be misleading unless one knows the spread of the normal range.

DR. TERRY: I would like to raise a note of caution about the interpretation of such data as these. Serum concentration may not actually drop off with age. Results of cross-sectional analysis may be interpreted quite differently if one looks at a cohort analysis and follows individuals through life. Persons now 70 years old with low serum IgG may also have had low IgG when they were 40, and persons now 40 years old with high IgG may still have high IgG when they are 70. This problem has turned up in cancer statistics, and one should start now to put away samples of serum so that individuals can be followed over a period of 40–50 years and any real changes in serum concentrations with time can be defined.

I would also like to ask Dr. Rowe to expand his comments on problems of quantitating sera that have myeloma or other anomalous immunoglobulins.

DR. ROWE: We and others have recognized difficulties in quantitation, for instance, of IgM in serum from patients with Waldenström macroglobulinemia, quantitative measurements and ultracentrifugal analyses of which do not agree. It is at least likely, *a priori*, that such differences as the restriction of antigenic determinants within myeloma proteins and macroglobulins may make for anomalies in quantitation. For instance, if the myeloma protein contains fewer antigenic determinants than its normal counterpart, then the antiserum is in effect a weaker antiserum, and one appears to obtain a higher value on the immunochemical analysis.*

---

*This argument does not apply if the antiserum is monospecific, as defined by Rowe, Anderson, and Skegg.–Ed.

H. BRUCE DULL, A. W. KARCHMER, *and*
MORRIS T. SUGGS

Surveillance of Immunoglobulins in the United States

Immunobiologics have become a fundamental resource of preventive medicine in the United States. This has occurred primarily in the last 25 years, with accelerating development of effective vaccines, improved technology of processing blood products, and increased provision of resources to stimulate the use and evaluation of immunobiologics.

Knowledge of the uses of immunobiologics and evaluation of their effectiveness are essential to the full interpretation of the progress of disease control. Therefore, when reliance is placed on artificially induced immunity, active and passive, there is a corresponding obligation to monitor the availability, uses, and value of immunobiologics.

We intend in this report to review data on the use of gamma globulin in the United States. Surveillance of gamma globulin is considerably less mature than surveillance of vaccines, on which more specific data have been collected for a longer time. Nevertheless, there is value in available information as an example of the usefulness of surveillance.

SOURCES OF DATA

Data for this report are derived from two principal sources: the Biologics Surveillance Program of the National Communicable Disease Center

(NCDC), Atlanta, Georgia, and a recent survey of immunoglobulin programs in state and metropolitan health departments.

The Biologics Surveillance Program, begun in 1962, was developed by the NCDC for several reasons: the rapid increase in use of biologics and evidence that even greater increases would follow the development of new vaccines; the national and local promotion of disease-control programs, such as oral polio vaccination and globulin prophylaxis against infectious hepatitis; and national and state legislation, in particular the Federal Vaccination Assistance Act of 1962, that added financial resources for comprehensive immunization of children. The Biologics Surveillance Program documented one aspect of this crescendo—the supply and distribution of biologics.

The Program is a voluntary collaboration between the NCDC and the 18 major producers (including both pharmaceutical manufacturers and state health-department laboratories). Data have been collected on 13 vaccine antigens and four human immunoglobulins. Each producer's information is confidential and is published only when at least three manufacturers report on the same product.

The second source of data is a 1968 survey of state and metropolitan health departments' policies and practices regarding distribution of gamma globulin. The survey sought information on gamma globulin of human and animal origin during the 5-year period, 1963–1967. It is obvious that a survey of public-health uses cannot be construed as a sampling of national practice, but it should reflect the principles of gamma globulin use generally accepted by the medical community. The data thus permit one to observe trends, carry out simple analyses, and make limited interpretations. Sufficient information can be retrieved to indicate the inherent value of surveillance, particularly if information can be collected consistently and comprehensively.

RESULTS

During the 6 years, 1963–1968, a net annual distribution of 6.2–11.6 million milliliters of all gamma globulins of human origin was reported to the Biologics Surveillance Program by 11 producers (Figure 1). The output of these 11 producers constitutes most of the national supply for military and civilian use.

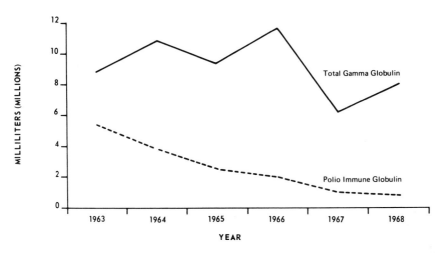

FIGURE 1   Net distribution of human gamma globulins by 11 major producers in the United
States, 1963–1968.

The volume of gamma globulin distributed in 1968 was less than that
in 1963, but the decline has been irregular.

Although it is impossible to correlate national distribution of gamma
globulin with *specific* disease requirements, some observations can be
made. The three communicable diseases against which gamma globulin
prophylaxis is most widely used—measles, hepatitis, and rubella—have
declined to relatively low levels in the last few years. Measles control
and its eventual eradication through vaccination have been nationally
promoted since 1965. Well over 35 million doses of vaccine have now
been administered. Some measles vaccines were recommended for use
with small doses of gamma globulin to diminish side reactions, and
gamma globulin was used prophylactically in infants exposed to the
disease. Both of these demands are now much reduced. The dramatic
results of measles-control efforts are evident in current case reports,
which are less than 5% of the average before measles vaccines were
widely used. The last national peak occurrence of hepatitis was in 1961,
when more than 72,000 cases were reported. There was a gradual decline in cases to less than half that number in 1966 and only a moderate
increase in the following 2 years. The rubella epidemic of 1964 was
probably the largest since the 1930's, but cases of rubella declined
sharply thereafter, and they remain at relatively low levels.

The total influence of these three diseases on demand for gamma globulin helps to explain the shape of the gamma globulin distribution curve but cannot account for the peak in 1966. It is likely that various factors influenced the peak, not all of them related to timely requirements. For example, it was in July 1966 that the American National Red Cross discontinued providing gamma globulin free of charge to health agencies in the United States. There may have been a coincident "stockpiling" from 1966 supplies. An even more important event in 1966 was a reportedly large military order for gamma globulin to continue programs of hepatitis prophylaxis. The rather abrupt decline in distribution in 1967 makes it even more evident that the 1966 peak was artifactual.

For historical interest only, we have included in Figure 1 the rapid decline in distribution of the portion of gamma globulin marketed as poliomyelitis immune globulin (human). It shows how a product's "pertinence" declines with the disease—even when very little was probably used for polio prophylaxis.

Our data do not indicate which of the major health and medical groups are the predominant users of gamma globulin. It would seem that the private practice of medicine constitutes the biggest, the military and other federal agencies intermediate, and state and local health departments the smallest.

How gamma globulin is used in the United States cannot be examined directly. However, survey data from health departments of all 50 states, New York City, and Washington, D.C., give us some indications, at least for communicable-disease control. Information from the 52 health departments is presented in Table 1. It contrasts the numbers of departments in 1963 and 1967 that distributed gamma globulin; human immune globulins for tetanus, pertussis, and measles; and antitoxins or sera of animal origin for prevention or therapy of diphtheria, tetanus, and rabies.

Of the 52 health departments, 38 (73%) indicated that they did distribute gamma globulin in 1967. That was a slight decline from the 44 departments (85%) that distributed it in 1963. In contrast with this decline is an increase in the number of health departments that provided human immune globulins by 1967—particularly tetanus immune globulin (human), offered by only three departments in 1963 but by 10 in 1967. The evident preference for human globulin is also reflected in two departments' discontinuing distribution of the antitoxin. (In 1968, two

TABLE 1   Public-Health Distribution of Gamma Globulins in the United States, 1963 and 1967;
Survey of 52 Health Departments[a]

	No. Health Departments Distributing	
Globulin Distributed	1963	1967
Gamma globulin (human)	44	38
Immune globulin (human)		
Tetanus	3	10
Pertussis	3	5
Measles	1[b]	3[b]
Antitoxin–antiserum (animal)		
Diphtheria	20	20
Tetanus	21	19
Rabies	17	18

[a]50 states, New York City, and District of Columbia.
[b]17 other departments distributed standard gamma globulin for measles prophylaxis.

additional states discontinued tetanus antitoxin in favor of the human
globulin.) Five departments provided pertussis immune globulin (human)
in 1967, and three supplied measles immune globulin (human); 17 others
made standard gamma globulin available for measles prophylaxis. Diphtheria and tetanus antitoxins and antirabies serum were offered by about
35–40% of the departments in 1967, essentially the same as in 1963.

Health departments that distributed gamma globulin during 1963–
1967 reported providing an annual average of between 0.5 million and
1.3 million milliliters. This volume generally represented less than 10%
of the national total reported to the Biologics Surveillance Program. The
year of peak gamma globulin distribution by health departments was
1964, and not 1966, as in national data. The reason will be suggested
later.

Among the 38 health departments distributing gamma globulin in
1967, all 38 provided it for family contacts of hepatitis cases, 31 (82%)
for pregnant women exposed to rubella during the first trimester, and
17 (45%) for measles prophylaxis. As already indicated, three additional
departments distributed measles immune globulin (human).

Seventeen of the surveyed health departments distributed gamma
globulin predominantly for hepatitis and rubella prophylaxis during
1963–1967 and also reported cases of these two diseases. (Rubella has
been nationally reportable only since 1966.) Figure 2 compares the vol-

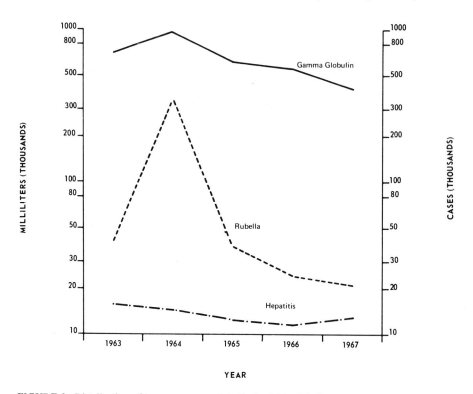

FIGURE 2 Distribution of human gamma globulin by 17 health departments (Alabama, Alaska, Colorado, Connecticut, Delaware, District of Columbia, Georgia, Illinois, Iowa, Kentucky, Maryland, Massachusetts, Michigan, New Hampshire, New York City, New York State, and Wisconsin) and reported cases of rubella and hepatitis, 1963–1967.

umes of gamma globulin provided by those departments with the numbers of reported hepatitis and rubella cases. Between 400,000 and nearly 1 million milliliters of gamma globulin were distributed annually. The peak distribution occurred in 1964, and there was an overall decline of nearly 40% from 1963 to 1967.

The numbers of rubella cases varied greatly. Reports ranged from nearly 350,000 during the 1964 epidemic down to 21,000 in 1967. Although reported rubella cases are primarily in children, they represent an increased risk for pregnant women and, therefore, a demand for gamma globulin prophylaxis. The frequency of hepatitis in 1963–1967 was relatively uniform, case reports ranging from 11,000 to 16,000.

Prophylaxis for family contacts probably used proportional amounts of
gamma globulin. It was therefore the 1964 rubella epidemic that best
accounts for the 50% increase in gamma globulin distribution above the
expected level in that year. In spite of the questionable value of gamma
globulin prophylaxis for preventing fetal anomalies after maternal rubella
infection and recommendations against its injudicious use, these data
suggest that gamma globulin was used widely for rubella in 1964.

Not only disease requirements, but fiscal and policy judgments as
well, accounted for the overall decline in the volume of gamma globulin
distributed by the 17 departments. Without free gamma globulin from
the Red Cross, more stringent controls on its distribution were undoubtedly imposed in many areas. Also, effects of the previously mentioned
measles immunization campaign were being realized during 1965–1967.
Eleven of the 17 departments provided small amounts of gamma globulin for measles prophylaxis. The frequency of measles in the 11 areas
had declined by 1967 to approximately 6% of the 1963 level, and consequently there was a diminished need for gamma globulin.

In brief summary of Figure 2, the health-department survey of gamma
globulin distribution showed a clearly disease-related orientation, particularly with respect to the 1964 rubella epidemic. The overall decline
in the volume of gamma globulin provided by the departments is consistent with the patterns of rubella, hepatitis, and measles in recent
years.

Turning now to immune globulins of animal origin, namely those for
diphtheria, tetanus, and rabies, data from the health departments offer
examples of the sorts of insights that surveillance information can give.

The amount of diphtheria antitoxin (primarily of equine origin) provided by 12 health departments that supplied data are compared with
their reported diphtheria cases in Figure 3. During the 4 years from
1963 to 1967, diphtheria cases declined to approximately 30% of the
1963 level (106 to 31 cases). However, the amount of diphtheria antitoxin distributed by the health departments declined by only about half
(19.4 to 10.8 million units). This discrepancy might be explained in several ways: increase in dose of antitoxin per case, greater reliance on the
health department for supplying antitoxin, underreporting of cases,
misdiagnosis and therapy, or combinations of these. One cannot be sure,
but the alternatives should stimulate further investigation of diphtheria-
control programs.

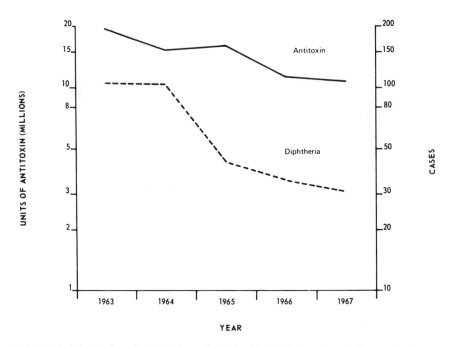

FIGURE 3   Distribution of diphtheria antitoxin by 12 health departments (Connecticut, Florida, Georgia, Hawaii, Illinois, Maryland, Michigan, Minnesota, New York City, New York State, North Carolina, and Virginia) and reported cases of diphtheria, 1963–1967.

Another kind of surveillance data involves tetanus prophylaxis, in which a new product has become popular since 1963. Figure 4 shows a nearly 60% decline from 1963 to 1967 in units of tetanus antitoxin provided by 15 health departments that supplied comparable data.

It also shows about a 23-fold increase in the amount of tetanus immune globulin (human) distributed during the same period. Although the increased popularity of this human globulin is dramatic, it still constituted less than 25% of the total units of passive tetanus prophylaxis supplied by these health departments in 1967 (an equivalent of more than 75 million units). In terms of total tetanus prophylaxis during the 4 years from 1963 to 1967, there has been an overall decline of 60%. Because most tetanus antitoxin or human globulin is given prophylactically, one can infer that the decreased demand may represent several related changes, including more active tetanus immunization, more judicious use of animal antisera, and more conservative interpretation of injuries considered to be tetanus-prone.

Rabies prophylaxis can also be explored somewhat with our data. The volume of antirabies serum provided by 16 health departments in 1963–1967 is presented in Table 2. It has declined by more than half during those 4 years, a period when many specialist groups encouraged using serum plus vaccine for optimal management of severe bite injuries thought to involve rabies exposures. The decline suggests that fewer persons are being considered for antirabies treatment. How many fewer might be estimated by assuming an average treatment to be 3,000 units of antirabies serum (1,000 units per 40 lb). Therefore, from 1963

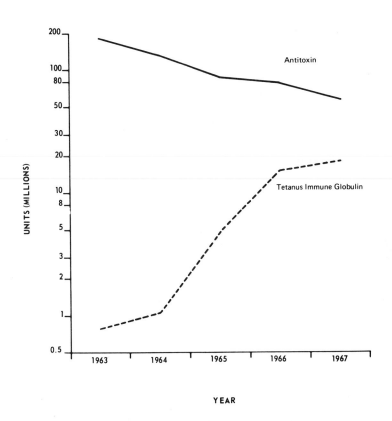

FIGURE 4 Distribution of tetanus antitoxin by 15 health departments (Alaska, Connecticut, Georgia, Hawaii, Illinois, Kentucky, Maryland, Michigan, New Hampshire, New York City, New York State, North Carolina, Pennsylvania, Vermont, and Virginia) and distribution of tetanus immune globulin (human) by seven health departments (Alaska, Illinois, Maryland, Michigan, New York City, New York State, and Virginia), 1963–1967. [Units of tetanus immune globulin (human) multiplied by 10 for equivalency.]

TABLE 2   Public-Health Distribution of Antirabies Serum, 1963–1967; Survey of 16 Health Departments[a]

	1963	1964	1965	1966	1967
Antirabies serum distributed, thousands of units	1,518	1,519	1,424	883	742
Estimated no. treatments[b]	506	530	475	294	247

[a]Alaska, Connecticut, Florida, Georgia, Hawaii, Idaho, Illinois, Iowa, Maryland, Minnesota, New Hampshire, New Jersey, Pennsylvania, South Carolina, Vermont, and Virginia.
[b]Based on average 3,000 units per treatment.

through 1967, the number of individual treatments can be estimated to have declined from approximately 500 to fewer than half that many.

Vaccinia immune globulin (human) (VIG) has been provided by the American National Red Cross for approximately 7 years through a special "consultant network." Consultants interpret each reported case and decide whether globulin should be given. Data provided to the NCDC on VIG distribution by fiscal year show that in 1963, 7,255 ml of VIG were distributed; in 1964, 8,645 ml; in 1965, 8,080 ml; in 1966, 8,305 ml; in 1967, 8,295 ml; and in 1968, 9,710 ml. The relatively constant amount of VIG distributed annually implies a uniform rate of occurrence of conditions for which the gamma globulin is used. Data from the VIG consultants corroborate that approximately 700 persons receive VIG each year (a dose of approximately 10–15 ml per patient). These data have been particularly important in assessing the complications of vaccinia vaccination in the United States and, as such, demonstrate another kind of usefulness of immunoglobulin surveillance.

SUMMARY

Immunobiologics have become fundamental in the practice of preventive medicine in the United States. Reliance on artificial immunization as a basis of communicable-disease prevention and control levies a commitment on health workers to pursue active surveillance of results. Data on supplies and distribution of gamma globulin have a very relevant role in this surveillance.

The Biologics Surveillance Program of the NCDC and a 1968 survey of 50 state and two metropolitan health departments provided the basis for a review of policies and patterns of gamma globulin use.

In the 6 years from 1963 through 1968, between 6.2 and 11.6 million milliliters of gamma globulins of human origin were distributed in the United States by the 11 major producers. There has been an overall but irregular decline. Decline in the communicable diseases for which gamma globulin is commonly used—hepatitis, rubella, and measles in particular—undoubtedly influenced the decline in recent years. "Stockpiling" may have accounted for peak distribution in 1966 and reduced demand in 1967.

Of the 52 health departments that provided data on their gamma globulin programs, 38 distributed gamma globulin in 1967, predominantly for hepatitis but also for rubella and measles prophylaxis. Seventeen provided information for 1963 through 1967 on volumes of gamma globulin distributed and on the occurrence of rubella and hepatitis, for which most of their supply was used. Peak distribution of gamma globulin in 1964 clearly reflected the impact of a rubella epidemic in that year.

Distribution of diphtheria antitoxin has declined, with reported cases of diphtheria, in the 4 years from 1963. However, the relative decrease in the amount of antitoxin used was less than the decrease in reported diphtheria cases.

Tetanus antitoxin distribution declined appreciably in 1963–1967, and there was a dramatic increase in preference for tetanus immune globulin (human). The human immune globulin accounted for approximately 25% of total tetanus prophylaxis provided by health departments in 1967.

Antirabies serum supplied by health departments declined in volume by more than half from 1963 through 1967, suggesting that fewer persons were considered to be at risk of rabies infection.

Vaccinia immune globulin (human) distributed by the American National Red Cross through a special consultant network has shown little fluctuation in its pattern of use since 1963. This suggests a constant rate of the conditions for which VIG is indicated, principally those related to vaccinia virus infections.

We acknowledge the assistance of Mrs. Jo Dean Sanders, of NCDC, in tabulation and presentation of data.

ROY WOODS *and* FRED HYMES

The National Cancer Institute's Immunoglobulin Reference Center

In recognition of the desirability of a central agency to assist investigators engaged in immunoglobulin research and of the need for increased research in this area, the National Institutes of Health in 1965 established by contract the Immunoglobulin Reference Center under the supervision of Dr. John L. Fahey and Dr. William Terry of the Immunology Branch of the National Cancer Institute (NCI). In collaboration with numerous investigators, the *modus operandi* to be outlined here was evolved.

The activities of the NCI Immunoglobulin Reference Center may be conveniently divided into six general categories: immunodiagnostic and reagent assistance; quantitative determinations of immunoglobulin levels; maintenance of an immunoglobulin anomalous-protein serum bank; training programs to assist investigators in the development of skills relative to quantitative determination of immunoglobulin levels, reagent production, and interpretation of immunoglobulin abnormalities; internal and collaborative research activities; and special studies.

IMMUNODIAGNOSTIC AND REAGENT ASSISTANCE

Immunodiagnosis

The Immunoglobulin Reference Center assists investigators throughout the world in the detection of qualitative immunoglobulin abnormalities.

374

Specimens are received and analyzed immunoelectrophoretically to determine the presence or absence of a qualitative immunoglobulin abnormality and the immunoglobulin H- or L-chain class to which the anomalous protein belongs. After completion of the analysis, a written report of test results is submitted to the investigator. If the specimen presents an unusual pattern, follow-up studies are performed to elucidate the nature of the abnormality. This immunodiagnostic service is available to all physicians and investigators in the United States and other countries.

Reagent Assistance

The Immunoglobulin Reference Center recognizes the desire of a number of investigators to perform analyses themselves and the need of research investigators for high-quality antisera that have been raised against and rendered specific for the various human and mouse immunoglobulin H and L chains. The Center supplies 2- to 3-ml aliquots of these reagents, including anti–human IgG, IgA, IgM, IgD, κ, and λ and anti–mouse IgG1, IgG2$_a$, IgG2$_b$, IgA, and IgM. It is our hope that these reagents will be used as standards for the assessment of the specificity and relative potency of reagents acquired commercially or prepared in the investigators' own laboratories. It is not the policy of the Center to provide specific antisera for routine use, but rather to begin to move in the direction of the standardization of reagents of this type.

The Center recognizes that there are experimental models that often require the use of mouse plasma-cell tumors. The Center therefore assists investigators in establishing their own mouse plasma-cell colonies by supplying them with tumors that secrete proteins representative of the five mouse H-chain immunoglobulin classes.

QUANTITATIVE DETERMINATION OF
IMMUNOGLOBULIN LEVELS

In characterizing the clinical status of various patients, it is often desirable to know the concentration of their serum immunoglobulins. The Immunoglobulin Reference Center carries out determinations in selected cases. After receipt of the specimen, a written report of the results is submitted to the investigator.

Gamma globulin replacement therapy has been used increasingly, often without prior determination of immunoglobulin concentration. This use of gamma globulin therapy can be optimized by the availability of quantitative tests of immunoglobulin concentration. It is hoped that this aspect of our functions will permit a more discriminating selection of patients for such therapy and will contribute to a knowledge of the effect of various disease processes on immunoglobulin levels and the frequency distribution of κ and λ chains among the immunoglobulins that are produced.

MAINTENANCE OF THE IMMUNOGLOBULIN ANOMALOUS-PROTEIN SERUM BANK

The Immunoglobulin Reference Center recognizes the need for a serum bank that contains representatives of the various immunoglobulin abnormalities. Such a serum bank serves not only as a central depository for sera of various types but also as a source of material for investigators involved in problems related to the structure and clinical use of immunoglobulins. The serum bank is now being used in studies dealing with the antibody activity of myeloma proteins and with quantitative and qualitative changes in nonimmunoglobulin serum proteins in association with the presence of myeloma proteins of various types. An analysis of the anomalous sera that have been received by the Center is shown in Table 1. These results add to previous reports dealing with the relative

TABLE 1   Relative Frequency of κ and λ Chains in Serum Myeloma Proteins of Various Classes

Diagnosis[a]	Number	Relative Frequency, %
GMP (κ)	383	64
GMP (λ)	216	36
AMP (κ)	139	69
AMP (λ)	62	31
WM (κ)	117	84
WM (λ)	22	16
DMP (κ)	1	25
DMP (λ)	3	75

TABLE 1 (continued)

Diagnosis[a]	Number	Relative Frequency, %
BJ (κ)	111	54
BJ (λ)	96	46
GMP (κ) with BJ (κ)	43	43
GMP (λ) with BJ (λ)	58	57
AMP (κ) with BJ (κ)	10	50
AMP (λ) with BJ (λ)	10	50
WM (κ) with BJ (κ)	0	0
WM (λ) with BJ (λ)	0	0
DMP (κ) with BJ (κ)	2	19.5
DMP (λ) with BJ (λ)	14	80.5

[a]GMP = IgG myeloma protein; AMP = IgA myeloma protein; WM = Waldenström macroglobulin; DMP = IgD myeloma protein; BJ = Bence Jones protein.

distribution of κ and λ chains in various myeloma proteins. In accord with previous studies, these results indicate that the occurrence of κ and λ chains appears to be related to the anomalous-protein H-chain type. Studies with normal immunoglobulins[1] indicate that the relative frequencies of the L chains in myeloma proteins parallel those in normal immunoglobulins of the various H-chain classes.

TRAINING PROGRAMS

Since its inception, the Immunoglobulin Reference Center has assisted investigators from six countries in the development of skills in specific antiserum production, quantitative determination of immunoglobulin levels, and interpretation of immunoelectrophoretic patterns of immuno-globulin abnormalities. Trainees are received at the Center and usually remain for a week. Attempts are made to tailor the training programs to fit the specific needs of each trainee. Because the number of trainees that can be assisted is limited, applicants are advised to make inquiries at least 3 months in advance of their anticipated time of availability for participation in this program. The program is conducted jointly by the

Immunoglobulin Reference Center and the Immunology Branch of the NCI. Participants are expected to defray their own travel and living expenses incidental to participation in the program.

INTERNAL RESEARCH ACTIVITIES

The senior personnel who are associated with the Immunoglobulin Reference Center are engaged in a number of research projects. They include the search for genetic markers on IgG4 myeloma proteins and investigation into the possible existence of additional immunoglobulin subgroups, the study of intraspecies and interspecies relationships among immunoglobulin classes, structural studies of γ chains, the study of antibody activity of myeloma proteins, development of immunoadsorbents, and the study of subgroups of mouse immunoglobulins.

SPECIAL STUDIES

The Immunoglobulin Reference Center has participated and is presently involved in a number of collaborative studies with individual investigators. These "special studies" have concerned immunoglobulin levels in twins, the effect of radiation from the atomic bomb on the immunoglobulin levels of citizens of the Marshall Islands, immunoglobulin levels in patients suffering from African Burkitt's lymphoma, the effects of various pathologic conditions on serum levels of IgD, and collaboration with the World Health Organization and other laboratories in the establishment of an international reference preparation for use in the quantitation of human immunoglobulin levels.

SUMMARY

The NCI Immunoglobulin Reference Center uses immunoglobulins in three general ways: the development, use, and dispensation of high-quality reagents for the detection of qualitative and quantitative immunoglobulin abnormalities; the establishment of a training program for the development of skills in reagent production and the interpretation of immunoglobulin abnormalities; and the execution of continuing research programs related to immunoglobulin structure and function. It is hoped that, through these kinds of activities, a variety of methods will emerge that will permit more effective clinical uses of immunoglobulins.

To continue to provide those services and to expand our research efforts, both internal and collaborative, the Immunoglobulin Reference Center must rely on cooperation from investigators who deal with patients having immunoglobulin abnormalities.

REFERENCE

1. Connell, G. E., and R. H. Painter. Fragmentation of immunoglobulin during storage. Canad. J. Biochem. 44:371–379, 1966.

FRED JOHNSON

Status of Supply of Gamma Globulin and Capacity to Produce It

The supply of immune serum globulin has generally been adequate, but there have been periods when the advent of a new hyperimmune globulin has been marked by a severe shortage. An example is tetanus immune globulin, which was introduced in 1958 and was so scarce for 6 years that its distribution was limited to California. Large-scale commercial hyperimmunization, along with the development of routine plasmapheresis, has largely solved the problem of producing adequate amounts of many hyperimmune globulins.

There has long been the specter of an acute shortage of gamma globulin if it were recommended for prophylaxis against posttransfusion hepatitis. A prophylactic regimen requiring approximately 30 ml for every transfusion in the United States would, in theory, consume approximately 60 million milliliters of gamma globulin every year. However, this has not come to pass; instead, supplies of gamma globulin accumulate to such a degree that the economy of plasma-component therapy is being threatened.

When plasma is fractionated, the various fractions are obtained in rather constant proportions. The relative yields of the clinically useful plasma fractions are shown in Table 1. This does not represent the con-

380

TABLE 1   Yields of Plasma Fractions

Prepared from		No. Packages	Size of Package	Quantity	Fraction
1 liter of plasma		0.3	500 units	150 units	Antihemophilic factor
		0.4	500 units	200 units	Factor IX complex
		1.2	1.0 g	1.2 g	Fibrinogen
		2.6	10 ml	26 ml	Gamma globulin, 16.5%
	Either, but not both	1.6	50 ml	80 ml	Normal serum albumin, 25%
		2.1	250 ml	525 ml	Plasma-protein fraction, 5%
1 placenta		0.31	10 ml	3.1 ml	Gamma globulin, 16.5%
		0.20	50 ml	10 ml	Normal serum albumin, 25%

centration of these proteins in plasma. From a single pool of plasma, it is possible to obtain antihemophilic factor, factor IX complex, fibrinogen, and gamma globulin in the proportions indicated. In addition, it is possible to obtain either albumin or plasma-protein fraction as indicated, but not both. The yields of gamma globulin and albumin obtained from placentas are also shown.

If patients cooperated in planning their afflictions, therapy with plasma components could be ideal, and cost could be reduced. Unfortunately, need is not proportional to yield. At one time before the development of synthetic fibrinolytic inhibitors, the demand for fibrinogen almost dominated plasma procurement, and other fractions were left over. Later, for a brief period before the development of vaccines for poliomelitis and measles, gamma globulin was the dominant fraction used, and the other fractions were left over. At that time, industry began fractionating placentas. Today, owing partly to the Vietnam war but largely to the regulations against pooled stored plasma, albumin and plasma-protein fraction are in greatest demand, and gamma globulin is left over.

Plasma procurement is the major expense encountered in production: the price structure requires that industry sell from each processed lot all of two fractions and most of a third. The situation is now precarious because of the excessive demands for plasma-protein fraction and albumin, when industry has been allocating somewhere between one third and one half of the plasma-procurement costs to gamma globulin. This problem does not occur when gamma globulin is produced from placentas. Because gamma globulin is the dominant fraction, and albumin a by-product, placentas can be purchased to meet estimated sales of gamma globulin.

Figures on current production and supply are estimates, because no producer is willing to say how much is being produced or how much it can produce. There are nine producers of gamma globulin in the United States. About 750,000 liters of plasma were fractionated last year, yielding some 19,000,000 ml of gamma globulin. About 2,500,000 placentas were fractionated, yielding an additional 7,000,000 ml of gamma globulin. There were 3.4 million births last year; about 70% of the placentas were used, and that is probably about as high a percentage as is economically desirable. All this amounted to a total production of 26,000,000 ml of gamma globulin. Distribution in the United States was 18,000,000 ml, leaving an excess of 8,000,000 ml. There are an estimated 1,400 kg of dry gamma globulin in storage, equivalent to 9,000,000 ml. Apparently, about 8,000,000 ml per year is being disposed of abroad, mostly in the dry state, in an attempt to recover the dollars spent for that portion of the plasma allocated to gamma globulin.

The American National Red Cross contracts with four or five laboratories to fractionate outdated plasma. In general, the contracts provide that the laboratories will produce a limited amount of packaged fibrinogen and all of Cohn's fraction V as packaged albumin or plasma-protein fraction. Gamma globulin is processed only to the dry powder and is held in that state until the national office requests the laboratory to furnish a particular number of 10-ml or 2-ml vials for the Red Cross stockpile. That is always done from the oldest dry powder on hand. At least one of the contract fractionators still has on hand a portion of the dry gamma globulin from the 1965–1966 contract and the total amount of the dry gamma globulin from the 1966 through 1968 contracts.

A close estimate of the amount of gamma globulin stockpiled by the Department of Defense is not available. However, it is apparent that it is not particularly large.

The ability of industry to produce more gamma globulin, if needed, depends on increased fractionation capacity and increased procurement of plasma and placentas. As mentioned, an additional 8,000,000 ml per year could be available now. With a simple increase in plasma procurement and without augmenting the fractionation facilities, industry could make available an additional 4,000,000 ml per year. Thus, industry could promptly meet an additional demand of 12,000,000 ml per year. Any demand beyond this point would require additional fractionation facilities, but these could be provided quickly. About 1,000,000 more placentas per year could be procured and would provide an additional 3,000,000 ml. Thus, an additional demand of 15,000,000 ml could be met. Procurement of plasma by plasmapheresis could probably be increased by an additional 300,000 liters per year (but at a significant increase in cost); and another 8,000,000 ml could be provided by this method. Thus, it is feasible for industry to provide, by conventional means, 23,000,000 ml of gamma globulin in addition to the 18,000,000 ml now being used annually in the United States.

It is apparent that for the last few years industry has not concerned itself with trying to increase supplies of gamma globulin. The major problem is to provide specific standardized immunoglobulins that are safe and effective. In some patients, acquired immunity to a genetically foreign type of gamma globulin has become apparent. We do not know how many specific allotypes will be found to be clinically significant. We hope there will be few, but we will have to learn how to separate or exclude those few. In addition, industry has to provide separate, standardized immune globulin preparations against a variety of antigens. Presently available in the United States are preparations standardized against measles, pertussis, mumps, tetanus, vaccinia, and $Rh_{(o)}$. Limited to clinical investigation are immune globulins standardized against rubella, malaria (*Plasmodium falciparum*), and Pseudomonas. The World Health Organization has recommended that immune globulins standardized against diphtheria, varicella (or herpes), botulism, and rabies also be made available.

The production of 13 or more standardized IgG immunoglobulins comprising only compatible allotypes would be a great accomplishment. In addition, IgA, IgM, and, possibly, IgE should be made available. Certainly, IgG free of IgA should be provided. Of more immediate importance, gamma globulin should undergo no fragmentation during storage, and prevention of fragmentation in storage has almost been accomplished. Gamma globulin should also undergo no aggregation during preparation or storage. That is probably the most urgent problem facing industry today. All IgG should be of the 6.7S type, without aggregates, and be capable of being administered either intravenously or intramuscularly without reactions. Finally, all this has to be accomplished without any changes in methods that could conceivably result in contamination with the hepatitis virus.

SAM T. GIBSON

Federal Requirements for Acceptance of New Immunoglobulin Products

Biologic products that are to be sold on the open market, which is the ultimate goal of making them available to everyone, are under the control of the Division of Biologics Standards (DBS) of the National Institutes of Health (NIH). The basis of this operation was the statute that arose out of tragedy. In 1900, just 25 years after Pasteur had associated bacteria with disease, and 9 years after the first antitoxin was produced in animals, some children who received diphtheria antitoxin in St. Louis died because of tetanus contamination. Aroused by this avoidable tragedy, the District of Columbia Medical Society petitioned Congress, and on July 1, 1902, the Virus, Antitoxin, and Serum Act was passed. It outlined a system of licensing establishments—at that time anyone who had a horse (and everyone did) could enter this thriving new business—and establishing conditions under which products were essential. Anyone who wished to offer for sale, barter, or exchange in interstate commerce or to import or export any biologic material as described in the Act would have to have a license, be inspected, and meet agreed-upon standards. This led to repeated inspection and individual licensing of the products.

The Act was signed in the same year that Dr. Landsteiner was publishing the discovery of the fourth blood group; this helps to put into perspective the kind of statute under which we are working. I think all the licensees are acquainted with the working of DBS. Most have heard about it in a general way. As a result of another tragedy, the DBS was reorganized in 1956 into a division with institute status at NIH. It comprises seven laboratories and a staff of about 300. Its activities are divided between routine testing of samples before release, inspecting, issuing new licenses, revising old ones, developing new standards with the help of interested people in science and industry, and engaging in research work pertinent to carrying out a mission of control and providing pure, potent, and safe products.

It is obvious that, in order to obtain a license, a manufacturer or person must already be in business, because the agency wants to examine the routine for manufacture and see samples and test them. How do you get into business without a license? It is very simple. A manufacturer either operates within a state, free from any federal interference, or, if he wishes to acquire clinical data, applies for permission to do so.

Still a third tragedy provided the mechanism under which new drugs are developed. After the thalidomide experience, the Harris-Kefauver amendments to the Food and Drug Act were passed, in 1962, and under them there is a provision for investigation of new drugs. Under this provision, a person who wishes to study a new drug presents data—in the case of potentially licensable biologic products, to the Director of the DBS. The qualifications of the investigator, the facilities available for study, the data on which one thinks he is justified in progressing to studies in man, and the plan of study are considered; if it is felt that adequate safeguards are built into the plan, the investigation proceeds, and it may involve interstate or foreign work as one wishes.

The first phase of investigating a new drug in man, based on animal work, would involve 1 to 10 patients, and the second, 10 to 300. If all goes well, the final stage before licensing would involve anywhere from 300 to a million patients. The use of a million patients is not meant to represent something forbidding. Changes in the manufacture of poliomyelitis vaccine, for example, would require somewhere between one and two million trials for authorization. So one is dealing with a variety of figures.

When sufficient data are presented to satisfy the Director of the DBS that the product should be available for general distribution on an unrestricted commercial basis, a license is issued.

I think this conference has presented a summary of current problems. It has stimulated us to move ahead, each in his own way, some in acquiring additional data, others in expediting the handling of these data, still others in developing ways of checking on changes in processing. I hope that before another conference we will make significant progress in solving the problems of improving present products by developing ways to avoid, or at least control, the aggregation and degradation of gamma globulins. We may find that it is to our advantage to manipulate, rather than eliminate.

There is need for a better correlation between *in vitro* and *in vivo* measurements of activity. Whether this involves routine turnover study or other methods, the problem is urgent. I think that a precise and simple method of measuring $Rh_{(o)}$ activity in gamma globulin is also necessary.

The isolation or identification of the factors that distinguish gamma globulin from placental sources from that from venous sources is urgent so that we can decide quickly whether new standards are necessary. At the moment, both are prepared and sold under the same regulations. It may be that these regulations need modification before any change in method is possible.

Of course, characterization of reactions so that they may be eliminated and sensitization avoided is still necessary, although the major progress in this field can be accomplished by clinical education, rather than by changes in manufacture.

The new products are new products. I think that it must be shown that the intravenous preparations can do something more than just be given intravenously, and that, having been given intravenously, they will last long enough to accomplish something. Obviously, we have to isolate more subfractions, and the materials for special use that Dr. Johnson listed are needed. These projected studies will lead to further progress in our effort to present the American public with biologic products that are pure, potent, and safe.

Authors and
Other Participants

Akers, Thomas G., University of California School of Public Health, Berkeley, California

Alexander, Benjamin, New York Blood Center, New York, New York

Anderson, S. G., Division of Biological Standards, National Institute for Medical Research, London, England

Ashworth, J. N., Travenol Laboratories, Inc., Los Angeles, California

Ballieux, Rudy E., University Hospital, Utrecht, The Netherlands

Beentjes, S. P., Central Laboratory of the Netherlands Red Cross Blood Transfusion Service, Amsterdam, The Netherlands

Bellanti, Joseph A., Georgetown University School of Medicine, Washington, D.C.

Blaese, R. Michael, National Cancer Institute, National Institutes of Health, Bethesda, Maryland

Brachott, Daniel, Ministry of Health, Jerusalem, Israel

Briggs, N. T., Walter Reed Army Institute of Research, Washington, D.C.

Brummelhuis, H. G. J., Central Laboratory of the Netherlands Red Cross Blood Transfusion Service, Amsterdam, The Netherlands

Brunell, Philip A., New York University Medical Center, New York, New York

Bryan, John A., National Communicable Disease Center, Atlanta, Georgia

Buckley, Charles E., III, Duke University Medical Center, Durham, North Carolina

Camp, Frank R., Jr., U.S. Army Medical Research Laboratory, Fort Knox, Kentucky

389

Chanock, Robert M., National Institute of Allergy and Infectious Diseases, National
    Institutes of Health, Bethesda, Maryland
Clarke, Frank, Lederle Laboratories, Pearl River, New York
Conrad, Marcel E., Walter Reed Army Institute of Research, Washington, D.C.
Crain, Joan D., Children's Hospital Medical Center, Boston, Massachusetts
Dauber, Leonard G., U.S. Army Medical Research Laboratory, Fort Knox, Kentucky
    (present address: The Hospital of the Albert Einstein College of Medicine,
    Bronx, New York)
Deutsch, H. F., University of Wisconsin, Madison, Wisconsin
Diamond, L. K., University of California San Francisco Medical Center, San Francisco,
    California
Dull, H. Bruce, National Communicable Disease Center, Atlanta, Georgia
Edsall, Geoffrey, Massachusetts Department of Public Health and Harvard School of
    Public Health, Boston, Massachusetts
Edwards, Earl A., Naval Medical Research Unit No. 4, Great Lakes, Illinois
Ellis, Elliot F., Denver, Colorado
Fahey, John L., National Cancer Institute, National Institutes of Health, Bethesda,
    Maryland
Fischer, J., Behringwerke A.G., Marburg (Lahn), Germany
Fortwengler, H. Philip, Jr., U.S. Army Medical Research Laboratory, Fort Knox,
    Kentucky
Fudenberg, H. Hugh, University of California San Francisco Medical Center, San
    Francisco, California
Geiger, H., Behringwerke A.G., Marburg (Lahn), Germany
Gibson, Sam T., Division of Biologics Standards, National Institutes of Health,
    Bethesda, Maryland
Giles, J. P., New York University School of Medicine, New York, New York
Good, Robert A., University of Minnesota, Minneapolis, Minnesota
Grady, George F., Tufts University School of Medicine, Boston, Massachusetts
    (present address: Massachusetts State Department of Public Health, Jamaica
    Plain, Massachusetts)
Heremans, Joseph F., Cliniques Universitaires Saint-Pierre, Leuven, Belgium
Hickman, R. L., Walter Reed Army Institute of Research, Washington, D.C.
Hymes, Fred, National Cancer Institute Immunoglobulin Reference Center,
    Springfield, Virginia
Ishizaka, Kimishige, Children's Asthma Research Institute and Hospital, Denver,
    Colorado
Janeway, Charles A., Harvard Medical School, Boston, Massachusetts
Johnson, Fred, Cutter Laboratories, Berkeley, California (deceased)
Kabat, Elvin A., Columbia University College of Physicians and Surgeons, New York,
    New York

Karchmer, A. W., National Communicable Disease Center, Atlanta, Georgia

Krijnen, H. W., Central Laboratory of the Netherlands Red Cross Blood Transfusion Service, Amsterdam, The Netherlands

Krugman, S., New York University School of Medicine, New York, New York

Kunkel, Henry G., Rockefeller University, New York, New York

LoGrippo, G. A., Henry Ford Hospital, Detroit, Michigan

Mannik, Mart, University of Washington Medical School, Seattle, Washington

Meiling, Richard L., The Ohio State University College of Medicine, Columbus, Ohio

Merler, Ezio, Harvard Medical School, Boston, Massachusetts

Mills, John, National Institute of Allergy and Infectious Diseases, National Institutes of Health, Bethesda, Maryland

Mosley, James W., National Communicable Disease Center, Atlanta, Georgia

Painter, Robert H., University of Toronto, Toronto, Ontario, Canada

Palmer, John W., Travenol Laboratories, Inc., Los Angeles, California

Peckinpaugh, Robert O., Naval Medical Research Unit No. 4, Great Lakes, Illinois

Pennell, Robert B., Blood Research Institute, Inc., Boston, Massachusetts

Perkins, John C., National Institute of Allergy and Infectious Diseases, National Institutes of Health, Bethesda, Maryland

Pike, Robert M., The University of Texas Southwestern Medical School, Dallas, Texas

Poulik, M. D., Wayne State University School of Medicine, Detroit, Michigan

Prato, Catherine M., University of California School of Public Health, Berkeley, California

Reed, Louis J., U.S. Army Medical Research Laboratory, Fort Knox, Kentucky (present address: The Hospital of the Albert Einstein College of Medicine, Bronx, New York)

Ringertz, Olof, National Bacteriological Laboratory, Stockholm, Sweden

Robbins, John B., Albert Einstein College of Medicine, Bronx, New York

Rosen, Fred S., Harvard Medical School, Boston, Massachusetts

Rowe, D. S., World Health Organization International Reference Centre for Immunoglobulins, Lausanne, Switzerland

Sadun, E. H., Walter Reed Army Institute of Research, Washington, D.C.

Schwick, H. G., Behringwerke A.G., Marburg (Lahn), Germany

Sgouris, James T., Michigan Department of Public Health, Lansing, Michigan

Skegg, Joyce, Division of Biological Standards, National Institute for Medical Research, London, England

Skvaril, F., Research Institute of Immunology, Prague, Czechoslovakia (present address: Swiss Centre for Clinical Cancer Research, Tiefenau Hospital, Bern, Switzerland)

Smolens, Joseph, Philadelphia Blood Center, Philadelphia, Pennsylvania

Soothill, J. F., University of London Institute of Child Health, London, England

Strober, Warren, National Cancer Institute, National Institutes of Health, Bethesda, Maryland

Suggs, Morris T., National Communicable Disease Center, Atlanta, Georgia

Sulkin, S. Edward, The University of Texas Southwestern Medical School, Dallas, Texas

Terry, William D., National Cancer Institute, National Institutes of Health, Bethesda, Maryland

Van Kirk, John E., National Institute of Allergy and Infectious Diseases, National Institutes of Health, Bethesda, Maryland

Waldmann, Thomas A., National Cancer Institute, National Institutes of Health, Bethesda, Maryland

Wall, Robert L., The Ohio State University College of Medicine, Columbus, Ohio

Ward, R., University of Southern California School of Medicine, Los Angeles, California

Watt, John G., Royal Infirmary, Edinburgh, Scotland

White, S. H., U.S. Army Medical Research and Development Command, Silver Spring, Maryland

Woods, Roy, National Cancer Institute Immunoglobulin Reference Center, Springfield, Virginia

Yount, William J., Rockefeller University, New York, New York

Index